Frontiers in Metabolism 2

Series Editor:
Keith Snell

For my parents, Sidney and Rachel Fell.

FRONTIERS IN METABOLISM 2

Understanding the Control of Metabolism

by David Fell

School of Biological & Molecular Sciences
Oxford Brookes University

PORTLAND PRESS
London and Miami

Published by Portland Press Ltd, 59 Portland Place,
London W1N 3AJ, U.K.

In North America orders should be sent to Ashgate Publishing Co.,
Old Post Road, Brookfield, VT 05036-9704, U.S.A.

Copyright ©1997 Portland Press Ltd, London

ISBN 1 85578 047 X ISSN 1353 6516

British Library Cataloguing-in-Publication Data
A catalogue record for this book is available from the British Library

Although, at the time of going to press, the information contained in this publication is believed to be correct, neither the author nor the publisher assumes
any responsibility for any errors or omissions herein contained. Opinions expressed in this book are those of the author and are not necessarily held by the
publishers.

All profits made by the sale of this publication are returned to The Biochemical
Society for the promotion of the molecular life sciences.

Typeset and printed in Great Britain by Cambridge University Press

Contents

3 Enzyme activity: the molecular basis for its regulation

4 Traditional approaches to metabolic regulation

5 **Metabolic Control Analysis**

6 **Measuring control coefficients**

7 Control structures in metabolism

8 Conclusion

Preface

There is little doubt that the central areas of traditional biochemistry (such as metabolism, metabolic regulation and enzymology) are currently unfashionable and generally regarded as problems long solved. They have been eclipsed by molecular genetics, which is not only able to identify the genes for protein components and their regulatory elements, but which also promises the means to change the genes and their control elements at will, to the point where it could truly be called biological engineering. In the press and on television, there are already debates about how we should use, and not abuse, the power we are expected to possess tomorrow to manipulate even complex multigenic, and environmentally influenced, characteristics such as human intelligence and resistance to disease. How simple it should be, then, to engineer a trait such as metabolism, where there are such clear and well-understood links from the genes to the enzymes to the metabolic pathways.

Why then have I written a book now about metabolism and its regulation, which returns to these central, unfashionable concerns of biochemistry and which only mentions molecular genetics in a subordinate role? The answer is that, even 20 years ago, a small number of researchers were convinced that there were fundamental flaws in the explanations that biochemists gave for the regulation and control of metabolism. Together, these critics created Metabolic Control Analysis as an alternative means to understand and explain these problems, and they have gradually been persuading more and more biological scientists to design and interpret their experiments in a different way. However, their criticisms and reworkings of traditional biochemical explanations are still not widely known and have, as yet, had little influence on the contents of the standard biochemistry textbooks, which still cling to the rejected concepts, usually without even mentioning the doubts and problems. The purpose of my book is, therefore, to present an introduction to Metabolic Control Analysis that places it in the context of the biochemical results and phenomena to which it must be applied. My hope is that this will provide a more accessible account of the major features of Metabolic Control Analysis than has previously been available, since most of the existing literature consists of reviews and original articles in research journals, or brief outlines of a few selected aspects.

My full case for why Metabolic Control Analysis deserves to be more widely known is contained in the rest of the book, but a representative illustration comes from genetic engineering itself. There have already been attempts to manipulate metabolism, and these have involved successfully changing the amounts or kinetic properties of certain target enzymes. These enzymes have been selected because traditional biochemical theory, and the textbooks, identify them as the key steps in the control of a metabolic process. Virtually none of these experiments has had the expected outcome: the technology exists, but traditional metabolic biochemistry does not provide the understanding needed to use it purposefully. Nor, it should be said, is Metabolic Control Analysis certain to be able to predict the outcome, though it can provide a framework in which the possibility of achieving a specific modification of metabolism by a particular genetic intervention can be assessed.

One factor that has undeniably worked against the wide acceptance of Metabolic Control Analysis is that it inevitably involves more mathematical concepts and numerical computation than is usual in metabolic biochemistry. This is inevitable because it is the essence of the Control Analysis case against the traditional concepts that they cannot be rigorously justified and are not adapted to the quantitative testing that would be necessary to discriminate between alternative explanations. Nevertheless, I have tried to limit the amount of mathematics that is used in this book, and to explain the meaning and interpretation of the essential equations. Sometimes I have placed additional mathematical material in boxes or appendices if it is not essential to the main lines of the argument. I have not, as a result, presented Metabolic Control Analysis in its fullest or most mathematically rigorous form, nor have I provided derivations of all its theorems: these can be found elsewhere. However, it would be a delusion for metabolic biochemists to imagine that the detailed behaviour of systems as complex as metabolic pathways can be predicted with the aid of a few qualitative, verbal principles. Other biological scientists studying comparably complex phenomena, such as population dynamics and genetics, or physiology, have long known this, and biochemistry is remarkable for its limited use of mathematical and theoretical analysis.

David Fell
Oxford, 1996

Acknowledgements

The ideas I present in this book draw on the work of a great many researchers and are only partly my own. Even the ideas I would claim as my own owe much to the influences of other scientists and colleagues, some of whom I wish specifically to identify.

Eric Newsholme first stimulated my interest in the control of metabolism with his excellent lectures and tutorials at the University of Oxford, even though I have not followed his approach nor, in the end, agreed with his conclusions.

Henrik Kacser's article *The control of flux*[119] (with Jim Burns) made me realize that a more rational approach to metabolic regulation was possible. Later, when I first started to publish my results in Metabolic Control Analysis, Henrik's encouragement gave me confidence to continue. His death, in March 1995, whilst still actively involved in research on Metabolic Control Analysis, even though officially in retirement, was a great loss to the field of Metabolic Control Analysis, of which he was a cofounder.

Herbert Sauro's unsuppressible curiosity when he was my research student led us to make our first discoveries in the theory of Metabolic Control Analysis. He also then began the development of the metabolic computer simulation package SCAMP, which has continued to be a useful tool in my research group ever since and which has contributed some of the simulations reported in this book.

My next research student, Rankin Small, helped continue the momentum of the work begun with Herbert and began the development of the Control Analysis of covalent modification systems, described in Chapter 7. Some of his subsequent work with Henrik Kacser influenced the ideas I put forward in the final chapter.

More recently, Simon Thomas has worked with me, first as a research student and then as a Leverhulme Special Research Fellow, on some of the ideas presented in the final two chapters and he drew my attention to some of the examples I have used there.

The elasticity calculus presented in the Appendix to Chapter 5 has been developed further and applied in computer programs by Simon Thomas, John Woods and Herbert Sauro.

A number of colleagues helped me by supplying various materials for the book. Kevin Brindle provided me with an original copy of Fig. 2.3. Jean–Pierre Mazat and Thierry Letellier provided me with the data and fitting functions for their inhibitor titrations in Fig. 6.16, but also, more importantly, much–appreciated hospitality in Bordeaux on several occasions for discussions about

Control Analysis. Christoph Giersch sent me a manuscript before publication and the data that appear in Figs. 6.18 and 6.19; we also had useful discussions about the related text.

I am grateful to all those who have commented on various parts of the book. Keith Snell, as editor of this series, read the whole text and made useful suggestions about presentation. Athel Cornish–Bowden corrected my errors in Chapter 3 on enzyme kinetics and also had helpful ideas about the presentation. Simon Thomas read much of the draft and helped to improve the text in several places. Others who have commented on the text include João Pedro Moniz Barreto, Stefan Schuster, John Woods and my wife, Mary.

Many other friends and colleagues have made an indirect contribution to this book through conversations, discussions and even critical scrutiny of my ideas, particularly at conferences. I cannot list them all, but three who have had a direct influence on material in the book are Athel Cornish–Bowden, Jannie Hofmeyr and Mark Stitt. Athel and Jannie have provided me with advance copies of several of their papers that relate particularly to material in the first chapter and the last two. Mark drew my attention to some of the illustrative material I have used from plant biochemistry.

I am also grateful to the undergraduates of Oxford Brookes University who were the unwitting guinea-pigs while I rehearsed the presentation of parts of this book.

In addition to those mentioned previously, the following authors have kindly given me permission to use their diagrams in this book: J. Katz; E. Chance; A. B. Tulp and Bert Groen.

I am also greatly indebted to the authors of the excellent public domain software that I have found so useful in preparing this book. Firstly, this manuscript was prepared using the LaTeX document preparation system by L. Lamport, itself a macro package for TeX by D. E. Knuth. Many other authors have contributed the parts that make this a working system, from the various TeX distributions on the different computers I have used and the auxiliary programs for making the bibliography, indexing, drawing diagrams and viewing the output (BIBTeX, MakeIndex, TeXcad and the DVI processors) to the additional packages for citation, drawing (PiCTeX) and inclusion of Postscript figures. Many of the graphs of data and functions were plotted with GnuPlot from the Free Software Foundation and viewed with GhostScript. Most of the text editing was done with various versions of MicroEmacs. I have received much help with finding, implementing and using this software from Herbert Sauro, John Woods and João Pedro Moniz Barreto.

David Fell
Oxford, 1996

Introduction: regulation and control

1.1 Regulation and control

Much of the detail of metabolism, represented by the interconversions of metabolites catalysed by enzymes, is known, and can be found in biochemistry texts and on metabolic maps. But biochemistry is a relatively young science and this detail has been discovered recently, mostly within the last seventy years. Our knowledge of this and other aspects of biochemistry and molecular biology reflects the success of the *reductionist* approach: the study of a whole system by detailed examination of the properties of its constituent parts, in the expectation that the behaviour of the system can be predicted once the properties of the parts are understood. In metabolism, the reductionist strategy has started with the discovery of the component pathways followed by that of the separate reactions in the pathways, and then passed to characterization and detailed study of the enzymes responsible for the reactions, and ultimately even to the identification of the genes that encode the enzymes. Knowing the routes and the molecules involved does not by itself, however, lead to an understanding of what determines the material flows in different pathways, nor of how the production and utilization of metabolites are kept in balance. The focus of metabolic research has therefore shifted to tackle these problems of regulation and control, though a number of different approaches have been adopted, as will be shown later.

First though, why is the study of regulation and control of metabolism important? The reasons include the following.

- To gain a more complete understanding of metabolism, under both normal and abnormal conditions. The former might be represented by healthy organisms in favourable conditions, and the latter by organisms affected by mutation, disease or hostile conditions. I will argue later that knowing the molecular mechanisms and interactions involved in regulation and control is not enough; we must be able to show in a convincing way how these lead to the observed metabolic responses of the organism.

- To understand the actions of hormones and drugs or other chemical agents that affect metabolism, for which it is necessary to understand how metabolism responds to various types of perturbation of enzyme activities.

- To aid the search for drugs that affect metabolism by identifying appropriate target sites for bringing about the required change.

- To enable biotechnologists to increase formation of the desired metabolic products, and decrease formation of unwanted secondary metabolites, in industrial processes for producing biological materials such as drugs, antibodies, enzymes or nutrients.

Indeed, our lack of understanding of metabolic regulation has been revealed by poor results from attempts to increase the rates of selected metabolic pathways. Genetic engineering techniques have advanced to an amazing extent, so it is now possible to change the activities of enzymes at will, but when this has been applied to the enzymes stated by biochemistry textbooks to be rate–controlling, there has often been no significant corresponding change in metabolism. Our ability to interfere with an organism's genetics has far outstripped our ability to predict the effects on its metabolism.

One of the difficulties in discussing regulation and control is that, in biology, there often appears to be no consistent distinction between the terms. Very often they are used interchangeably. If we try to be more specific about the terms, and to make our usage consistent with other areas of science and technology, such as engineering, we find a fundamental difficulty in drawing analogies between control systems in engineering and biology: in engineering we know the purpose the mechanism serves, but in biology we can only presume the function as a hypothesis, and we cannot be certain that there is not a range of other requirements that are to be met by it. For example, we know why there is a thermostat in a refrigerator, whereas we do not know why the regulation of glycogen metabolism has to involve all the molecular components that it does (see Chapter 7.4.3.3, p. 238). Nevertheless, it is important to discriminate between the terms *regulation* and *control*.

Regulation, both in technological and biological systems, is occurring when a system maintains some variable (e.g. temperature or concentration) constant over time, in spite of fluctuations in external conditions. [See, for example, the McGraw–Hill *Encyclopaedia of Science & Technology* (1982) and the Longman *Dictionary of Scientific Usage* (1979).] Regulation, in the sense of minimizing the effects of disturbances, is therefore linked to *homoeostasis*, the maintenance of a relatively constant internal state. For example, Jannie Hofmeyr & Athel Cornish–Bowden[106] recently defined metabolic regulation in terms of the performance of the metabolic system rather than the existence of particular mechanisms in the system. They stated that the effectiveness of metabolic regulation should be assessed from the way a metabolic system responds to environmental changes. For example, metabolic regulation could be a sensitive response of the rate of a metabolic pathway to environmental conditions whilst metabolite concentrations are kept near constant. In other circumstances, the notable feature of the performance might be the maintenance of near-constant metabolic rates (for example, of ATP synthesis) in the face of fluctuations in the environment. This underlines the problem that it might not be completely clear what aspect of a metabolic system is being regulated; this might be assumed or presumed, whereas in a technological system, this aspect of function would be an explicit feature of the design.

Control is used in technology to refer to adjusting the output of a system with time, perhaps to match some required profile (e.g. a time–varying input signal) or to obtain a desired response. [See Chambers' *Science & Technology Dictionary* (1974) and Longman's *Dictionary of Scientific Usage* (1979).] In common usage, control as a verb implies the ability to start, stop, direct or adjust something. Again these meanings can often not be applied literally to biological systems, because to do so would imply there is an identifiable and unique characteristic of the system under consideration, whereas we know that many metabolic pathways are multifunctional and that the ultimate requirement is that they are controlled in such a way as to ensure the fitness (in an evolutionary sense) of a species in its ecological niche. However, we can regard metabolic control as the power to change the state of metabolism in response to an external signal. Hofmeyr & Cornish–Bowden[106] similarly regard control as being measurable in terms of the degree of influence that an external factor has on the state of a metabolic system. The advantage of this definition is that metabolic control can be assessed in terms of the strength of any of the responses to the external factor without making any assumption about the function or purpose of that response. It also means control is a simpler, lower–level concept than regulation, because it does not require a judgement about the function of the system.

To complicate matters further, whether regulation or control is the appropriate term depends as much on the context and level of study as on the system under consideration. For example, vertebrate blood glucose is regulated by insulin and glucagon (homoeostasis), but these hormones achieve this by controlling the metabolism of various body tissues. In this example, we could say that the concentration of a metabolite is kept constant (regulated) by varying (controlling) the rates of metabolism, if we wanted to emphasize the homoeostatic and active aspects respectively of the two terms. Hofmeyr and Cornish–Bowden's definitions imply that we refer to the regulation of the blood glucose because it is the behaviour of a complete system, underlying which is the control that the hormones exert on specific components of the system, particularly the rates of metabolic pathways in various tissues.

1.2   Approaches to metabolic regulation

The study of regulation and control draws on a range of different approaches; the challenge is to combine these into a logically consistent whole. My aim in this book is to present the basics of these approaches and to suggest that Metabolic Control Analysis offers one way of achieving a consistent overview. What are the different strands that have to be combined? They are the views that result from studying metabolic biochemistry either at relatively high levels of organization and integration, the *system* level, or at much lower levels of organization, effectively at the *molecular* level.

Study at the system level typically involves whole pathways, organelles, cells or even organs. The topics belonging to the system level within this book are:

- methods of studying metabolism

    – measuring metabolites

    – measuring metabolic fluxes

    – measuring enzyme contents

- methods of identifying supposed 'rate–limiting steps'

- Metabolic Control Analysis: replacing the erroneous concept of the rate–limiting step

(Note that I have used *metabolic fluxes* rather than *metabolic rates*. Although the two expressions mean essentially the same, it is conventional in Metabolic Control Analysis to use flux to refer to a rate in a multicomponent system such as a metabolic pathway and to reserve rate for individual component steps, such as enzymes. I will maintain this distinction in the rest of this book.)

At the molecular level, the properties of individual molecular components of metabolic systems are characterized. Examples from later in the book include:

- enzyme kinetics

    – single–substrate enzymes

    – two–substrate enzymes

    – allosteric enzymes

- feedback inhibition

- covalent modification of enzymes

    – irreversible (degradation or activation)

    – reversible (phosphorylation etc.)

Researchers in the areas I have just crudely allocated into these two groups may resent my implication that, by studying a topic from one of them, they are distanced from biochemistry at the other level. They might point out that system–level studies have established that particular pathways have some means of responding to certain physiological or environmental stimuli, and that molecular–level studies have identified molecules that relay the signals and the enzymes on which they act. However, I still believe that to build a bridge between these two levels, to ensure that the knowledge and understanding we have at each can be combined as a consistent whole, is extremely difficult and has not received sufficient attention until recently. Even though the discovery of control molecules and signals has required work at the two levels (e.g. Chapter 7.4), I do not think I am proved wrong because there have been many unresolved disagreements about the physiological significance and role of many of the molecular events that have been discovered to have the potential for regulation and control. The relative lack of attention given to relating the two levels, and to developing an adequate theory able to resolve disputes, probably reflects the optimistic tendency in science to exaggerate the extent of our islands of knowledge and to stress the importance of work at their margins, whilst minimizing the significance of the relatively uncharted seas of ignorance that separate them. To explain how this applies to metabolic regulation, I will consider in the following sections three types of approach to the explanation of metabolic control and regulation. Although the aim of the book is to promote the advantages of the third type of approach, examples of the other two will be found, sometimes to show how current thinking has evolved from previous ideas, sometimes to criticize ideas that are still current, and sometimes because the third type of approach is incomplete and does not yet have a view to offer.

1.2.1 Molecular or reductionist explanations

The justification for the reductionist approach is that, once the properties of the component parts are known, it will be possible to explain the behaviour of the whole system. For the biochemist, the system might be a particular pathway, or the whole metabolism of a particular cell type, and what must be explained includes why there is a certain rate of flow through a pathway under some defined set of external conditions. Now, a metabolic map does not supply this sort of answer, any more than a town map reveals how much traffic can flow through the streets. Even if the information available includes the catalytic activity of the enzymes in the cell, and how the activities respond to signals from the concentrations of metabolites, the answer is still elusive, in the same way that the traffic flow problem is still a problem even if the map shows the relative widths of the streets and where the traffic signals are.

How feasible is it to construct an explanation of metabolism in terms of the properties of the parts? There can be thousands of enzymes and metabolites in a cell; if every enzyme interacted with all the metabolites, the number of separate interactions to be investigated would be in the millions. Fortunately, most of these interactions do not occur, and the most important ones are obvious: first of all, an enzyme must interact with its substrates and products, and then perhaps with certain other metabolites from its own pathway. Even so, for an enzyme such as glutamine synthase, which has three substrates, three products and nine significant effectors, the problem of obtaining an accurate description of its behaviour for all concentrations of these fifteen metabolites is huge. Michael Savageau[217] pointed out that it would be necessary to make 4^{15} or approx. 10^9 measurements in order to investigate all the possible interactions, even if only four different concentrations of each of the fifteen metabolites would be needed to characterize its response. Obviously, it is unlikely that complete descriptions of complex enzymes will ever exist, though the principal characteristics of many of the common enzymes, such as those in glycolysis and the tricarboxylic acid cycle, are known for several different cell types. Indeed, there have been attempts to build this information into computer models to simulate metabolism, particularly by David Garfinkel and his group working on the carbohydrate catabolism of mammalian heart muscle,[78] and by Barbara Wright and her co-workers on the carbohydrate metabolism of slime moulds[2,278] (Chapter 6.2). Whilst these models have had some success, in order to make their behaviour realistic it is usually necessary to change some of the values for some of the enzymes' properties, since the experimental values seem unsuitable, often for no very clear reason.[279]

In terms of my previous metaphor, reductionists are not worried about a sea of ignorance between the molecular level and system level of explanation, because they believe that in principle it will eventually be crossed with the boat of mathematical modelling and computer simulation, even though the record of successful crossings is not very good. It seems we are still a long way from being able to simulate metabolism easily and routinely on the basis of our present biochemical knowledge. If we cannot do this, can we be justified in claiming that our knowledge of the molecular properties explains the system-level behaviour in biochemistry? Up to a point we probably can, because the types of behaviour observed with real metabolic pathways are seen in computer simulations of metabolic systems composed of model enzymes with properties typical of real enzymes, even though we cannot easily reproduce the exact behaviour of a specific metabolic pathway.

1.2.2 Qualitative systems approach

In this approach, the information about the underlying molecular structure (e.g. existence of a feedback inhibition on an enzyme) is used in general terms only. That is, there is a qualitative, or at best semi-quantitative, decision as to whether a particular interaction is large enough to have a significant effect at the system level or not. A verbal description is then built up of how the enzymes and metabolites interact to give the system properties of the whole pathway, perhaps drawing on analogies with other disciplines such as engineering. The verbal model might be used to predict responses of the system to external events, but exact comparison with experimental observations is diffi-cult because these predictions are qualitative rather than precise. When different groups have produced different verbal models for the same phenomena, it has proved difficult to resolve the dispute in favour of one or the other because model performance cannot easily be objectively assessed. Nevertheless, such qualitative verbal models have been dominant in biochemistry as a whole and in metabolic regulation in particular. This is understandable in a young science studying complex little–known systems; it offers a starting point for the gener-ation of models of the system behaviour that can be refined and tested. What is disturbing is the apparent lack of any ambition to progress to more rigorous specifications of the models so that quantitative predictions emerge that can be compared with experimental results.

In terms of my metaphor, the qualitative systems approach tries to avoid falling into the sea of ignorance by never walking close enough to the water's edge to be able to see it clearly, and therefore does not know how far the sea extends. For each little island of knowledge, there are lots of travel guides that tell you what you might see there, but little in the way of maps to show how the different features are connected together.

1.2.3   Quantitative systems theory

A quantitative systems approach involves using information about the general features of the underlying molecular structure to build a formal (mathematical) description of the system properties, without attempting to incorporate a fully detailed model of all the behaviour at a molecular level. Instead, one of several theoretical schemes is used to build in a general description of the behaviour of metabolic systems. If this is combined with the measurement or calculation of some selected system parameters, the description can be made quantitative and compared with experimental observations. Generally, the quantitative descrip-tion is best close to a measured experimental state, and the larger the movement away from this state, the less exact the predictions become because the model is not sufficiently detailed to give an exact representation over a large range of conditions. The advantage of forgoing a precise model of the system is that the amount of information needed for these system-level models is much smaller than for complete molecular models, so it is more feasible to collect it experi-mentally. Even though the models are not highly precise, they are quantitative so it ought to be easier to decide whether different models give significantly different predictions and whether they are consistent with experimental obser-vations.

Thus it is accepted that there will be a degree of ignorance about whether the molecular properties account for the system behaviour, but that does not mean that there can be no link between the two levels of description and it is also possible to have a quantitative model. In this case, we are saying that we do not expect to have the islands of knowledge that correspond to our system components mapped internally in very great detail; however, more importance is attached to determining the position of each of these islands on the world map, so that we have a good impression of the global geography even though we accept that there is a lack of very specific detail.

1.3   An overview of mechanisms of regulation and control

One notable feature of metabolism is the very wide range of time scales over which changes can occur. In some cases, adjustments can happen within seconds or less, whereas in others they may be linked to seasonal changes or the life cycle of the organism. Underlying these events can be mechanistic steps, such as the binding of a hormone by a receptor, that take tiny fractions of a second, or the breakdown of unwanted enzyme occurring over hours or days. Not surprisingly, it is difficult to consider such disparate events simultaneously. So both theoretically and experimentally, it is usual to choose a time span to work on, and to try to arrange matters so that changes requiring longer periods of adjustment can be ignored and changes taking place on shorter time scales can be regarded as having reached completion almost immediately. For example, the laboratory measurement of an enzyme activity is usually performed so that the initial events of substrate binding to the enzyme on mixing are essentially instantaneous and the measurement is completed before the inevitable long–term depletion of substrate occurs to any significant extent.

In the regulation and control of metabolism, it is possible to group the operative mechanisms into three major classes on the basis of the relative lengths of time they take to bring about adjustments.

(1) **Long time scales**, *i.e.* of the order of hours or days in eukaryotes, though only a few minutes in prokaryotes. The mechanisms on these time scales typically involve the control of amounts of enzyme protein by:

  – the rate and degree of gene expression
  – the rate of enzyme degradation

Mechanisms for the first of these are known in great molecular detail in a number of cases, beginning with the work of Jacob and Monod on the control of the *lac* operon of *Escherichia coli*. Much less is known about the mechanisms of the second, though it is known that in mammals, for example, some enzymes have lifetimes of only a few minutes, whilst other enzymes in the same cells can last for days. Proteolytic breakdown of enzymes can be selectively targeted, for example with the ubiquitin system,[102] and can be initiated in response to specific stimuli. The dynamic range of these mechanisms can be very large; that is, the amount of enzyme protein in a cell can be varied between nothing and the level of the major metabolic enzymes such as those of glycolysis. This book will not deal with the molecular details of these mechanisms, examples of which are commonly given in many textbooks. However, the effects of the variations in enzyme amount that are caused in such ways have not been studied so systematically, and this will be considered later in the book. For example, it was over 20 years after Jacob and Monod's proposal of the *lac* operon before the contributions of the enzymes of the operon to the growth of the bacteria on galactose were assessed in detail (see Chapter 6.1.1.2 and Chapter 6.1.2).

(2) **Medium time scales**, *i.e.* of the order of minutes or a few seconds. A major mechanism for changes on this scale is the cyclic activation and deactivation of existing enzymes by covalent modification of the protein.

The Nobel Laureates E. G. Krebs and E. Fischer first demonstrated this in mammalian muscle for the activation of glycogen phosphorylase by phosphorylation (Chapter 7.4.1); since then, many eukaryotic enzymes have been found to be affected by phosphorylation and dephosphorylation, and more recently the process has been discovered in bacteria. There are also other types of covalent modification apart from phosphorylation (see Chapter 7.4.2, p. 227). In animals, the modification reactions may respond to hormonal or nervous signals, and are in fact the means whereby these signals can have relatively rapid effects on metabolism. The potential degree of change from the lowest enzymic activity to the highest (the dynamic range) is very large with this mechanism. This is because the inactive form of the enzyme can be almost completely devoid of activity, and virtually all the enzyme can potentially be converted to this state; on the other hand, when activation occurs, there can be essentially complete conversion of all the enzyme present in the cell to the active form. Examples of cyclic covalent modification schemes are considered later in this book (Chapters 7.4.3 and 7.4.4), together with an examination of the types of behaviour they can exhibit (Chapter 7.4.5).

(3) **Short time scales**, *i.e.* seconds or less. The mechanisms on this time scale are presumed to be the reversible binding of metabolites to enzymes, causing effects such as allosteric inhibition and activation (Chapter 3.5, p. 70).

The forces holding metabolites to enzymes are usually non–covalent and therefore relatively weak, but as the links can easily break and re-form, the equilibria are established extremely rapidly. On the other hand, the dynamic range of these effects on enzyme activity is limited, since inhibition and activation involving non–covalent binding are rarely 100% effective. The maximum activation is also limited by the amount of enzyme available, but it is not possible to have a large reserve of enzyme to compensate for this partial activation because then the inhibition effects would not be strong enough to slow the enzyme when it is not needed. These effects are considered in several places in this book; in the chapter on enzyme kinetics (Chapter 3.5) the molecular mechanisms of the effects are considered, whereas in Chapter 7.2 examples are given of the ways in which they implement feedback control systems.

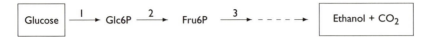

Figure 1.1 A metabolic pathway
This is part of the catabolic pathway from the source, glucose, available from the medium to the sink, the ethanol plus CO_2 which are released to the surroundings. At steady state, the rate of formation of glucose 6-phosphate (Glc6P) in the cell by reaction 1 is equal to its consumption in reaction 2 (assuming there are no other significant uses of Glc6P). Thus the rates of reactions 1 and 2 are the same. Similarly, since the rate of formation of fructose 6-phosphate (Fru6P) by reaction 2 is the same as its consumption by reaction 3, the latter also works at the same rate as reaction 1. The steady state in metabolite concentrations is therefore equivalent to a constant rate through the whole pathway.

The basis on which it is legitimate to concentrate on one of these time scales and to ignore the events and mechanisms on longer time scales is explored in the next section.

1.4   Basic theory of metabolism

1.4.1   Metabolic steady states

One of the characteristic features of living organisms is their ability to maintain a relatively constant composition whilst continually taking in nutrients from the environment and returning excretory products. These two aspects are necessarily linked: organisms can only keep their internal state constant by this flux of matter and energy through the metabolic pathways of their cells. This is termed *dynamic equilibrium* to distinguish it from chemical equilibrium, in which a constant state is reached when the net reaction fluxes die away. The concept of the steady state corresponds to a perfect dynamic equilibrium; we suppose that a metabolic pathway starts with a *source* of material that is derived at constant concentration from the environment (directly or indirectly) and finishes with an end product, *the sink*, that is kept at constant concentration by direct or indirect excretion into the environment. In most cases, this will lead to the development of a steady state, where the concentrations of the intermediates remain constant because their rates of formation have come to be in exact balance with their rates of degradation (Figure 1.1). This also requires that the flow through the pathway remains constant for the reasons explained in the figure legend. It is not inevitable that any sequence of successive enzymic reactions will always be able to reach a steady state in these circumstances, but the consequence of not reaching a steady state would be that one or more intermediate metabolites would continue to accumulate in ever increasing amounts. Such an increase would start to give a cell severe osmotic problems, and would be at odds with the general impression of dynamic equilibrium. Indeed, biochemists must have an expectation that a metabolic system tends to a reproducible state, since similar experimental results could only be obtained from day to day in this case. It would not generally be pos-

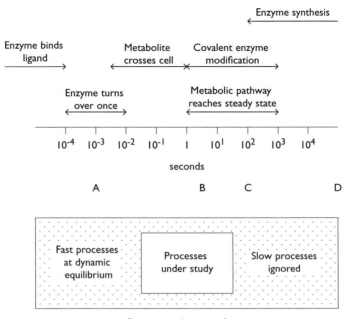

Figure 1.2 Metabolic time scales and the quasi-steady state
For different types of experiment, the experimental viewing frame is placed over the time axis in different positions, masking off the regions that are not being observed. For example, a fast reaction enzyme kineticist would centre the window of the frame above the letter A, a metabolic biochemist working on isolated cells or tissues might centre it in the range B to C, and a biochemist working on whole animals, or a nutritionist, might centre it above D. The time scales of various biochemical events are indicated as very approximate ranges.

sible with non–steady states, since the amounts of metabolites would depend very sensitively on the previous history of the sample to such an extent that it would be difficult to repeat any observation. (An exception to this would be the metabolic oscillations that are sometimes observed reproducibly; however, although these show regular fluctuations in concentrations and fluxes, their average values are constant.)

Nevertheless, an exact steady state is a mathematical abstraction. One reason for this is that as a pathway comes closer and closer to steady state, its rate of approach becomes ever slower, so that in theory it will only arrive there after an infinite amount of time. In practice this does not matter, because the limited accuracy of methods of biochemical measurement mean that a system that is more than 95% of the way to steady state is virtually indistinguishable from the steady state itself, and 95% attainment of the steady state could well occur in the preincubation phase of a metabolic experiment.

Even so, there is another limitation to the concept of a steady state: the environment, whether inside some laboratory glassware or in nature itself, is never completely constant, not least because of the action of metabolism. It is inevitable that the source materials of metabolic pathways will slowly deplete, and that excretory products will accumulate. Also, as mentioned in the previous section, there are other events that come into effect on longer time scales, such as induction or repression of enzyme synthesis. Another possibility is that minor metabolic pathways, such as those for the synthesis of adenine or nicotinamide nucleotides, cause slow changes in the amounts of coenzymes like ATP and NAD^+. If there are very slow changes in the concentrations of metabolites or the pathway flux caused by any of these factors, the pathway may still be regarded as being in *quasi steady state* provided the time scale of the changes is very much longer than the time taken by the pathway to approach steady state. In other words, if there are slow changes in one or more metabolites, this must mean that the rates of synthesis and degradation are not quite in balance, but if the degree of imbalance is only a small fraction of the rate of synthesis, then it may still be a good approximation to regard it as being at steady state. Figure 1.2 illustrates the way in which the quasi steady state is related to the time scale of the experimental observations. In the chapter on enzyme kinetics (Chapter 3), it is shown that exactly the same concept of quasi steady state is routinely accepted as a basis for interpreting experiments.

1.4.2 Thermodynamics of metabolic pathways

The study of the regulation and control of metabolic pathways is concerned with the factors that affect the rates of the pathways, so at first sight it might seem that thermodynamics can offer little insight. After all, in spite of its name, classical thermodynamics gives no information about the rates of processes; even worse, many of its formulae are only precise about systems that are at equilibrium or changing infinitely slowly. Nevertheless, thermodynamics as the science of energy relationships reveals the energy constraints to which pathways are subject and which, independently of the details of the enzyme kinetics, place some limits on possible steady states of a pathway. A more recent branch of thermodynamics, non-equilibrium thermodynamics (developed by the Belgian Nobel Laureate I. Prigogine in particular), does make explicit links between the rates of processes and their energetics. Furthermore, it is not enough for mechanisms of regulation and control just to bring about the necessary steady state fluxes through the pathways. Other constraints have to be satisfied as well, and these can be directly linked to the energetics of the processes. For example, Dan Atkinson[6,7] pointed out that the concentrations of most intermediary metabolites must be kept low, for otherwise, with thousands of different metabolites in a cell, the total volume they would occupy and their demand for water of solvation would be far greater than the space available in the cell. In addition, he argued that the low concentrations of metabolites ensure that non–enzymic side reactions between metabolites are minimized.

Classical thermodynamics deals principally with *closed systems*, defined as systems that can exchange energy but not matter with their surroundings. The only steady state that can develop under these circumstances is chemical equilibrium, when all net chemical change will have ceased. Living organisms, in contrast, are *open systems* that exchange energy and matter with their surroundings. This crucial difference allows the development of a dynamic equilibrium as a stable displacement from chemical equilibrium. (Non–equilibrium stable states are explained by non-equilibrium thermodynamics.)

According to classical thermodynamics, the change in free energy ΔG for a reaction at equilibrium is zero, but is non–zero if the reaction is displaced from equilibrium. (The Appendix to this chapter explains why the symbol ΔG is inappropriate for the concept of free energy, but it is retained here to be consistent with general usage.) If the reaction is taking place of its own accord (*i.e.* spontaneously, with no input of work energy such as an electric current) then it will have a negative free energy change and will be going in the direction towards equilibrium. Incidentally, non-equilibrium thermodynamics can show that metabolic pathways at dynamic equilibrium are indeed systems of spontaneous reactions. Where there is a net flow through a metabolic pathway, there must be a negative free energy change at each reaction step, every one of which must therefore be displaced from equilibrium. However, whereas successive reactions in an unbranched metabolic pathway must be going at the same rate in a steady state, there is no requirement that they all have the same free energy change, since this has no direct link with the kinetics. In fact, it is a matter of observation (see Chapter 4.2, p. 86) that the degrees of displacement from equilibrium of the reactions of a pathway are extremely variable. Before we consider the significance of this, let us first define the degree of displacement more precisely.

Consider the reaction:

$$A + B \rightleftharpoons C + D$$

The actual free energy of this reaction for a given set of concentrations of the substrates and products is $\Delta G'$ [where the prime indicates the (biological) standard condition of pH 7], related to the standard free energy $\Delta G^{o\prime}$ by the expression:

$$\Delta G' = \Delta G^{o\prime} + RT \ln \frac{CD}{AB} \qquad (1.1)$$

where R is the gas constant, T the absolute temperature and ln is the natural logarithm. The ratio of product concentrations to substrate concentrations is defined as the *mass action ratio*, Γ, *i.e.* :

$$\Gamma = \frac{CD}{AB} \qquad (1.2)$$

At equilibrium, $\Gamma = K_{eq}$, and $\Delta G' = 0$. Hence:

$$0 = \Delta G^{o\prime} + RT \ln K_{eq}$$

or

$$\Delta G^{o\prime} = -RT \ln K_{eq} \qquad (1.3)$$

Substituting Eqns. (1.2) and (1.3) into Eqn. (1.1) gives:

$$\Delta G' = -RT \ln K_{eq} + RT \ln \Gamma$$

which rearranges as:

$$\boxed{\Delta G' = RT \ln \left(\frac{\Gamma}{K_{eq}} \right)} \qquad (1.4)$$

The disequilibrium ratio, ρ, defined as Γ/K_{eq}, gives a measure of the displacement of a reaction from equilibrium. As Eqn. (1.4) shows, it is 1 at equilibrium when $\Delta G' = 0$, and is always less than 1 when $\Delta G'$ is negative, becoming small for large negative free energy changes. (This is because for logarithms in any base, $\ln 1 = 0$, and the logarithm of any number between 1 and 0 is negative, approaching $-\infty$ as the numbers approach closer to 0.)

For reasons to be considered below and in the next section, the value of ρ, the disequilibrium ratio for a reaction, is thought to determine whether it is a potential site for regulation and control. Accordingly, it is common to find that reactions are classified as either non–equilibrium or near–equilibrium reactions. The former are reactions for which ρ is very small, and the latter are those for which it is close to 1. Unfortunately there is no strong theoretical basis for deciding the demarcation point between these two classes, as will be discussed later (Chapter 4.2, p. 86, and Chapter 5.5.1, p. 126). However, there are many reactions where the classification is not disputed, and generally the non–equilibrium reactions are those which have a large negative standard free energy change, corresponding to a large equilibrium constant.

On the other hand, the undisputed near–equilibrium reactions tend to be those that have a small standard free energy change, corresponding to an equilibrium constant close to 1. This is not a surprising finding for a reason that has little to do with regulation and control. Most metabolite concentrations are in the micromolar to millimolar (10^{-6} M to 10^{-3} M) range. If concentrations were above this range, cells would have problems with the osmotic strength of the cytoplasm and the water requirement for solvating all the metabolites. In addition, higher metabolite levels would slow down the response rates of metabolism, because the large pools of metabolites would buffer the impact of sudden changes in enzymic activity caused by a control signal (an effect analysed in more detail by John Easterby in his studies of the transition times of metabolic pathways[62]). In contrast, if the concentrations were very low, enzymes acting on the metabolites would have to have a very high affinity for them, and whilst enzymes could no doubt evolve to have much higher affinities for their substrates, there are theoretical grounds for believing that this is incompatible with the development of high catalytic efficiency. Therefore it is likely that metabolites are on the whole constrained to be in the micromolar to millimolar region.

If this is so, then reactions with large equilibrium constants will have to be non–equilibrium reactions. For example, the first three reactions of glycolysis

(Figure 1.1) have equilibrium constants of approximately 4000, 0.4 and 1000 respectively, giving an overall equilibrium constant for the three reactions of 1.6×10^6. Given the concentrations of glucose, ATP and ADP in the human red blood cell, the fructose 1,6–bisphosphate concentration would have to be more than a million molar for these three reactions to approach near to equilibrium. In the case of reactions with small standard free energy changes, corresponding to equilibrium constants close to 1, a similar argument suggests that they have to be near to equilibrium. If such a reaction were non–equilibrium, this would mean that its products would be present in much lower concentrations than the substrates, and this effect would multiply if there were successive reactions with small standard free energy changes, each displaced far from equilibrium so that the metabolite concentrations would become progressively smaller. In one of the founding papers in Metabolic Control Analysis,[99] Reinhart Heinrich and Tom Rapoport in Berlin in 1974 were able to show by a mathematical proof that there is a natural tendency in a pathway at steady state for the reactions with the largest equilibrium constants to be the furthest displaced from equilibrium.

In conclusion, the simplest way that metabolite concentrations can be kept within reasonable bounds is for reactions with large negative standard free energy changes to be far from equilibrium, and for reactions with small standard free energy changes to be near to equilibrium. In addition, as Atkinson[7] pointed out, chemical energy can only be conserved by maintaining a reaction such as ATP hydrolysis far from equilibrium; free energy coupling in metabolism requires the existence of non–equilibrium reactions.

If these thermodynamic considerations are now combined with chemical kinetics, it is possible to show why non–equilibrium reactions are more likely than near–equilibrium reactions to have a determining influence on the rate of a metabolic pathway, using arguments developed by a number of biochemists in the 1960s.

Consider first the reversible reaction:

$$A \; \underset{v_r}{\overset{v_f}{\rightleftharpoons}} \; B$$

If we consider simple chemical kinetics, where the rate v_i of reaction i is a rate constant, k_i, times the reactant concentration, then $v_f = k_f A$ and $v_r = k_r B$. At equilibrium, there is no net change, so $v_f = v_r$, so:

$$k_f A = k_r B$$

and since $B/A = K_{eq}$:

$$\frac{B}{A} = \boxed{\frac{k_f}{k_r} = K_{eq}} \tag{1.5}$$

If we now consider this reaction when it is **not** at equilibrium, we can substitute this equation (Eqn. 1.5), and the definition of the mass action ratio (Eqn. 1.2) into the expression for v_f/v_r as follows:

$$\frac{v_r}{v_f} = \frac{k_r B}{k_f A}$$

$$= \Gamma \frac{k_r}{k_f}$$

$$= \boxed{\frac{\Gamma}{K_{eq}} = \rho} \qquad (1.6)$$

Now let us consider that this reversible reaction occurs in a metabolic pathway, which has reached a steady state in which there is a flow v_p along the pathway:

$$\xrightarrow{v_p} A \underset{v_r}{\overset{v_f}{\rightleftharpoons}} B \xrightarrow{v_p}$$

For the pathway to be at steady state, $v_f - v_r = v_p$, or $v_f - v_p = v_r$, so using Eqn. (1.6) gives:

$$\boxed{\frac{v_r}{v_f} = \frac{v_f - v_p}{v_f} = \rho}$$

Alternatively,

$$\frac{v_p}{v_f} = 1 - \rho$$

With $v_p > 0$, this shows that the reaction can only be near–equilibrium (*i.e.* with $\rho \simeq 1$) if $v_f \gg v_p$ so that $v_f \approx v_r$. A non–equilibrium reaction has a small ρ, and therefore the pathway rate, v_p, is comparable in size to the forward reaction rate v_f, and the rate of the reverse reaction, v_r, is relatively very small. (Although these relationships between ρ and the ratio of the reverse and forward reaction rates have been derived here using first–order chemical kinetics, the same expression is obtained for the *ratio* of the reaction rates if proper enzyme kinetic equations are used.[201])

Such calculations convinced biochemists that a near–equilibrium reaction is catalysed by an enzyme that is present in a great excess over the amount required to deliver the overall flux of the pathway, and that therefore it is not limiting the rate of the pathway. The non–equilibrium reaction, on the other hand, is a potentially limiting factor on the overall pathway flux, because the catalysed reaction rate is only slightly greater. Furthermore, many biochemists gained the impression from these equations for the ratios of rates that the reverse and net rates of a non–equilibrium reaction would not be significantly affected by changes in the product concentration. Unfortunately this is not true for enzyme–catalysed reactions because the values of the net and reverse rates do in general depend on product concentration, though as the proportional effect is the same on both, the ratio does not show this. As a result, product inhibition effects have been wrongly discounted unless they are unusually strong.

A second argument (originally put forward by another Nobel Laureate, Hans Krebs[140]) reinforced the view that non–equilibrium enzymes can be rate–limiting, but near–equilibrium enzymes cannot. Suppose more enzyme is added to catalyse a reaction that is already near–equilibrium; this will tend to increase the amount of product and decrease the amount of substrate to bring the reaction closer to equilibrium [as Eqn. (1.6) shows for an increase in v_f]. However, since the reaction is already close to equilibrium, if it is brought closer to equilibrium there will not be much change in the metabolite concentrations, nor will the reaction using the product be stimulated to go much faster so there is no reason to expect a great change in the pathway rate. On the other hand, for a non–equilibrium reaction, increasing the amount of enzyme could bring the reaction much closer to equilibrium, causing the product concentration to rise significantly, and stimulating the next reaction to go faster. Thus the change could propagate through the pathway to cause a significant change in pathway flux.

These arguments may seem persuasive and in many cases they probably have some validity. A potential weakness though is that they focus too closely on a single reaction in the pathway, and give insufficient weight to how the metabolite concentrations will change as the whole system responds to an attempt to change the rate at one step. Later we will see why these fears are justified (Chapter 5.5.1).

1.4.3   Principles of regulation and control

Until recently, what I termed the qualitative systems approach has been dominant in the attempt to formulate principles of regulation and control. That is, the theories were developed verbally, and little in the way of quantitative tests was undertaken to check their adequacy. Unfortunately, there is one seriously inadequate concept that has held a dominant position throughout the history of the study of metabolic regulation until relatively recently. Furthermore, because it has been so dominant, it is impossible to explain the motivation behind many of the experiments in metabolic regulation without referring to it. This troublesome concept is that of the *rate–limiting step*, originally proposed in the form:

> When a process is conditioned as to its rapidity by a number of separate factors, the rate of the process is limited by the pace of the slowest factor. (Blackman[18])

This concept has been described as a 'truism' and 'self–evident', and versions of it continue to be stated in biochemistry textbooks up to the present day. In many ways this is odd, because it is difficult to give a literal interpretation of the concept. As explained in the earlier section on the steady state (p. 10), a requirement of successive steps along a linear metabolic pathway is that they are operating at the same rate in the steady state, so none of them could be termed the 'slowest' step in the normal sense of the word. What was meant by the many advocates of the 'rate–limiting step' was that the rate of a pathway could be altered only by changing the activity of one particular enzyme in the pathway. On this basis, the study of the control of a pathway entailed the identification of the rate–limiting step. From time to time, doubts were expressed: why should the fact that the alteration of the activity of one enzyme can change the rate of a pathway mean that this cannot be true of another enzyme in the pathway? Attempts to analyse the kinetics of multi–reaction systems did not support the rate–limiting step; it was possible to show that the overall rate depended in principle on the kinetics of every reaction in the system. Until recently, these criticisms had little impact, but this is changing with the growing acceptance of Metabolic Control Analysis. From Chapter 5 on, the theoretical and experimental grounds for rejecting the rate–limiting step concept will be presented. In summary, it has been found that more than one enzyme can affect the rate of a pathway; although it is possible to imagine conditions where only one step affects the rate of a pathway, experimental studies show that this is not the usual case.

In studying the control of metabolism, we therefore have a problem. Much of the work that has been done has been interpreted in terms of the concept of the rate–limiting enzyme. This work cannot be disregarded, because it has given us methodologies for studying metabolic pathways, has provided evidence about what does happen in pathways as their rates change and has led to the discovery of many mechanisms that appear to have a role in the control of pathway rates. Since it is necessary to look back at this work, as I shall do particularly in Chapter 4, it is necessary to recognize that it was often motivated by the search for a rate–limiting enzyme. This search was conducted by looking for enzymes that had the characteristics of potential *regulatory enzymes*, and then attempting to gather evidence that one of these was the rate–limiting step.

The key characteristics of regulatory enzymes were variously given as:

- an enzyme that catalyses a non–equilibrium reaction (e.g. Newsholme & Start[171]),

- an enzyme that catalyses a non–equilibrium reaction and whose activity is controlled by factors other than substrate concentration. (e.g. Newsholme & Start;[171] Denton & Pogson[60]),

- ... the enzyme which responds to the original metabolic signal and thereby initiates subsequent changes in the activity of the remaining enzymes ...(after Newsholme & Start[171]).

The reasons for concentrating on non–equilibrium enzymes were explained previously. However, pathways often contain several non–equilibrium enzymes, so it was thought necessary to look for further features that distinguish between them. All enzymes will change their rate of reaction if their substrate concentrations are changed, unless they are already saturated (which is not usually the

case in a pathway). The second definition of a regulatory enzyme therefore
attempts to eliminate enzymes that can be regarded as responding passively
to a requirement to change rate because some other change in a pathway has
altered the rate of supply of substrate, but that lack any mechanism to initiate
a change in the pathway rate. The third definition goes further by stating that
there might be a number of enzymes that satisfy the second definition, but that
one amongst these must be the one that first reacted to some signal to change
the pathway rate. Chapter 4 describes the ways in which these characteristics
were identified in the various enzymes of a pathway.

The difference between the second and third definitions of regulatory enzymes given above implies that some of them could have functions other than
flux control. Bücher & Rüssmann[24] noted in 1963 that one of the remarkable
things about muscle glycolysis was that the pathway flux could change by a
factor of more than a hundred between the resting and working state with only
small changes in the relative concentrations of the metabolites. They linked
this *homoeostasis of cellular metabolite ratios* (as they termed it) to the requirement for *functional readiness* of the muscle on the basis that the time taken to
establish a new steady state when the flux is changed is shorter if the associated
changes in metabolite concentrations are small. This is because the time taken
to reach a new steady state includes the time taken to synthesize or remove
the metabolic intermediates. (This concept has since been verified in more
detailed analyses, first by John Easterby[62,64] and later by others.[157]) Bücher
& Rüssmann[24] therefore proposed that regulatory enzymes were involved as
much in homoeostasis of metabolite levels as in flux control and, for this reason, multiple sites of control were needed. Biochemists generally seemed to pay
little attention to this original suggestion of a requirement for multiple control
sites, but towards the end of this book, I will raise the topic again and look at
the reasons for believing Bücher & Rüssmann were right (Chapter 8.1, p. 257).
Their observations about homoeostasis of concentrations were noted though,
as reflected in Newsholme & Gevers' definition[169] of a regulatory enzyme as
one:

> . . . the activity of which is controlled by factors other than substrate
> availability, and the activity of which controls the rate of flux or the
> concentrations of metabolic intermediates.

Some biochemists, therefore, had recognized that there could be two types of
role for regulatory enzymes:

- the stabilization of the pathway to adapt its production or consumption
  of a particular metabolite to the rest of metabolism; this is metabolic
  homoeostasis, and often involves internal signals acting on the regulatory
  enzymes;

- the response to external signals that change the state of a pathway or metabolism in general (e.g. hormones, second messengers etc); this is control, again acting on regulatory enzymes.

Metabolic Control Analysis introduces coefficients that measure the potential of enzymes to fulfil the second of these roles. One of the reasons that some biochemists have been reluctant to give up the traditional characterization of regulatory enzymes is that these measures from Metabolic Control Analysis do show that some enzymes that clearly possess regulatory properties cannot control pathway flux. My reason for mentioning this is to underline my final point: these two aspects of regulation and control are distinct, and there is no reason to assume that they are both performed by the same regulatory enzymes. In fact, Metabolic Control Analysis gives grounds for believing that there is a basic incompatibility between these two roles. The traditional approaches to the search for rate–limiting enzymes, on the other hand, offer no clear criteria for distinguishing between them.

1.5 Summary

(1) Regulation is homoeostasis, or the maintenance of constant conditions in the face of external perturbations.

(2) Control is the ability to make changes as necessary.

(3) Regulation and control are properties of metabolic systems of great complexity and the unsolved challenge is to link our knowledge of molecular details to system–level explanations in a convincing yet feasible manner.

(4) In metabolism, different mechanisms for regulation and control exist on different time scales:

- On long time scales, amounts of enzyme are changed by enzyme synthesis and degradation.
- On medium time scales, the activities of ready–formed enzyme are altered by covalent modification.
- On short time scales, the activities of enzymes alter in response to changes in metabolite concentrations.

(5) Metabolic pathways generally tend to a steady state, a dynamic equilibrium where rates of formation of intermediates equal their rates of breakdown and concentrations remain constant. Individual reactions are displaced from chemical equilibrium, but reactions with small standard free energy changes tend to be close to equilibrium and reactions with large standard free energy changes tend to be far from equilibrium.

(6) Enzymes that catalyse reactions that are far from equilibrium are thought to be more important in regulation and control than those whose reactions are near to equilibrium.

(7) In the past, analysis of regulation and control has concentrated on identifying the supposed rate–limiting enzymes for each pathway, but this concept is unsatisfactory in many respects.

(8) Regulatory enzymes can function to regulate intermediate concentrations or to control flux.

1.6 Appendix: Free energy changes

There are serious objections to the use of ΔG to represent the free energy change in a biochemical reaction for reasons that have been given by Rick Welch in New Orleans.[271] When ΔH is used to represent the enthalpy change of a reaction, it indicates the difference in enthalpy between the reactants and products, measured by the heat change on complete conversion. The free energy value given for a (bio)chemical reaction in solution is not a difference between initial and final states after complete conversion, but the rate at which the free energy is changing during the conversion of reactants to the products at the current values of their concentrations. It should really be represented as $\partial G/\partial \xi$, where ξ is a measure of the extent of the reaction in terms of moles converted. This is also equal to $-A$, where A is the *chemical affinity* used in non-equilibrium thermodynamics to characterize the driving force on a reaction. Unfortunately, this more appropriate terminology is not familiar from standard biochemical texts, so the usual, misleading, symbol will be used here.

Further reading

Atkinson, D. E. (1977) Cellular Energy Metabolism and its Regulation, Academic Press, New York

van Dam, K. (1986) *Biochemistry is a Quantitative Science.* Trends Biochem. Sci. **11**, 13–14

Kacser, H. (1987) *Control of Metabolism.* In The Biochemistry of Plants (Davies, D. D., ed.) Vol. II, pp. 39–44, Academic Press, New York

Problems

(1) Phosphofructokinase catalyses the reaction:

$$\text{Fru6P} + \text{ATP} \rightleftharpoons \text{Fru1,6P}_2 + \text{ADP}$$

The following substrate and product concentrations were measured in the perfused rat heart:

Metabolite	Tissue content ($\mu mol/g$ of dry tissue)
Fru6P	0.154
Fru1,6P$_2$	0.042
ATP	21.70
ADP	2.49

Rat heart contains 5.67 cm^3 of H$_2$O/g of dry weight; 50% of this water is intracellular and 50% extracellular. Calculate the intracellular concentrations of the metabolites, and then the mass action ratio, Γ. The equilibrium constant K_{eq} is 1.0×10^3. Calculate the ratio Γ/K_{eq} and thus conclude the degree of displacement from equilibrium.

(2) Glucose-6-phosphate isomerase catalyses the reaction:

$$Glc6P \rightleftharpoons Fru6P$$

for which the equilibrium constant is believed to be in the range 0.36–0.47. Under control conditions, the contents of the two intermediates in perfused rat hearts were determined as 290 and 63 nmol/g of wet weight respectively. Given that rat heart contains 0.43 cm^3 of intracellular water per g of wet weight, what are the concentrations of these metabolites in the cytoplasm? What is the mass action ratio, Γ, for the reaction, and what can be inferred about its displacement from equilibrium?

2

Methods for studying metabolism and its regulation

2.1 Introduction

Although my aim in this book is to describe a new approach to the interpretation of control and regulation in metabolism, the experimental methods that are needed are exactly the same as those traditionally used in biochemistry. This chapter therefore introduces the experimental measurements that have been used in the past to develop explanations of control and regulation and that continue to be used in the growing body of experimental studies in Metabolic Control Analysis.

There are four main issues that have to be addressed before carrying out most experiments in metabolism:

- the choice of the particular experimental system in which the metabolism is to be studied;

- the problems of measuring metabolite concentrations *in vivo*;

- the problems of making meaningful measurements of the activities of the relevant enzymes;

- deciding how to measure the metabolic fluxes.

Each of these issues is considered in turn in the following four sections.

2.2 Experimental systems

In principle, the choice of experimental system could start with the organism in which to study the metabolic activity of interest but, in practice, the range of this element of choice can be very limited from the beginning. The reasons for this, though, are varied. Some will relate to the extrinsic motivations for studying a particular metabolic pathway in the first instance. For example, if the aim is to explore the differences between an aspect of human metabolism in health and disease, and if suitable human cell or tissue samples cannot readily be obtained ethically, then it will almost certainly be necessary to use animal material. The animal would need to be no larger than necessary to supply sufficient material for study (since larger animals are more expensive to feed and house humanely), have a metabolism sufficiently similar to humans for the results to be relevant, and have been sufficiently studied in the past that the results can be placed in context. It is also an advantage if inbred strains are available that have a restricted range of individual variation. In most cases, this points to the small rodents. Another aim might be to study the metabolism of an organism of economic importance, for example an animal or plant used as food, or a microorganism that produces a valuable chemical such as a drug, and in this case there is no real choice. What I am implying, of course, is that the extrinsic motivation to study a particular organism arises from the existence of an organization prepared to fund biochemists to carry out the experiments. (Unfortunately, there are few sources of funding for carrying out basic research propelled by an intrinsic motivation to understand metabolic regulation better, in spite of the evidence that the funded applied research is handicapped by the limitations in our basic understanding.)

Given, then, that a choice of organism has been made, or forced, there still remains the choice of how it, or parts of it, are to be used. Here are a range of options (not all of which are appropriate to all organisms).

2.2.1   Whole multicellular organisms

At this level of study, examples of the types of experiment that can be done include the effects of diet or environmental conditions on the tissue contents of enzymes and measurement of the overall patterns of conversion of nutrients into various end products. While the organism is alive and actively metaboliz-ing, the methods of investigation must cause little perturbation. For example, with animals, non–invasive methods such as analysis of respiratory gases, urine and faeces can be used, or else minimally invasive methods such as taking blood samples or small tissue samples with a biopsy needle. Other possibilities can include the tracking of the metabolism of compounds that have been labelled isotopically, for example by substituting hydrogen with its radioactive isotope tritium (^{3}H) or carbon with its radioactive isotope ^{14}C and monitoring the distribution of radioactivity. Recently, the technique of nuclear magnetic reso-nance (NMR), which produces characteristic spectra of chemicals based on the magnetic properties of certain atomic nuclei (including hydrogen, phosphorus and the carbon isotope ^{13}C), has been scaled up to allow non–invasive measure-ments of metabolites *in vivo* on human limbs or whole small animals. (More details of NMR spectrometry are given later, in Section 2.3.2.)

After the death of the organism, the full range of analytical biochemical techniques can be applied to tissue samples, but this obviously terminates the experiment with that individual, and different individuals must be analysed to determine the effects of different experimental conditions.

The **advantage** of whole-organism studies is that metabolism is taking place under physiologically normal conditions.

The **disadvantages** are as follows:

(1) Physiologically normal conditions for multicellular organisms mean that there are metabolic interactions between tissues, which usually have different metabolic specializations. Observations will show the net result of these interactions, as modulated by the effects of hormonal and nervous stimuli (which may be difficult to control).

(2) Metabolizable substrates must reach the site of their metabolism, and the products escape, by crossing the natural permeability barriers. Since these are selective, this reduces the scope for introducing artificial substrates or changing the amounts of intermediates that are normally confined within the cells.

(3) The natural biological variability of the organisms on which the experiments are performed means that it is necessary to carry out replicate experiments to determine the mean behaviour and to perform statistical tests to establish the significance of any observed differences between control and experimental conditions. This increases the number of experimental subjects that have to be used, which increases the time taken and the cost and, in the case of animal experiments, raises the ethical dilemma of minimizing the number of individuals used whilst adequately verifying the findings.

2.2.2 Isolated tissues and organs

The metabolism of a specific part of a multicellular organism can be studied in isolation if it can be maintained in a viable state.

The **advantages** that this offers include the following.

(1) The metabolic responses of the tissue can be studied in the absence of interactions with other organs.

(2) It is easier to control the concentrations of nutrients, hormones and so on to which the tissue is exposed. And yet

(3) The functional integrity of the tissue is retained.

The **disadvantages** of studying whole organs include the following.

(1) The supply of nutrients and removal of excretory products can be technically difficult, particularly with animal tissues in the absence of a functioning blood circulation. The simplest solution is to use naturally thin

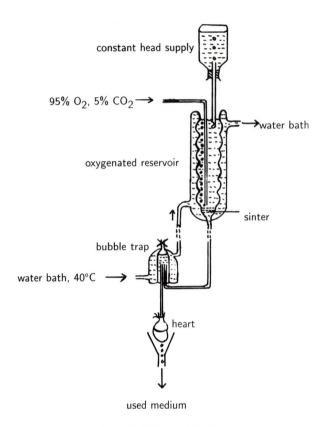

constant head supply

95% O_2, 5% CO_2 →

→ water bath

oxygenated reservoir

sinter

bubble trap

water bath, 40°C →

heart

used medium

Figure 2.1 Apparatus for perfusion of isolated rat heart
The components are not to scale.

tissues and to rely on exchange of materials with the surroundings by passive diffusion. Examples of suitable thin tissues include plant leaves and the diaphragm muscle and epididymal fat (the fat around the testes) of rats. With larger animal organs it is necessary to replace the blood circulation by *perfusion* of an oxygenated nutrient solution through the blood vessels. This is technically more difficult and requires more equipment (see Figure 2.1). Liver and heart are two organs often studied in this way.

(2) Tissues and organs themselves are often heterogeneous, with different cell types exhibiting different metabolic functions and responses.

(3) Most of the permeability barriers that restrict experiments in whole organisms are still intact in the isolated organs.

(4) Biological variability will still result in the need for replicate experiments and statistical analysis. If, as with animal liver and heart, there is only one such organ per animal, the number of experimental subjects needed is no lower than with whole-animal studies. Where there is more than

one organ per organism, then the numbers needed are reduced because control and test experiments can be performed on matched organs from the same organism.

2.2.3   Tissue slices

With tissues that are too thick for diffusion to be an efficient means of supplying nutrients and removing waste products, another option is to cut from them uniform slices of the order of 1 mm thick. This works well with potato tubers and the kidney cortex of rats, for example, but is less successful with liver as the slices prove to be less viable.

The **advantages** are as follows.

(1) The procedure is technically simpler than organ perfusion, since the slices just have to be incubated in oxygenated nutrient solution as the nutrient supply is by diffusion.

(2) Fewer individuals are used than in whole-animal studies because many slices can be taken from one organ and this also reduces the effects of biological variability since control and test treatments can be compared on slices from the same organ.

There are some **disadvantages**, as follows.

(1) There is inevitably cell damage at the cut surfaces, and substances released from the damaged cells may affect the undamaged ones.

(2) The permeability barrier formed by the cell membranes is still in place.

2.2.4   Isolated cells

If the initial choice of organism was a microorganism, this will be the first relevant option. However, it is increasingly an option in plant and animal studies also. Of course, there are only a few types of animal cell that exist naturally in a free state; red blood cells and sperm are examples, but they have extremely specialized metabolism. Certain types of cancer cell have been established as cultures that can be grown readily in laboratory conditions and are available from cell culture collections. However, cancer cells show significant metabolic differences from the normal cells from which they are derived and, whilst this is important in its own right for the study of cancer as a disease process, they cannot be used as a reliable guide to the metabolism of normal cells. Most differentiated animal cells will not grow indefinitely in culture conditions, although some relatively undifferentiated precursor cells may grow, most readily as cell monolayers attached to a surface. In general, animal cells die after about 20 to 40 cell divisions (a limitation on the growth of cultures often termed the Hayflick limit). Undifferentiated cells persist in plants throughout their lives and can often be grown as cell suspensions. In plants, even differentiated cells may dedifferentiate and grow well, whereas differentiation is largely irreversible in animal cells.

Techniques have also been developed for isolating cells from animal organs. For example, in 1969 Berry & Friend[16] in Australia devised the method commonly used these days for obtaining individual cells, hepatocytes, from mammalian liver in high yield. Their innovation was to perfuse the liver with an oxygenated solution containing proteolytic enzymes that attack the intercellular ground substance and the adhesion factors on the cell surfaces. After a short while, the tissue loses its integrity and can be dispersed to yield free cells. Similar techniques have been applied to other tissues, for example, giving fat cells (adipocytes) from fat tissue. In most cases, these isolated cells will not grow in culture and can only be maintained for relatively short periods.

Compared with the other systems examined so far, the **advantages** of using isolated cells include the following.

(1) Diffusion is entirely adequate for nutrient supply provided that the cell suspension is kept adequately mixed and there is sufficient surface area for gas exchange (where necessary). The equipment required is therefore relatively simple.

(2) Many samples can be taken from the same batch of cells, and since each sample might typically contain 10^5–10^7 cells, inter–sample variation should be minimal. This should reduce the number of experiments needed to establish statistically significant findings. Variability between different experiments, and between different laboratories, can be reduced if clones of cells are used.

(3) In studies of animal metabolism, many fewer experimental animals will be needed. This may be just because of the previous reason, but in the case of cell culture, the material from the original animal is multiplied up many times. However, it should be noted that most animal cell culture media need the inclusion of some foetal calf serum to supply the growth factors without which most isolated animal cells die. (In plant cell cultures, coconut milk supplies the needed factors.)

The **disadvantages** of studies on isolated cells are as follows.

(1) The amounts of cellular material are small, particularly in relation to the amount of suspension medium, so it is necessary to have efficient techniques for separating the cells and sensitive analytical techniques for assaying their contents.

(2) The cell membranes still pose permeability barriers.

2.2.5 Permeabilized cells

Cells can be made permeable to small molecules by partial removal of lipid from their plasma membranes by treatment with aqueous solutions of organic solvents or non-ionic detergents and still remain metabolically active. The treatment has to be brief and carefully controlled so that the holes made in the membrane are too small to allow the enzymes to leak out. In an early experiment of this type, Serrano, Gancedo & Gancedo[225] permeabilized yeast cells and showed that it was possible to measure the kinetics of hexokinase retained within.

The **advantages** of using permeabilized calls are the same as those of isolated cells plus the greater access to the cell interior, which allows the addition of metabolites that would not normally cross the membrane.

The **disadvantages**, apart from those associated with isolated cells generally, include the following

(1) The dilution or loss of key metabolites of low molecular mass.

(2) Possible uncertainty about the extent of damage to the cells and the degree of loss of enzymes etc.

2.2.6 Cell–free systems

One of the first experiments in metabolic biochemistry was when the Buchner brothers ground up a paste of yeast cells with sand and demonstrated that ethanol formation from sugar could take place in a cell extract. Hans Krebs' experiments that led to his discovery of the tricarboxylic acid cycle used homogenates of pigeon breast muscle, so metabolically competent, cell–free systems obtained by mechanically breaking tissues and cells have a long history. A more recent variant is to take isolated, purified components, such as individual enzymes, and to combine them to form a working, though limited, replica of a particular segment of metabolism.

The **advantages** are the simplicity and reproducibility of the procedure and the lack of permeability barriers. The **disadvantages** are as follows.

(1) The variable degrees of loss of (eukaryotic) cell structure, such as the separate compartments formed by intracellular organelles and any possible cytoskeletal structure. Whether this is significant for the pathway under study would have to be a matter for experiment.

(2) The possible dilution of key metabolites and enzymes if the cells are lysed or homogenized (as is usual) in a liquid medium.

2.2.7 Isolated organelles

Just as there is metabolic specialization amongst the tissues of multicellular organisms, so there is in the organelles of eukaryotic cells. Therefore, it is often

desirable to obtain a particular organelle in a pure state by subcellular fractionation (usually by differential or zonal centrifugation) in order to determine
its metabolic capabilities in the absence of interactions with the cytoplasm and
other organelles. For example, oxidative phosphorylation is most usually studied on preparations of isolated mitochondria by the techniques described in
more detail later in the book (Chapter 6.5, p. 191).

The **advantages**, apart from that of isolating a particular metabolic subsys-
tem of the cell, are similar to those of studying isolated cells (indeed, mitochondria and chloroplasts are comparable in size to bacterial cells).

The **disadvantages** are as follows.

(1) The degree of damage during isolation and the purity of the samples are
    difficult to assess. Some types of damage are inevitable and reproducible.
    For example, the biochemist's microsomes are extensively disrupted frag-
    ments of endoplasmic reticulum. Again, the mitochondria of many cell
    types are large extended structures present in small numbers (unlike those
    from the animal liver cells that are used as their most frequent source)
    and presumably fragment into smaller pieces during isolation.

(2) The cellular environment is replaced by an artificial one, although this
    does offer greater opportunity for experimental manipulation.

(3) The membranes of some organelles act as permeability barriers restricting
    access.

2.2.8   Isolated enzymes
The next lower level of study is the enzymes themselves. Techniques for purification of enzymes have been developed throughout the 20th century, and many
are now prepared on an industrial scale and marketed. Obviously, an individual
enzyme is hardly a metabolic system in its own right. However, studies of the
properties of isolated enzymes have an important role in the study of metabolic
regulation and will be introduced in Chapter 3.

2.3   Measurement of metabolites

In any approach to understanding the inner workings of metabolism it is essential to know the concentrations of the intermediary metabolites while the
pathway is in operation and to know how they change in circumstances that
affect the rate of the pathway. In making these measurements there are several
distinct problems which I will describe in turn.

2.3.1   Fixing concentrations
Only a small number of analytical techniques allow the estimation of *in vivo*
concentrations of metabolites. Examples include the use of fluorescence spectrophotometry to measure NADH concentrations, dual beam spectrophotometry

to measure the concentrations of redox components of the mitochondrial and chloroplast electron transport chains, and NMR spectrophotometry (which unfortunately can take up to 45 min to take a single spectrum, and even then can only measure the more concentrated metabolites with an error of about 10%). Most other methods of analysis therefore require release of metabolites from cells and take some time to complete. For these methods, the problem they all have in common is how to prevent changes in metabolite concentrations between the time a sample is taken for analysis and the results recorded. The goal is to stop all the enzymic reactions rapidly and simultaneously to get an instantaneous snapshot of the concentrations. How rapidly this needs to be depends on the amount of metabolite in the cell relative to the rate at which it is produced or consumed; the amount divided by the rate gives the *turnover time*. Typical values range from several seconds to milliseconds in the worst cases (such as oxaloacetate in the tricarboxylic acid cycle — for which the situation is virtually hopeless).

Methods that have been used to *quench* metabolism rapidly include the following.

(1) Sudden pH change, e.g. by mixing with perchloric acid ($HClO_4$), which is a powerful protein denaturant. This is particularly suitable for cell-free systems that can be rapidly injected into a well–mixed solution of the acid. It can be used with cells, but will be slower because of the lag time whilst the acid penetrates the cells. One of the motives for using perchloric acid is that the resulting solution can be neutralized with KOH, and the perchlorate removed because potassium perchlorate precipitates from cold solutions.

(2) Rapid freezing at liquid N_2 temperatures. This relies on the rapid drop in temperature first slowing enzymic reactions and then stopping them as the system solidifies. Freezing rates are very rapid if cell–free solutions or cell suspensions are sprayed into the liquid nitrogen. Larger objects such as isolated organs cannot be frozen sufficiently rapidly unless they are very thin. This is because the nitrogen boils and forms an insulating layer of bubbles over their surface. For isolated organs, such as heart muscle, the technique of freeze–clamping is used instead. In this, two blocks of metal (aluminium or copper) with a high heat conductivity and mounted on long scissor–like handles (a Wollenberger clamp) are cooled in liquid nitrogen. The organ is then squashed between the two metal blocks. The temperature of a guinea pig kidney has been measured to fall from 38 to 0 °C in 90 ms and to −160 °C in 0.5 s when frozen in this way. Whatever the way in which the samples have been frozen, they are ground to a powder whilst still frozen, and then thawed by rapid mixing with perchloric acid so that enzymic activity does not recover as the metabolites are taken into solution.

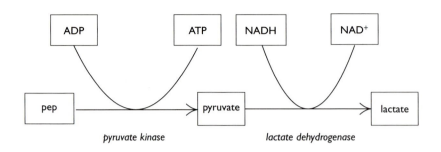

Figure 2.2 A coupled enzyme assay
Lactate dehydrogenase alone can be used to assay pyruvate in a sample by the fall in NADH concentration. If pyruvate kinase and ADP are then added, the coupled assay can be used to measure phosphoenolpyruvate (pep). Alternatively, if pyruvate kinase and pep are added, ADP can be assayed.

(3) Mixing with organic solvents. Again this relies on the denaturing effect of the solvent to stop enzyme activity. For example, Melvin Calvin used hot methanol to stop metabolism in *Chlorella* algae in his experiments to determine the photosynthetic carbon pathway by determining the rate of appearance of ^{14}C in intracellular metabolites from CO_2, which was one of the earliest studies to make use of radioisotope labelling.

2.3.2   Low concentrations in complex mixtures

Most intermediary metabolites occur in cells at concentrations in the micromolar to millimolar range amongst a mixture of thousands of other substances, some of which will be chemically similar. Measurement of their concentrations therefore requires sensitive methods that are either intrinsically selective or that include a separation step. The following are examples of techniques that have proved useful.

(1) Enzymic analysis, often using spectrophotometric or fluorimetric detection. Here the selectivity of the analysis is provided by choosing an enzyme with a narrow specificity for the metabolite to be assayed. Of course, this only helps if the products of the reaction are easier to detect than the metabolite itself. A common strategy is to use dehydrogenases so that the reaction consumes or produces NADH or NADPH, both of which can be detected spectrophotometrically and, with about a thousand times greater sensitivity, fluorimetrically. If the metabolite of interest is not acted on by a dehydrogenase, *coupled enzyme assays* can be used, where a sequence of two or three enzymes ends with a dehydrogenase reaction. An example is shown in Figure 2.2. Many other detection techniques can be linked to the enzyme assay. One that provides particularly high sensitivity for measuring metabolites in very low concentrations is luminescence. This involves the detection of the weak pulse of light produced by the light–emitting enzymes, the luciferases. Luciferase derived

from fireflies acts on ATP, thereby detecting it and reactions that produce it, whilst bacterial luciferase reacts with NADH and so can be used with coupled enzyme assays involving NAD–linked dehydrogenases.

(2) Chromatographic separation and quantification. The requirements for separation of complex biological mixtures have long been a driving force in the development of chromatographic methods, and most techniques have had some application in the separation of metabolic intermediates. The most useful methods are those which are linked to some form of quantitative detection and these days the most versatile method is HPLC. This is based on apparatus designed to force solvents at high pressure through strong, finely divided support particles that can carry one of a variety of selective stationary phases that are responsible for the separations. Relatively high flow rates allow separations to be achieved in around 10 min, and a variety of highly sensitive detectors have been developed to monitor substances in the column eluate. Most metabolic intermediates carry ionic charges and can be separated by ion-exchange or reverse-phase columns.

(3) Immunoassay methods. These exploit the specificity and high affinity of binding by antibodies, but first it is necessary that the metabolites can act as antigens and elicit an immune response, which is not straightforward since most metabolites are small molecules that are not intrinsically immunogenic. If they are attached to a larger immunogenic molecule, then a response to them can sometimes be stimulated. Immunoassay methods are capable of extremely high sensitivity and have been used for metabolites that are present at particularly low levels and that are difficult to assay by other techniques, such as the second messenger, cyclic AMP.

(4) NMR spectrometry. Most spectrophotometric techniques, for example visible/ultraviolet spectrophotometry, are not sufficiently selective to be applied to a complex mixture of metabolites in order to identify and assay specific components. The exception is NMR spectrophotometry. This detects certain atomic nuclei that have a magnetic moment by means of their absorbance and emission of high-frequency radio waves when they are placed in very strong magnetic fields generated with super–conducting electromagnets. The magnetic field and radio frequency combination that leads to absorption by an atomic nucleus is subtly influenced by the valence shell electrons surrounding the nucleus, so that nuclei in different chemical compounds absorb in different parts of the spectrum. Helpfully for biologists, the nuclei of two common elements, hydrogen (^{1}H) and phosphorus (^{31}P), are magnetic and give a signal. The rare isotope of carbon, ^{13}C, also gives a signal, though this is extremely weak at the levels of this isotope found naturally in organic material. However, by using compounds enriched in their content of this stable isotope, it is possible

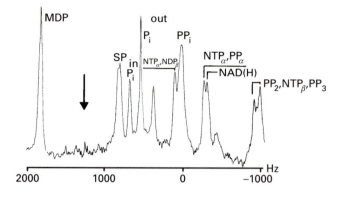

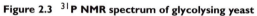

Figure 2.3 ^{31}**P NMR spectrum of glycolysing yeast**
This spectrum was recorded *in vivo* by Kevin Brindle & Susan Krikler [(1985) Biochim. Biophys. Acta **847**, 285–292, Figure 1; reproduced with permission from the publishers]. MDP, reference signal; P_i^{in}, cytosolic phosphate; P_i^{out}, extracellular phosphate; SP, sugar phosphates; NTPγ, γ–phosphate of nucleotide triphosphates, etc; PP$_1$ terminal phosphate of polyphosphates; PP$_2$ and PP$_3$, penultimate phosphates of polyphosphate. The result is the average of 512 spectra collected over 40 min.

to monitor its spread through a metabolic pathway. NMR is so selective that it can be used to detect and measure metabolites *in vivo* without any need to quench metabolism and separate the metabolites (Figure 2.3). The disadvantage is that the sensitivity of the technique is not quite as high as is needed. It can measure down to fractions of a millimolar, but this is only enough to detect the more abundant intermediary metabolites (though this does include important compounds like ATP). In addition, the signals from phosphorus and carbon are very weak, and may have to be collected for half an hour or more. Finally, the equipment needed to make these measurements is very expensive to buy, and costly to use because the super–conducting magnets have to be kept near absolute zero all the time with a supply of liquid helium (in a vacuum flask itself surrounded by liquid nitrogen).

2.3.3   Compartmentation

Tissues and cells contain a number of liquid compartments separated by selectively permeable membranes. Most metabolites will not be present at a uniform concentration in every compartment, and whilst average values may show significant changes with experimental conditions, they cannot accurately represent the concentrations to which a particular enzyme is exposed within the compartment in which it is found.

The first distinction to be made is between intracellular and extracellular fluid compartments. Obviously these are both present in tissues, but less obviously, they are also present in samples of packed cells obtained from cell suspensions by centrifugation or filtration, since these techniques always leave some medium around and between the cells. We can assume that most metabolites are present only in the intracellular compartment, but that when substances are present in the extracellular compartment, their concentrations there can be determined by assay of the bulk medium in which the cells or tissues were incubated. The key to the problem of determining intracellular concentrations is then to determine the relative volumes of water in these two compartments. A common approach is to determine the total volume of water in the sample and then subtract the volume of extracellular water. The total water content can be measured by the loss of weight of a sample on gentle drying, though this is not compatible with sample preparation for metabolite assays. Another possibility is to add tritiated water, $[^3H]H_2O$, to the medium. A measurement of the radioactivity from the tritium in a sample will then indicate its total water content, since the tritiated water will distribute uniformly and rapidly through the system. The extracellular water content can be determined by adding a substance to the incubation medium that can be readily measured, is not naturally present in the cells and is unable to enter them across the cell membrane. Large polysaccharides, such as inulin, labelled with radioactive ^{14}C are often used.

A more difficult problem is to determine the distribution of metabolites within cells. In most cells, the cytoplasm will be the largest aqueous compartment, so if a metabolite is reasonably uniformly distributed within the cell, the average concentration obtained by dividing its content in the sample by the intracellular water content will be close to the cytoplasmic concentration. (Plant cells are more of a problem as the vacuole is the largest intracellular volume.)

Few techniques allow the direct observation of metabolite distributions in eukaryotic cells. NMR may be able to resolve and measure cytoplasmic and mitochondrial ATP because the ^{31}P spectra are pH–dependent and the pH difference between these two compartments can be sufficient to separate the peaks. Photometric measurements can be made on microscope images, but either the cells must be fixed and stained for the metabolite in such a way that it does not redistribute (for example by rapid freezing) or the measurements must be made on living cells (for example, using the natural fluorescence of compounds such as NADH, or fluorescent indicators and labels, such as aquorein, which is sensitive to calcium concentrations).

Rapid animal cell fractionation techniques have been developed to measure mitochondrial metabolite levels, which are the ones most likely to show significant differences from cytoplasmic concentrations in animal cells. One of these was developed for hepatocytes by Zuurendonk & Tager[283,284] in Amsterdam in the laboratories from which some of the major experimental advances in Metabolic Control Analysis were to emerge a few years later. In their method, a tube for a small centrifuge that accelerates very rapidly is filled with a small volume of perchloric acid solution overlaid by a layer of inert silicone oil. On top of this is laid a medium containing the metal–chelating agent EDTA and the detergent digitonin. Digitonin attacks cell membranes according to their cholesterol content, which is much higher in plasma membranes than in mitochondrial membranes. In a short period of exposure, therefore, the outer membranes of the cell lyse, but the mitochondria remain intact. The whole tube is cooled on ice before the cell sample is added to the top layer and mixed; 10–15 s later, the centrifuge is started and the mitochondria are rapidly spun down through the oil into the perchloric acid. The centrifuge is stopped and the top layer containing the cytoplasm is acidified. The lower layer is assayed to give the metabolite concentrations in the mitochondria and the top layer those in the cytoplasm. The separation of the mitochondrial and cytoplasmic compartments is 80–90% efficient, and changes in the cytosolic adenine nucleotide levels by continuing metabolism are minimized by the low temperature and the EDTA, which removes essential Mg^{2+} ions.

2.3.4   Free and bound metabolites

Some of the metabolites in cells will, at any one time, be bound to proteins, in particular to the enzymes that act on them. The fraction that is bound varies depending on the concentrations of the metabolite and the binding protein and the affinity of the binding reaction. Only the free metabolite in solution contributes to the concentration that is 'seen' by enzymes, but the majority of analytical methods measure the total amount of metabolite. Whether there is a significant difference between the free and total concentrations varies on a case-by-case basis. In muscle cells, for example, there is a measurable amount of total ADP, but the evidence is that most of this is bound to the myosin ATPase. Probably around half of the cellular content of the second messenger cyclic AMP is bound to cyclic AMP–dependent protein kinase.

Various sorts of experimental evidence support these statements.

(1) NMR measurements. For technical reasons, the NMR signals from metabolites that are bound to large molecules are not usually visible in the spectra and only molecules in free solution are detected. NMR showed that ADP was undetectable in muscle cells, whereas the measured total concentrations were high enough to have been visible. Unfortunately, the limited sensitivity of NMR measurements means that they cannot provide information on the metabolites at low concentration that might be most affected by binding to proteins.

(2) Determination of the binding characteristics of e.g. a cell homogenate. This can be undertaken in the same way as binding experiments on enzymes (see Chapter 3.4), except that there is a possibility that the metabolite might be converted by enzymes in the homogenate. (This could be averted by removing essential coenzymes and cofactors.) This was one of the ways that the binding of cyclic AMP was assessed.

(3) Estimation using measured concentrations of the known major binding proteins and the dissociation constant. All the necessary information may not be easy to collect with sufficient accuracy to make a reliable calculation, but it is often possible to assess whether sufficient binding is

likely to occur for further investigation to be warranted. In both specific cases I have cited (binding of cyclic AMP by protein kinase and muscle ADP by myosin) such calculations indicated the likelihood of significant binding.

(4) Calculation of the concentration assuming the metabolite is in equilibrium with other metabolites that are unbound. The assumption that the enzyme catalysing the reaction involved is sufficiently active to bring the reaction near to equilibrium is obviously difficult to test when the metabolite concentration measurements are themselves in question. However, ADP concentrations calculated from the equilibrium constant of the creatine kinase reaction and the measured concentrations of ATP, creatine and creatine phosphate are much lower than measured total ADP concentrations.[164,258] Thus discrepancies in such calculations, or equivalently the observation of consistently unusual disequilibrium ratios involving a particular metabolite, can offer evidence that there is a problem.

2.4 Measurement of enzyme activity

Measurements of enzyme activity are invariably involved in the experimental investigation of metabolic regulation and control, yet it is often not clear how these measurements should be made in order to provide relevant evidence. I will not describe basic techniques of enzyme assay here; let us assume that assay methods exist for the enzymes of interest and consider some of the remaining problematical issues.

2.4.1 Assay conditions

Many enzyme assays were developed and optimized to aid detection of the enzyme and to carry out kinetic investigations for identifying the catalytic mechanism (see Chapter 3). The resulting assay conditions were not necessarily intended to reproduce *in vivo* conditions. For example, the pH of an assay may have been chosen because it is the optimum pH for enzyme activity, or because it is the pH at which the change in light absorption used for the assay is at a maximum, or because the equilibrium constant of the reaction is more favourable, or because it is the value at which the enzyme is most stable. Resemblance to intracellular pH will have come low down the list of priorities. Similar considerations may have swayed the choice of the assay temperature.

Does this matter? If the aim of the measurements is to detect relative changes in the amount of active enzyme in different physiological states, then probably not. If the aim is to compare the measured enzymic activity with the rate of metabolism (one of the traditional stages in the search for regulatory enzymes — see Chapter 4.4), then it would be better if pH, temperature and the ionic environment were as close as possible to *in vivo* values.

2.4.2 What to measure

Similar difficulties surround the choice of substrate concentrations at which to measure the activity. If high concentrations (relative to the K_m values) are used, the measurement approximates to the limiting rate (or maximum velocity), V. Again, this may be a useful measurement if the aim is to detect variations in the amount of active enzyme. It is of limited use otherwise, since few enzymes are exposed to such high substrate concentrations *in vivo*, and act in the presence of the reaction products, which are rarely included in assay mixtures. (See Figure 3.5 to see how much difference the products can make.) It is doubtful whether many enzymes *in vivo* are acting at more than a few per cent of their limiting rates.

2.4.3 Control of other factors affecting *in vivo* activity

Finally there are the miscellaneous factors that are the stuff of biochemists' nightmares because, if they affect the enzyme in question, but have escaped detection or not been adequately controlled, they could render the results meaningless. Some of the possibilities are as follows.

(1) Existence of unknown effectors. If the enzyme samples contained variable amounts of such an effector, then the results would be uninterpretable. This was found to have happened in 1980 in a metabolic pathway that has been known for most of this century: glycolysis. Van Schaftingen, Hue & Hers in Belgium discovered that the most powerful activator of phosphofructokinase was the previously unknown compound fructose 2,6–bisphosphate.[253,254] It acts as a messenger of hormone action. Ignorance of this effector has almost certainly resulted in erroneous conclusions about the regulation of glycolysis, since much has been made of the apparent (and unusual) product activation of mammalian liver phosphofructokinase by fructose 1,6–bisphosphate, but this is probably an artifact caused by binding of the product at the site for the effector. When fructose 2,6–bisphosphate is present at *in vivo* levels, activation by fructose 1,6–bisphosphate is much less significant and is often outweighed by its action as a normal product inhibitor,[255] as is the case for yeast phosphofructokinase.[11,186] Strangely, one of the criticisms of Metabolic Control Analysis has been that it would lead to the wrong conclusions if there were undiscovered effectors. Apart from the obvious point that all previous explanations of whatever form would be in danger of being wrong if there were undiscovered effects, the criticism seems to overlook the fact that it is a key characteristic of science to discard old explanations and embrace new ones when fresh discoveries are made.

(2) Degree of activation by cyclic covalent modification reactions. One of the ways that enzyme activity is altered *in vivo* is by enzyme–catalysed modification reactions (see Chapter 7.4). These can either interconvert

the enzyme between active and inactive forms or change its kinetic properties more subtly. The difficulty is ensuring that the degree of modification does not change from its *in vivo* level when the sample is taken for enzyme assay. For obvious reasons, it is not possible to use protein denaturation to inhibit the modification reactions, as is done for metabolite assays. Instead, the modification reactions have to be stopped by removal of necessary cofactors or the use of specific inhibitors. For example, glycogen synthase and glycogen phosphorylase have been extracted in an unchanged state by homogenizing freeze–clamped tissue with a buffer containing EDTA and KF^{125} as part of the study mentioned in Chapter 4.4 (Figure 4.4).

(3) Possible effects from loss of intracellular structure by homogenization and dilution. Enzymes are often assayed at concentrations thousands of times lower than their concentration in the cell. The assay environment is a simple aqueous solution. In the cell, enzymes are in a protein–rich environment, and may bind to other enzymes, membranes, glycogen particles or cytoskeletal elements. Investigations are still continuing into how common such interactions are and whether they have major implications for enzyme activity.

2.5 Measurement of metabolic fluxes

Measuring fluxes is a problem that can be either very easy or very hard. The easy part is measuring the fluxes of uptake of materials by the metabolic system or of output of end products, since these can be determined by the rates of disappearance or appearance of the relevant compounds. Of course, it may be necessary to look carefully to find all the products. For example, if yeast cells are metabolizing glucose, measurement of ethanol production and either oxygen consumption or CO_2 production will define the rates of anaerobic fermentation to ethanol and aerobic catabolism. These will probably account for a large part of the glucose consumption, but other minor end products could include glycerol, storage compounds such as trehalose and glycogen, and yeast cell biomass if the cells are growing, all of which could be measured to provide a balance sheet for the fate of glucose.

The more complicated problem is determining metabolic fluxes in the internal parts of metabolism, where the branches and cycles create multiple routes between an input and output metabolite. Sometimes it is possible to infer the pathway usage by calculating a pattern of pathway fluxes that accounts for the mass balances between the inputs and outputs and ensures that all the internal metabolites (including coenzymes such as NAD^+) have rates of formation equal to their rates of consumption. However, this does require very extensive and

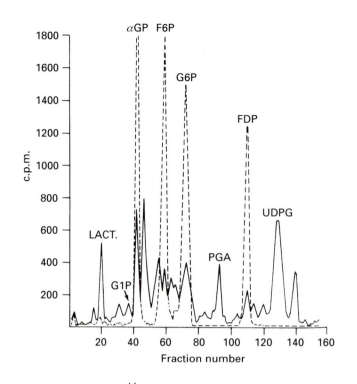

Figure 2.4 Ion-exchange HPLC of ^{14}C–labelled metabolites in rat hepatocytes
Chromatograms of extracts from cells incubated with [U–^{14}C]glucose. The broken lines show the positions of ^{3}H–labelled markers. LACT., lactate; G1P, glucose 1–phosphate; αGP, 3–phosphoglycerol; F6P, fructose 6–phosphate; PGA, 3–phosphoglycerate; FDP, fructose 1,6–bisphosphate; and UDPG, UDP–glucose. Reproduced with permission from Figure 3 of Katz et al. (1977), J. Biol. Chem. **253**, 4530–4536.

accurate measurements of all the inputs and outputs of the system, as well as full knowledge of the pathways that are potentially active.

The most common method of determining internal fluxes experimentally is by isotopic labelling. The system under investigation is incubated for a while to allow it to reach a metabolic steady state. One or more of the input metabolites is then replaced by material in which one or more atoms have been labelled by substitution with a rare isotope of the element (e.g. ^{2}H or ^{3}H for ^{1}H, ^{13}C or ^{14}C for ^{12}C, ^{15}N for ^{14}N, ^{32}P for ^{31}P). Isotopically labelled compounds are metabolized at essentially the same rate as the natural compounds. (Although there can be slight differences, they will be too small to be significant in these experiments, except perhaps in the case of hydrogen isotopes.) If the pathway is at steady state before a small amount of label is added; the spread of label follows simple linear kinetics, even though the enzyme kinetics of the steps involved are generally non–linear. Fluxes can be calculated from measurements of the degree of labelling of particular metabolites (their specific radioactivities) against time. In the past, the calculations tended to use simple approximations, based on assumptions about the relative rates of different parts of metabolism.

Nowadays, the best practice is to use a computer to find the best–fit solution to the results.[19] For example, Jacob Blum's group at Duke University, North Carolina, have determined networks of component metabolic fluxes in the catabolic pathways of the ciliate *Tetrahymena pyriformis*[19] and the gluconeogenic pathways of rat hepatocytes.[10,58,190] Barbara Wright's group in Montana have built up an extensive picture of the carbohydrate and amino acid metabolism during differentiation of the slime mould *Dictyostelium discoideum* by computer modelling of their isotopic tracer studies.[130,280]

More information about fluxes, especially of internal cyclic pathways, can be obtained from the experiments if the rates of spread of the isotope into individual positions in the compound are measured, and not just its overall activity.

The simplest and cheapest method of measurement is of the radioactivity associated with unstable isotopes such as ^3H and ^{14}C. The metabolites to be analysed must first be separated from other compounds carrying the isotope, and the total amount of labelled and unlabelled compound must be measured by conventional methods so that the degree of labelling (the specific radioactivity) can be determined. An example of the separation by ion-exchange HPLC and radioactive counting of glycolytic metabolites in an experiment[128] to measure fluxes in glucose metabolism in rat hepatocytes is shown in Figure 2.4. If the position of the isotopic label in the compound is to be determined, the compound must be broken up by enzymic or chemical means and the radioactivity of the fragments measured. For example, Blum's group measured the radioactive labelling in the C–1 position of glucose in their studies on gluconeogenesis in rat hepatocytes by enzymically cleaving this carbon atom from a sample of the glucose using the enzymes hexokinase, glucose–6–phosphate dehydrogenase and 6–phosphogluconate dehydrogenase. The carbon atom is released as CO_2 which is collected and has its radioactivity counted.[58]

Isotopic tracer studies can be carried out with stable (*i.e.* non–radioactive) isotopes if a mass spectrometer is used to make the measurements. A major advantage of using stable isotopes rather than radioactive ones is that they allow metabolic and nutritional investigations that would otherwise be unethical to be carried out safely on humans. Mass spectrometry separates molecules and molecular fragments on the basis of molecular mass with sufficient sensitivity to distinguish molecules containing the rare isotope from those containing the natural one, so that the relative proportions of labelled and unlabelled molecules can be measured in the same spectrum. Often the mass spectrometer is used as a detector after a chromatographic separation of the sample by gas–liquid chromatography or HPLC, though it is not essential to purify the target compound completely since the mass spectrum will separate the impurities. Furthermore, since compounds break down in a reproducible way into fragments in the mass spectrometer, the extent of labelling at particular positions in the molecule can be determined from the mass spectrum of the fragments. For example, the relative fluxes of gluconeogenesis and glucose phosphorylation in rats after 17 h

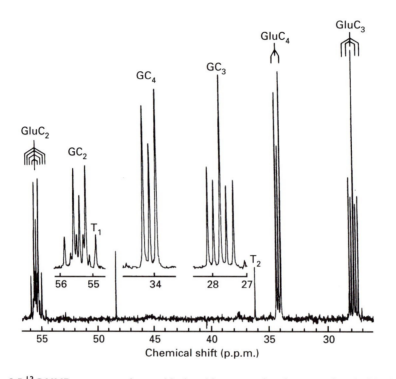

Figure 2.5 ^{13}C NMR spectrum of a perchloric acid extract of rat heart perfused with glucose and [2-^{13}C]acetate

GluC$_2$, (GC$_2$) etc are the groups of lines corresponding to carbon atoms 2, 3 and 4 of glutamate (*i.e.* oxoglutarate). The spectrum is the average of 2000 scans collected over more than an hour. T$_1$ and T$_2$ are carbon atoms 1 and 2 of naturally abundant taurine. Reproduced with permission from Fig. 3, Chance et al.[36]

fasting were estimated by the relative rates of incorporation of deuterium (^{2}H) from heavy water ([^{2}H]H$_2$O) on to the C–6 and C–2 carbon atoms of glucose respectively.[227] Mass spectrometry, like radioactivity measurements, has much higher sensitivity and precision than NMR measurements of isotopic labelling. The major disadvantages compared with radioisotope studies are the much higher cost and greater complexity of the apparatus.

NMR can be used to detect the spread of ^{13}C through a pathway. Since individual carbon atoms give separate lines in the spectrum, the position of labelling in the molecule is determined at the same time (Figure 2.5). As mentioned previously, the method can be applied to live metabolizing specimens, though the low sensitivity of detection of ^{13}C means that it takes a long time to collect a measurement — a clear disadvantage when the degree of labelling is changing. For these purposes, it is better to collect samples as for other types of metabolic experiment and then take the spectra of the extracts. Then the measurement time is unimportant, and better accuracy can be achieved. The results are best interpreted by fitting to a computer model of the metabolism. For example, citric acid cycle fluxes in perfused rat hearts were measured and interpreted in this way by Chance et al.[36] in the experiment illustrated in Figure 2.5. The kinetics of the pentose phosphate pathway in human red blood cells were also analysed by ^{13}C NMR by Kuchel's group in Sydney, Australia, combined with computer modelling of the enzyme reactions involved.[17] Computer modelling is not always necessary, as in Sheila Cohen's measurements of the relative rates of the pyruvate kinase reaction to gluconeogenic flux in perfused livers of normal and diabetic rats using *in vivo* NMR studies of the redistribution of label from the substrate [3–^{13}C]alanine.[46]

NMR can also measure the rates of individual steps in metabolism *in vivo* in favourable circumstances by magnetic labelling using a technique called magnetization transfer. The sample is irradiated with radio waves of the specific frequency that is absorbed by certain atoms of a particular compound, for example the terminal phosphate of ATP. This causes the magnetic axis of the nuclei to change their alignment in the magnetic field of the instrument, and if the irradiation is strong enough, most of them will become aligned in the same direction. If one of these atoms is transferred by a reaction into another chemical grouping, it takes its alignment with it for a while, until it spontaneously flips back. If enough of the atoms are transferring to this other compound at a rate comparable to the rate at which the magnetic alignment is lost, they affect the spectral line recorded from the new compound in a manner that allows the rate of transfer to be recorded. There are a number of ways the measurements can be taken, but one of the simplest measures the rate at which the atoms transfer from the compound whose spectrum is being measured to the compound being irradiated (perhaps rather counterintuitively, since at first sight it looks as though it is the transfer in the other direction that is being measured.) Unfortunately, this potentially powerful technique is limited in its applicability by the sensitivity of NMR in general, and also by the time window in which the technique operates, for it can only detect processes that occur within a fairly narrow band of reaction rates. For example, Kevin Brindle measured the rate at which inorganic phosphate was being incorporated into ATP in yeast *in vivo* by irradiating the γ-phosphate of ATP and measuring the spectrum of phosphate.[22]

2.6 Summary

(1) Methodologies exist to study metabolism in systems at all levels of organization:

- whole multicellular organisms;
- isolated tissues and organs;
- tissue slices;
- isolated cells;
- permeabilized cells;

- cell–free systems;

- isolated organelles;

- isolated enzymes.

(2) Measurement of metabolite concentrations can be demanding because of the low values and the complex mixtures that have to be analysed. Even then, there are further problems of experimental design and interpretation in order to ensure the results are representative of *in vivo* concentrations at the site of interest. These include:

  - the need to prevent changes in metabolite levels during preparation and analysis of samples;

  - the need to relate the measured metabolites to known cellular and subcellular compartments of known volume;

  - the difficulty of testing whether the metabolite exists mainly in the free state or not.

(3) The measurement of enzyme activities also raises difficult issues about the relevance of *in vitro* measurements to *in vivo* conditions.

(4) Measurement of overall metabolic fluxes is often a simple analytical problem of measuring rates of change of input and output metabolites. Measuring internal fluxes, however, can require ingenious use of isotopic tracer methodologies, using detection by radioactivity, NMR or mass spectrometry.

Further reading

Denton, R. M. & Pogson, C. I. (1976) Metabolic Regulation, Chapman & Hall, London

Wilson, K. & Walker, J. (eds.) (1994) Principles and Techniques of Practical Biochemistry 4th edn., Cambridge University Press, Cambridge

Fraenkel, D. G. (1992) *Genetics and intermediary metabolism.* Annu. Rev. Genet. **26**, 159–177

Bergmeyr, H. V. (ed.) (1983) Methods of Enzymatic Analysis, 3rd edn., vols. 1 & 2, Verlag Chemie, Weinheim

Zuurendonk, P. F., Tischler, M. E., Akerboom, T. P. M., van der Meer, R., Williamson, J. R. & Tager, J. M. (1979) *Rapid separation of particulate and soluble fractions from isolated cell preparations.* Methods Enzymol. **56**, 207–223

Badar–Goffer, R. & Bachelard, H. (1991) *Metabolic Studies using* ^{13}C *NMR spectroscopy*. In Essays in Biochemistry (Tipton, K. F., ed.), vol. 26, pp. 105–119, Portland Press, London

Cohen, S. M. (1989) *In vivo studies of enzymatic activity.* Methods Enzymol.
    177, 417–434
Cohen, J. S., Lyon, R. C. & Daly, P. F. (1989) *Monitoring intracellular meta-
    bolism by NMR.* Methods Enzymol. **177**, 435–452

3

Enzyme activity: the molecular basis for its regulation

3.1 Introduction

A description of metabolic regulation at the molecular level must include an account of how the rates of the enzyme–catalysed reactions vary with the concentrations of the metabolites in the cell. The metabolites that most obviously affect any enzyme are its substrates, and the best–known model for enzyme action on a substrate gives rise to the Michaelis–Menten equation. The dominance of this model in the context of metabolism is unfortunate, for, as I will show, it is over–simplified for our purposes and can too easily be misapplied. This chapter starts by reviewing Michaelis–Menten kinetics and then presents some of the other aspects of kinetics relevant to metabolic regulation, in particular:

- the effects of a product on enzyme rates;

- the kinetics of enzymes with two substrates;

- binding of metabolites by enzymes;

- the kinetics of enzymes whose rates are affected by metabolites other than their substrates and products.

3.2 Michaelis–Menten kinetics

The Michaelis and Menten model of enzyme action was developed to describe how the initial rate of reaction of an enzyme–catalysed conversion of a single substrate to product(s) varied with substrate concentration. 'Initial rate' is used here to specify that this is the rate at the beginning of the reaction before substrate has been depleted and product has started to accumulate; therefore it is not necessary to consider the possibility that the product binds to the enzyme, far less that catalysis of the reverse reaction occurs. There are two aspects of the model that limit its applicability to metabolism in a cell:

- the majority of enzymes have more than one substrate (it is only amongst the hydrolases and isomerases that single substrates are the norm);

- an enzyme in a metabolic pathway is always operating in the presence of its product(s), which are generally the substrates for other enzymes in the cell.

Nevertheless, the Michaelis–Menten model, and the later derivation of the same equation by Briggs and Haldane using a steady–state method, introduce a number of useful concepts. Most importantly, the model does describe the key outcome of initial rate studies on the variation of the rate of reaction with substrate concentration: the rate depends non–linearly on substrate concentration (in contrast with the usual linear dependence seen in chemical kinetics) and exhibits saturation (Figure 3.1) at high substrate concentrations. The Michaelis–Menten equation that successfully describes such a curve is:

$$v = \frac{SV}{S + K_m} \qquad (3.1)$$

where V is the *limiting rate* (or maximum velocity, V_m) and K_m is known as the *Michaelis constant*. The original derivation of this equation by Michaelis and Menten in 1913 depended on the assumption that the enzyme (E) and substrate (S) reacted together to form an enzyme–substrate complex (ES) that in turn broke down to form free enzyme and product (P), all according to the laws of ordinary chemical kinetics, *i.e.*

$$\text{E} + \text{S} \underset{k_{-1}}{\overset{k_1}{\rightleftharpoons}} \text{ES} \overset{k_2}{\longrightarrow} \text{E} + \text{P} \qquad (\text{Scheme 3.1})$$

They assumed that the reactions between E, S and ES were so rapid that the process was virtually at equilibrium (the *rapid equilibrium* assumption), with the position of equilibrium essentially undisturbed by the much slower reaction whereby ES broke down to E and P. If we draw an analogy with the problem of understanding what determines the rate of a whole metabolic pathway, then Michaelis and Menten were effectively declaring the breakdown of ES to product to be the *rate–limiting step* of catalysis. Under these conditions, K_m in Eqn. (3.1) is equal to the equilibrium constant for the dissociation of ES to E and S.

Briggs and Haldane later showed that the same equation could be derived without any assumption about the relative rates of the reactions or their closeness to equilibrium. They used what they called the *steady state assumption*; that is, they assumed that the rate of formation of the ES complex becomes equal to its rate of breakdown shortly after mixing of the enzyme and substrate

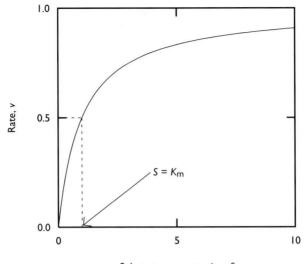

Figure 3.1 Dependence of enzyme rate on substrate concentration
The K_m and V have arbitrarily been set to 1 for the purposes of illustration.

(*cf.* Chapter 1.4.1). In Scheme 3.1, there is a single reaction forming ES, which by the normal laws of chemical kinetics takes place at a rate $v_f = k_1 E S$ (i. e. rate equals a rate constant times the concentration of each reactant). There are two routes of breakdown, one to E and S, the other to E and P; thus the breakdown rate, v_b, is given by $v_b = k_{-1} ES + k_2 ES$. By equating the rates of formation and breakdown, rearranging the equation and making a few substitutions, the Michaelis–Menten equation can be derived, as shown in most biochemistry texts. The effects of their change in assumptions relative to those of Michaelis and Menten is buried in the interpretation of K_m: in the Michaelis–Menten derivation, K_m equals the dissociation constant for ES, or k_{-1}/k_1; in the Briggs–Haldane derivation, $K_m = (k_{-1} + k_2)/k_1$.

I have highlighted the distinction between these two derivations to emphasize that neither of them is a factual description of enzyme activity; they are conceptual and mathematical models. Any particular experimental observation that the rate of an enzyme-catalysed reaction depends on the substrate concentration in the way predicted by the Michaelis–Menten equation merely demonstrates that either model is an adequate mathematical description of the phenomenon for our purposes. We must look to other lines of evidence (such as the existence of enzyme–substrate complexes) to support the molecular details of the theory. Another characteristic of the models is that they are mathematical approximations; both derivations assume that the substrate concentration is very much higher than that of the enzyme, which is generally true in laboratory experiments, but not always true in the intracellular environment. In addition, it is clear in the case of the Briggs–Haldane derivation that the equation is an approximation because the steady state assumption is not true on very short time scales (before the steady state concentration of ES builds up). Indeed it is only approximately true the rest of the time because there is a continual slow decline in ES, corresponding to the gradual slowing down of the rate of reaction as the substrate is exhausted, which in turn means that the rate of formation of ES must be very slightly less than its rate of breakdown. Generally we can expect that the errors introduced by these approximations will be much smaller than the inherent observational inaccuracies in our experiments. This should not make us forget that we have chosen to use a simple model that is adequate for our purposes rather than a more elaborate one that would accurately reflect the underlying molecular mechanisms. It is also worth noting that the derivation involves the same assumptions of a time hierarchy of events that is necessary in considering metabolic pathways, along with the same decision to ignore events on very short and very long time-scales (*cf.* Chapter 1.3, p. 8).

For a more realistic molecular model of enzyme action, we could take into account the reversibility of enzyme catalysis: the enzyme can catalyse the conversion of product to substrate, so it must be able to form an EP complex as well as an ES complex. The pathway from ES to EP passes through a transient, intermediate form, the transition state ET, so if we also include this in initial rate conditions where product is absent, Scheme 3.1 would become:

$$\text{E} + \text{S} \underset{k_{-1}}{\overset{k_1}{\rightleftharpoons}} \text{ES} \underset{k_{-2}}{\overset{k_2}{\rightleftharpoons}} \text{ET} \underset{k_{-3}}{\overset{k_3}{\rightleftharpoons}} \text{EP} \overset{k_4}{\longrightarrow} \text{E} + \text{P} \qquad \text{(Scheme 3.2)}$$

There is a lot more work involved in solving the initial rate equation, and the result is to some extent disappointing because it turns out to be in the same form as the Michaelis–Menten equation, except that K_m is now an expression involving all seven rate constants.

3.2.1 The measurement of K_m and V

The advantage of describing an enzymic reaction by the Michaelis–Menten equation is that it is possible to predict the rate at any substrate concentration just by knowing the two parameters K_m and V. The equation corresponds to a rectangular hyperbolic relationship between the rate and the substrate concentration (Figure 3.1) with a limiting value, or *asymptote*, at infinite concentration corresponding to the limiting rate, V. The substrate concentration giving a rate half this limiting value is the K_m. However, plotting the results in this form is not a very practicable method for determining the parameters because an enzyme kinetics experiment does not give the curve directly; instead it gives a small set of rate measurements made at particular starting concentrations of substrate. Furthermore, these discrete points on the graph include experimental errors which move them off the curve, and it is not possible to sketch an accurate rectangular hyperbola that passes as closely as possible to the points.

In most branches of science until recently, the usual solution to the problem of analysing a non–linear relationship like the Michaelis–Menten equation was

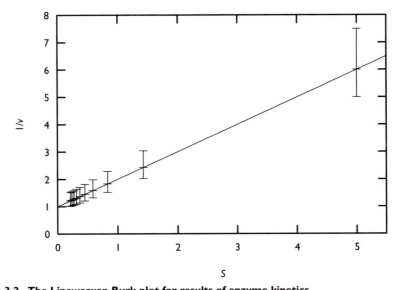

Figure 3.2   The Lineweaver–Burk plot for results of enzyme kinetics
The K_m and V have again been set to 1. The substrate concentrations are equally spaced. The vertical bars show the range where an experimental point might be found because of errors assumed proportional to the value of the rate.

to rearrange the equation to give a linear relationship, so that the points could be plotted as a graph and the best straight line drawn through them. It is very unfortunate that the most popular linearization for enzyme kinetics has been that proposed by Lineweaver and Burk:

$$\frac{1}{v} = \left(\frac{K_m}{V}\right)\frac{1}{S} + \frac{1}{V} \tag{3.2}$$

This corresponds to the equation of a straight line, $y = mx + c$, with $y = 1/v$, $x = 1/S$, the gradient $m = K_m/V$ and the y-intercept $c = 1/V$ (Figure 3.2). The problem with this method is that using the reciprocals of v and S causes extreme stretching of the axes at low substrate concentrations. This is illustrated in Figure 3.2 by showing what happens to a set of equally spaced concentration values. The experimental errors in the rate determinations are differentially amplified in the same way, so that small errors in the slow rates at low concentrations give a much bigger displacement of the point than an equivalent error at high concentrations. The line that is drawn through a set of actual experimental points is therefore unduly influenced by the chance placing of the low-concentration results, which makes this method perform consistently badly in comparison tests alongside other methods. The problem is not merely one of a poor subjective choice of line by the experimenter; using linear regression to calculate the best–fit line does not help unless the points are heavily weighted to compensate for the bias.

The best results with graphical linearization methods come from the plot of

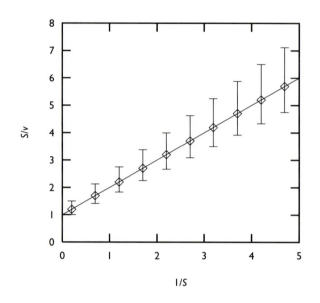

Figure 3.3   The Hanes plot for results of enzyme kinetics
The K_m and V have again been set to 1. The same equally spaced substrate concentrations are shown as in Figure 3.2. The vertical bars show the range where an experimental point might be found because of errors assumed proportional to the value of the rate.

S/v against S (the Hanes or Woolf plot) according to the following rearrangement of the Michaelis–Menten equation:

$$\frac{S}{v} = \frac{1}{V}S + \frac{K_m}{V}$$ (3.3)

This equation corresponds to a line of slope $1/V$, with y–intercept K_m/V and x-intercept of $-K_m$ (Figure 3.3). There is no distortion of the substrate concentration spacing, since this is used unaltered as the x-axis, and the errors in the velocity measurements are not unduly exaggerated or suppressed in any part of the graph. The use of linear regression to determine the best-fit straight line is therefore justifiable. This graph can equally as well be used to diagnose inhibition effects as the Lineweaver–Burk plot. For example, a competitive inhibitor (which increases the apparent K_m of the enzyme for its substrate but leaves the limiting rate unchanged) gives a parallel line on the plot above that of the uninhibited enzyme. Because of the favourable characteristics of this plot, it will be used later in the chapter for the analysis of two–substrate enzyme kinetics.

There are two other approaches to determining K_m and V that illustrate other issues in the fitting of equations to experimental results. The first, made possible only by the availability of computers to perform the large amount of repetitive calculation, is direct fitting of the equation to the experimental results, as suggested by Wilkinson[275] in 1961. This avoids the distortion involved in

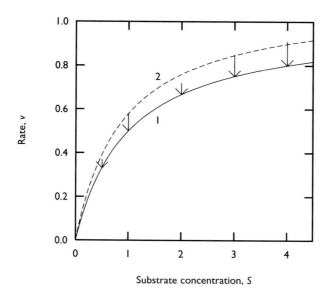

Figure 3.4   Computer fitting of enzyme kinetics results
Curve I is the rectangular hyperbola predicted by the initial estimates of K_m and V. The arrows represent the distances from the observed rates to this curve. As explained in the text, new estimates of the parameters are made giving the better curve 2.

generating a linear graph from a non–linear function. Some objective criterion of the best fit to the results has to be used. Often, just as in linear regression for fitting straight lines to results, the chosen criterion is that the sum of the squares of the distances of the points from the curve has been minimized (see Figure 3.4) but, unlike linear regression, the calculation cannot generally be done in one step. It is necessary to start with an approximate estimate of K_m and V. For each substrate concentration used, these estimates are used to calculate an expected rate from the Michaelis–Menten equation, and the difference between this expected rate and the experimental value is taken and squared. One of a number of possible mathematical approaches is then used to examine how these discrepancies would respond to alterations in the estimates, and a prediction is made of a change in the values of K_m and V that would give a better overall fit to the results. However, this prediction is based on an approximation, so the new values of K_m and V are used as new estimates, and the whole procedure is repeated. This iterative improvement is continued until the suggested changes are too small to be worth bothering with, at which point the current values are reported, usually along with estimates of their standard errors. Under most circumstances, this method performs better than graphical methods, though there are some pitfalls. Firstly, the procedure will attempt to continue even if the experimental results do not fall on a rectangular hyperbola, so the user must take responsibility for checking that the fitted curve is an acceptable description of the experimental results. Secondly, if the initial estimates are inappropriate, or the results contain some points that are grossly in error (sometimes because they have been mistyped into the computer!) the procedure may fail to converge on a best–fit answer and get hopelessly lost. Details of the mathematical implementation of this process are not given because of the wide availability of ready-written computer packages, both freely distributed and commercial, that carry out non–linear least squares fitting, either for any equation in general or for enzyme kinetics in particular.

The final approach is the direct linear plot method of Eisenthal and Cornish–Bowden.[65] Although this was devised as a simple graphical method, there are computer implementations of it. This will not be described in detail because its application to two–substrate kinetics is not widely used. However, in essence it consists of taking all possible pairs of measurements. Suppose the pair is v_1 measured at substrate concentration S_1 and v_2 at S_2; then these values can be considered as a pair of simultaneous Michaelis–Menten equations that can be solved for K_m and V. The graphical version is a simple method of solving the equations. The estimates of K_m and V from all possible pairs are then taken in order, and the median values taken as the result. The significance of this is that the method does not make any assumptions about the nature or type of error in the measurements, whereas least–squares methods are implicitly based on the assumption that the errors are normally distributed. In addition, the direct linear plot is less sensitive to occasional very bad points, or outliers, which unduly influence the results obtained by other methods. Outliers will arise occasionally in any experiment, just by a rare chance conspiracy of all the contributing factors; everyone feels the temptation to delete them, but it is difficult to justify this on statistical grounds.

The optimal design of an enzyme kinetics experiment for determining K_m and V has been investigated with a slightly surprising result.[67] If it is already known that the enzyme obeys the Michaelis–Menten rate law, then the best design is to repeatedly measure just two points. One should be at as high a substrate concentration as possible to give a rate close to V. The best value for the other should be below K_m, but depends on how the measurement errors vary with the rate. Since the latter is often not known, Athel Cornish–Bowden recommends using one-fifth of the expected K_m value.[49] If the experiment must also assess whether the Michaelis–Menten equation is applicable, then a range of substrate concentrations should be used covering over 75% of the velocity range. This requires that the highest velocity is at least 16 times the lowest observed velocity, and will require a range of substrate concentrations from less than 1/10th of the suspected K_m to more than 4 times the K_m.

3.2.2 Product inhibition
Most measurements of enzyme kinetics are based on initial rate measurements, where only substrate is originally present, and the measurement is completed before much product has accumulated. On the other hand, all enzymes in cells operate in the presence of their products, and the lack of information

about the effects of product on the enzyme rate frequently limits our ability to predict the behaviour of metabolic pathways. For reasons to be discussed later (Chapter 6.2, p. 163 and Chapter 6.3.4, p. 187), even apparently weak product inhibition can have a significant influence on pathway behaviour and cause significant differences compared with the less probable case that there is no inhibitory effect at all.

There are two contributions to the effect of product on an enzyme reaction. First, an enzyme is a catalyst, and cannot change the equilibrium constant for the conversion of substrate to product, which is governed by the difference in free energies between them. Therefore, since it catalyses the conversion of substrate to product, it must also be a catalyst for the conversion of product to substrate; affecting one of the rates without affecting the other would change the position of equilibrium. Secondly, since the enzyme can act as a catalyst of the reverse reaction, product must presumably bind at the active site as a first step. Therefore, even for a reaction with a large equilibrium constant in favour of product formation, where the rate of the reverse reaction from product to substrate will be relatively very small, there could still be a significant inhibition of the enzyme by the product that is bound at the active site, blocking the binding of the substrate. This inhibition is likely to be of the competitive type, at least for single substrate enzymes.

The rate equation for a single substrate enzyme in the presence of its product can be derived in a similar way to the usual Michaelis–Menten equation to give:

$$v_{net} = \frac{(V_f/K_{m,S})\,(S - P/K_{eq})}{1 + S/K_{m,S} + P/K_{m,P}} \qquad (3.4)$$

where v_{net} is the net rate (positive for formation of P), V_f is the limiting rate in the forward direction, $K_{m,S}$ and $K_{m,P}$ are the K_m values for substrate and product and K_{eq} is the equilibrium constant for the reaction. [This equation can be found in other forms in some books because there is also a V_r for the limiting rate in the reverse direction; however, one of the parameters can always be eliminated because of the constraint imposed by the equilibrium constant known as the Haldane relationship: $K_{eq} = V_f K_{m,P}/(V_r K_{m,S})$.] An illustration of the way the net rate of the reaction varies with both S and P is shown in the three-dimensional plot of Figure 3.5. The exact details of the form would depend on the relative values of the constants and the equilibrium constant. It is clear though that once both substrate and product are present, the response of an enzyme cannot necessarily be visualized by thinking about where, on a rectangular hyperbola, the substrate concentration would fall relative to the $K_{m,S}$. Later we will look at how we can characterize the position on this three-dimensional graph that corresponds to particular intracellular concentrations of S and P when we look at the concept of elasticity (Chapter 5.3). For the moment, note how the diagram shows that a substrate concentration above the K_m value does not guarantee that the enzyme rate is approaching V; that will de-

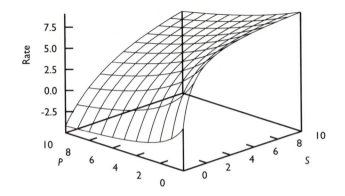

Figure 3.5 Simultaneous dependence of enzyme rate on both substrate and product
The parameters in Eqn. (3.4) have been set to: $K_{m,S} = 1$; $V_f = 10$; $K_{m,P} = 2$; $K_{eq} = 4$.

pend on the product concentration and the equilibrium constant. An example where this has been overlooked is at the enzyme aldolase in the glycolytic pathway. In certain cells, the concentration of substrate (fructose 1,6-bisphosphate) is greater than the K_m, and this has been erroneously interpreted to suggest that the enzyme is working near to its limiting rate.

3.3   Two–substrate enzymes

Approximately three quarters of all enzymes have two substrates, given that coenzymes, such as NAD and ATP, count as substrates for this purpose. The proportion of two substrate enzymes would be higher if water were to be counted as a substrate, for it is a reactant in the reactions catalysed by the hydrolases such as trypsin and β–galactosidase, but it is not usual to do so because of its very high concentration for enzymes that work in an aqueous environment. Besides, it is difficult (though not impossible) to vary its concentration. Some enzymes have three substrates, and many have a requirement for a cofactor, particularly a metal ion, that affects the rate in a similar way to a substrate. Not all metal cofactor requirements involve a direct interaction of the metal and the enzyme; kinases typically require Mg^{2+} for activity, but this is because their true substrate is an ATP–Mg complex ($ATP^{4-} \cdot Mg^{2+}$) that forms spontaneously and reversibly between ATP and Mg at physiological pH. Thus counting the number of substrates and deciding what they really are may need more scientific detective work than at first appears. Nevertheless, whatever they happen to be, there are two substrates for the majority of enzymes, and in this section we shall look at the kinetics of this important group. Of course, in the cell, these enzymes work in the presence of their products (of which there will also be two in very many cases), but I will not deal with the effects of products in this section because this introduces unnecessary complications. Let it suffice to say that the enzyme will catalyse a forward and a reverse reaction, and the numerator of the rate equation will contain a positive and a negative term, similar to the single-substrate case [Eqn. (3.4)].

The obvious kinetics experiment to perform when a two–substrate enzyme is first investigated is to keep one substrate constant and to vary the concentration of the other. The most common result from such an experiment is that the enzyme behaves just like a single–substrate enzyme, and the rate of reaction plotted against the concentration of the varied substrate gives a hyperbolic curve. Indeed, it is usually possible to calculate a corresponding K_m and V, although these will generally turn out to be dependent upon the concentration chosen for the other substrate. Nevertheless, the similarity of the behaviour to that expected from the Michaelis–Menten model suggests that the formation of enzyme–substrate complexes is involved. This immediately poses a problem: it is quite easy to think of several ways that enzyme–substrate complexes could form for two–substrate enzymes. Suppose that the reaction is:

$$A + B \rightleftharpoons P + Q \qquad \text{(Scheme 3.3)}$$

Even though we are only considering the reaction from left to right, in the absence of products, the following might all be possibilities:

- a three-body collision;

- a compulsory-order mechanism;

- a random-order mechanism;

- a double–displacement mechanism.

Of these, a three-body collision is unable to explain catalysis because the simultaneous collision of the enzyme molecule and the two substrates A and B would be a relatively rare event.

The compulsory-order mechanism would occur when the enzyme molecule has a binding site for one of the substrates (say A), but not the other; when this substrate binds, a conformational change in the enzyme (as proposed in Koshland's *induced fit* model of enzyme action) generates the binding site for the second substrate, B. The *ternary complex* EAB therefore forms by an obligatory sequence and is converted to the ternary product complex, EPQ, by the catalytic action of the enzyme. The product complex then breaks down to release products, thus:

$$E + A \rightleftharpoons EA$$

$$EA + B \rightleftharpoons EAB$$

$$EAB \rightleftharpoons EPQ$$

$$EPQ \longrightarrow E + P + Q \qquad \text{(Scheme 3.4)}$$

The random-order mechanism also forms the ternary complex EAB in two stages, but occurs when the enzyme has binding sites for both substrates so that either one may bind before the other (though not necessarily with equal probability).

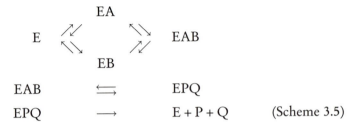

$$\text{EAB} \quad \rightleftharpoons \quad \text{EPQ}$$

$$\text{EPQ} \quad \longrightarrow \quad \text{E} + \text{P} + \text{Q} \qquad \text{(Scheme 3.5)}$$

The double-displacement mechanism differs from the previous two in that a ternary complex is not formed. Instead, a chemical entity that is transferred between the two substrates is temporarily parked on the enzyme molecule by the first substrate, and then collected by the second substrate to complete the catalytic cycle:

$$\text{E} + \text{A} \quad \rightleftharpoons \quad \text{EA}$$

$$\text{EA} \quad \longrightarrow \quad \text{EX} + \text{P}$$

$$\text{EX} + \text{B} \quad \rightleftharpoons \quad \text{EXB}$$

$$\text{EXB} \quad \longrightarrow \quad \text{E} + \text{Q} \qquad \text{(Scheme 3.6)}$$

The scheme shows that B and P are related in that they both must have an attachment point for X, and A and Q are related in that they both consist of something linked to X (A = P + X and Q = B + X).

Similar strategies and assumptions to those used in the derivation of the Michaelis–Menten equation are used to obtain the equations that describe how the initial rate of a two–substrate enzyme varies with the concentrations of the substrates, though the algebra becomes more lengthy. As a result, methods were devised to simplify the derivation, such as the graphical King–Altman method[133] (details of which can be found in some of the books listed in the further reading at the end of the chapter). To a first approximation, all three mechanisms lead to equations that are particular cases of a general equation of the form:

$$v = \frac{VAB}{K_{iA}K_B + K_B A + K_A B + AB} \qquad (3.5)$$

The meanings of the different parameters in this equation are as follows. V is, just as for single-substrate enzymes, the limiting rate approached as the concentrations (but this time of both the substrates) increase to very high values. Suppose the concentration B is fixed at a very high level and A is varied; Eqn. (3.5) above can have both top and bottom lines of its right-hand side divided by AB to give:

$$v = \frac{V}{\dfrac{K_{iA}K_B}{AB} + \dfrac{K_B}{B} + \dfrac{K_A}{A} + 1} \tag{3.6}$$

We can suppose that B can be raised high enough that the terms in the denominator of the equation that are divided by B become very much smaller than the others, so that we can ignore them and get the approximation:

$$v \approx \frac{V}{\dfrac{K_A}{A} + 1} = \frac{VA}{K_A + A} \tag{3.7}$$

This is the same as the single substrate Michaelis–Menten equation [Eqn. (3.1)], with A instead of S and K_A in place of K_m; in other words, when B is fixed at a high value and A is varied, the enzyme behaves like a single-substrate enzyme, and K_A is the K_m for A under these conditions. By exchanging A and B, we can conclude that at high A, the rate will vary with B like a single-substrate enzyme with K_B being the K_m under these circumstances. Thus K_A and K_B can legitimately be regarded as the K_m values for these two substrates, except that we only know this to be true when the concentration of the other substrate is very high, which is unlikely to be the case in intracellular conditions for most enzymes. What happens at lower concentrations of the other substrate? To illustrate this, let us consider very low concentrations of B. As B decreases, the numerator term of Eqn. (3.5) becomes smaller because the whole of it is multiplied by B; the denominator, however, only shrinks to a certain extent. The denominator terms mutiplied by B certainly become smaller and smaller, but the terms without B are unaffected and, since the different terms are added together, the denominator cannot be smaller than $K_{iA}K_B + K_BA$, so that at very low concentrations of B, Eqn. (3.5) approximates to:

$$v \approx \frac{VAB}{K_{iA}K_B + K_BA} = \frac{\left(V\dfrac{B}{K_B}\right)A}{K_{iA} + A} \tag{3.8}$$

This means that the enzyme again behaves like a Michaelis–Menten enzyme when A is varied. Comparison with Eqn. (3.1) shows that the apparent limiting rate, V_{app} is given by $V_{app} = VB/K_B$, and the K_m is K_{iA}. At intermediate concentrations of B, it is possible to show that the apparent K_m for A is between K_A and K_{iA}. Thus although it is possible to study a two–substrate enzyme by holding one substrate constant and varying the other, the results have limited value. It is necessary to determine the values of all four parameters V, K_A, K_B and K_{iA} to calculate how rapidly the enzyme will work at any particular concentrations of A and B. How the parameters are found is described next.

Table 3.1 Two-substrate kinetics: schematic set of results

Concn. of B	Concentration of A				
	A_1	A_2	A_3	A_4	A_5
B_1	$v_{1,1}$ $\dfrac{A_1}{v_{1,1}}$	$v_{1,2}$ $\dfrac{A_2}{v_{1,2}}$	$\cdots$		
B_2	$v_{2,1}$ $\dfrac{A_1}{v_{2,1}}$	$\cdots$			
B_3	$\cdots$				
B_4					$\cdots$
B_5				$\cdots$	$v_{5,5}$ $\dfrac{A_5}{v_{5,5}}$

The upper entry in each cell is the observed rate and the lower is the derived value for plotting Figure 3.6.

3.3.1 Experimental investigation

Since the way in which the velocity of a two substrate enzyme varies with one substrate is likely to depend on the concentration of the other, the experimental design must involve simultaneous variation of the two substrates. In addition, this must be done on a regular grid of combinations of the two substrates (Table 3.1) if graphical analysis of the results is going to be used. If a sufficiently wide range of both concentrations is used, the range of velocities observed will be very large, with the lowest, $v_{1,1}$, being as little as one-hundredth of the highest, $v_{5,5}$. It is not neccesary to fill the grid completely, and if computer analysis of the results is to be used, it can be sparsely filled.

The graphical methods of analysing these results involve primary and secondary graphs: the results are plotted first against one substrate concentration, and measurements taken from that graph are plotted against the second substrate concentration to make the secondary graphs. The method given in many books is a variant of the Lineweaver–Burk plot; for the reasons given earlier, this method is liable to error, and the two–substrate analogue of the plot of s/v against s, originally described by Cornish–Bowden, is preferable[49]). In this case, one of the substrates is chosen as the independent variable (x-axis) of the primary plot, say A from the table of results (Table 3.1). The table is then rewritten with the entries consisting of A/v values, so that the entry in the top left hand corner, for example, is $A_1/v_{1,1}$.

These values are then plotted on a graph of A/v against A, and a line drawn through each set of points from the same row of Table 3.1, i.e. for sets of points measured at the same value of B (Figure 3.6). The y-axis intercept and slope of the line is measured for each value of B. The intercepts give values

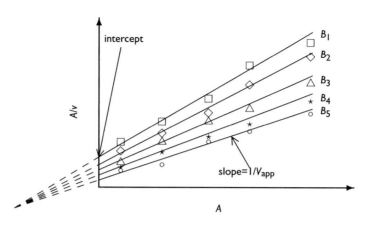

Figure 3.6   Primary plot of two substrate enzyme kinetics results
Each line on the plot corresponds to points measured at a set value of B as in Table 3.1. The slope (corresponding to $1/V_{app}$) and intercept ($K_{A,app}/V_{app}$) of each line are measured for use in the secondary plots (Figure 3.7).

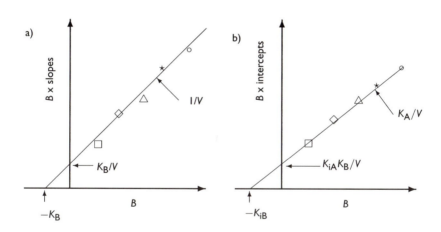

Figure 3.7   Secondary plots of two substrate enzyme kinetics results
The point symbols are those of the corresponding line of Figure 3.6 from which they were derived. a) The secondary plot from the slopes gives K_B and V. The units of the y–axis are concentration/rate units. b) The secondary plot from the intercepts leads to K_A and K_{iA}. The units of the y–axis are (concentration)^2/rate units.

of $K_{A,app}/V_{app}$, where these are the apparent values of K_m and V that fit the variation of rate with A at each of the values of B. The slopes have values of $1/V_{app}$. Two secondary plots are then constructed. The first of these involves plotting each slope value times the value of B at which it was measured against B (Figure 3.7a). The slope of this plot gives $1/V$, and the y-axis intercept is K_B/V. (The x-axis intercept is $-K_B$.) The other secondary plot is each intercept value from the primary plot times the value of B at which it was measured against B (Figure 3.7b). The slope of this plot is K_A/V, and since V has already been determined, this gives K_A. The intercept on the y-axis is $K_{iA}K_B/V$, and since K_B/V has been determined, this gives K_{iA}.

The values of the parameters obtained by this graphical analysis can themselves be reported as the properties of the enzyme. These days, they can also be used as the initial estimates in an iterative computer-fitting procedure, and the results from this are then taken as the best estimates of the parameters. In this case, the ultimate worth of the graphical analysis is that it gives visual confirmation that the results do fit the two-substrate equation. (If they do not, there will be systematic deviation of the points from a straight line.)

What can the results tell us about the mechanism of the enzyme? We need to look at this for each mechanism in turn.

3.3.2   Compulsory-order mechanism

Enzymes following the compulsory-order mechanism obey the general form of the two substrate rate equation [Eqn. (3.5)]. If A is the first substrate to bind, then K_{iA} is actually equal to the dissociation constant of the EA complex. Without other evidence, it is not possible to tell which substrate binds first from the initial rate kinetics experiments described above. Furthermore, the results can equally be used to calculate a K_i term (*i.e.* K_{iB}) for the other substrate even though, if B is the second substrate to bind, the EB complex is not formed when enzyme and B are mixed together, so that a dissociation constant for the EB complex cannot be measured. Therefore if a purified sample of the enzyme is available, a comparison of the kinetic results with binding studies (see p. 65) may show that the enzyme obeys a compulsory-order mechanism. Another experiment that can be used to diagnose this mechanism is possible if there are a number of different substrates on which the enzyme can act. For example, alcohol dehydrogenases will act on alcohols with carbon chains of different lengths, though generally at different rates with different substrates. Suppose that there are a number of substrates of the B type: B1, B2 etc. If the kinetics are determined using A and each of these substrates in turn, K_{iA} is the same whichever B substrate is used. On the other hand, if the kinetics are studied with a number of different variants of the A substrate, K_{iB} will vary with the nature of the A substrate. This is because the binding of the first substrate cannot be affected by the nature of a substrate that has not yet bound, whereas the binding of the second substrate is obviously influenced by the molecule already at the active site.

Aspartate transcarbamylase catalyses the reaction:

carbamoyl phosphate + aspartate $\rightleftharpoons$ carbamoyl aspartate + phosphate

The enzyme has some very interesting properties that will be discussed later in the section in connection with allosteric enzymes (Chapter 3.5), but its kinetic mechanism is ordered. Carbamoyl phosphate binds first, followed by aspartate. Products also leave in an ordered fashion: carbamoyl aspartate first, then phosphate. Binding studies did detect aspartate binding to the enzyme, though with a slightly high K_d. The binding of non–reactive aspartate analogues, such as succinate and malate, has been found to be greatly enhanced by the presence of carbamoyl phosphate.[82]

3.3.3 Random-order mechanism

The random-order mechanism gives rise to potential problems for our analysis. The general two–substrate rate equation [Eqn. (3.5)] can be derived for it by the 'rapid–equilibrium' method, that is, the equivalent of Michaelis and Menten's original method, assuming in this case that E, A and B are close to equilibrium with EAB because the binding reactions are relatively faster than the catalytic conversion of EAB to products. However, if no assumption about the relative rates of reaction are made and the rate equation is derived by the steady state assumption (as in the Briggs–Haldane method for single-substrate enzymes), a more complicated equation is obtained, containing terms in A^2 and B^2. This equation does not necessarily predict hyperbolic curves of rate against substrate concentration, nor straight lines in the graphical analysis described above, though these are both observed as long as the rate constants for certain steps of the mechanism have appropriate relative magnitudes. Now there is certainly a significant minority of enzymes that do not give hyperbolic rate curves but, in most cases, the reason for this is not that they obey a special form of the random-order mechanism, but because of cooperative binding that will be described later (p. 70). In practice, it seems that most enzymes working by the random-order mechanism do actually follow the two–substrate rate equation. One characteristic of the random order mechanism is that binding of both substrates to the enzyme will be demonstrable in binding studies, with the dissociation constants for the EA and EB complexes being K_{iA} and K_{iB} respectively. Unlike the compulsory order mechanism, these K_i terms would not be expected to be invariant if different forms of the other substrate were used in the kinetic studies.

The effects of products in inhibiting the reaction can distinguish between compulsory-order and random-order mechanisms. Whether the inhibition by each product with respect to each substrate is of the competitive or non-competitive type gives a set of results that differs between the two mechanisms.

One difficulty in distinguishing between the random-order and compulsory-order mechanisms is that in kinetic experiments, the dividing line may be fuzzy. Although a random order enzyme may bind either substrate first, it is unlikely that both routes will be equally probable. If one route is always dominant under the conditions investigated, then the enzyme is effectively compulsory order, even though on the longer time scales of a binding experiment, the binding of both substrates to the enzyme might be demonstrable. This might explain why some enzymes have been difficult to classify, with different laboratories reaching opposite conclusions. The hexokinase of yeast is one example where contradictory conclusions were reached by different groups: some favoured an ordered mechanism in which glucose bound first, whereas others thought that the mechanism was random. However, the probable explanation is that the enzyme follows a steady state (rather than rapid equilibrium) random mechanism, in which only the binary complexes, enzyme–glucose and enzyme–ATP, are near to equilibrium with the enzyme.[202] (In these conditions, the random-order mechanism could show hybrid characteristics with the compulsory-order mechanism.)

3.3.4   Double-displacement mechanism

The double-displacement mechanism shows a clear difference from the other two mechanisms in that the term $K_{iA}K_B$ is not present in the denominator of the rate equation [Eqn. (3.5)]. This is because there is no ternary complex, EAB. As a result, in the primary plot (Figure 3.6), all the lines cross on the y-axis at a value of K_A/V.

The double-displacement mechanism is common in group-transfer reactions, such as those catalysed by the transaminases that transfer amino groups between oxo acids. The amino group is held on the pyridoxal phosphate that is a prosthetic group in these enzymes.

Another feature of enzymes working by this mechanism is that they bring about partial reactions in the presence of just one substrate. With small amounts of enzyme, the amount of product formed may not be detectable as the enzyme is unable to complete its catalytic cycle in the absence of the second substrate, and the net reaction stops when all the enzyme has been converted into the modified form. If larger amounts of enzyme are available, it may be possible to detect and characterize the modified form of the enzyme. However, even when the amount of enzyme is small, so that the net product formation is also small, the equilibrium between substrate and product is being catalysed, and it is possible to detect this reaction by isotope exchange. Thus, suppose the partial reaction with one substrate AX is:

$$E + AX \rightleftharpoons EX + P$$

If isotopically unlabelled AX and labelled product P* are added to the enzyme, then the reverse reaction of the above equilibrium will include.

$$EX + P^* \longrightarrow E + A^*X$$

After a while, if AX is recovered from the reaction mixture, it will be found to be isotopically labelled.

An example of both these features is given by the three–substrate three–product enzyme pyruvate carboxylase:

$$\text{pyruvate} + \text{ATP} + \text{HCO}_3^- \rightleftharpoons \text{oxaloacetate} + \text{ADP} + \text{P}_i$$

This has two partial reactions: in the first, ATP and HCO_3^- react with the enzyme to form an enzyme–CO_2 complex (in which the CO_2 is attached to the prosthetic group biotin), and in the second, the enzyme–CO_2 complex reacts with pyruvate to form oxaloacetate. The enzyme–CO_2 complex has been isolated after incubation with $H^{14}CO_3^-$ to demonstrate the first partial reaction, and the exchange of ^{14}C from pyruvate into oxaloacetate has been detected to show the second partial reaction.[252]

3.4 Binding characteristics of enzyme sites

The aim of steady state approaches to enzyme kinetics is to avoid explicit interpretation of the kinetics in terms of possibly invalid assumptions about the role of the substrate-binding equilibrium. Nevertheless, sometimes it is easier to interpret an enzyme's properties in terms of its binding equilibria with its substrates. In some of these cases, direct measurements of the binding equilibria are able to confirm that the kinetically measured properties are in fact direct consequences of the binding behaviour. Before considering some more complex enzyme kinetic behaviour, it is therefore necessary to consider the types of binding that are observed between enzymes and substrates (or inhibitors or products). The binding of substances (generically known as *ligands*) by enzymes is, in essence, no different from the binding of molecules by transport proteins, of hormones by receptors, or of antigens by antibodies, except that there is the possibility of chemical reaction at the binding site. However, for two–substrate enzymes (apart from the double displacement type), there is no reaction if only one substrate is present, so it is perfectly feasible to study the binding in isolation.

3.4.1 Identical independent binding sites

The simplest binding curve is given by a protein P that has just a single type of binding site for a ligand L. If there is only one binding site per molecule of P, the binding equilibrium is:

$$P + L \rightleftharpoons PL$$

Here PL is the protein–ligand complex, and its concentration is equal to that of the *bound* ligand, L_b. The equilibrium constant for this reaction is commonly expressed in terms of the *dissociation constant*, K_d, defined as:

$$K_d = \frac{PL}{L_b}$$

where K_d has the units of concentration. Furthermore, when the total protein P_t is divided equally between free protein, P, and protein–ligand complex, $PL = L_b$, K_d equals the free ligand concentration L. Although the dissociation constant has the advantage that its value corresponds to the concentration of ligand needed to fill half the binding sites, it has the disadvantage that strong binding (or high ligand affinity) corresponds to low values of K_d, and weak binding corresponds to high values. (The equilibrium defined in the opposite direction is the association constant, K_a; $K_a = 1/K_d$, and large values correspond to strong binding, but the units of K_a are the reciprocal of concentration.) The equation for K_d can be rearranged with substitution of $P_t = P + L_b$ to give:

$$L_b = \frac{P_t.L}{K_d + L}$$

This is analogous to the Michaelis–Menten equation (not surprisingly, as it was the origin of their derivation) and therefore defines a rectangular hyperbolic binding curve.

Many enzymes are composed of a number of identical subunits (most commonly four). Binding will involve the formation of complexes with $1, 2 \ldots n$ molecules of L at various stages of the binding curve:

$$P + L \leftrightharpoons PL \leftrightharpoons PL_2 \cdots \leftrightharpoons PL_n$$

If the binding sites do not interact in any way, then defining the concentration of bound ligand, L_b as $L_b = PL + 2PL_2 \cdots + nPL_n$ leads to essentially the same equation:

$$L_b = \frac{nP_tL}{K_d + L} \tag{3.9}$$

Thus the binding curve can be characterized by the values of n and K_d, and this is done by measuring L_b at various concentrations of L. Sometimes it is easier to determine the fraction of binding sites occupied, the fractional saturation, $\overline{Y}$, where

$$\overline{Y} = \frac{L_b}{nP_t} = \frac{L}{K_d + L} \tag{3.10}$$

in which case it is still possible to determine K_d.

The analysis of the results of binding experiments has parallels with that of enzyme kinetics. There are graphical methods based on the linearization of the binding equation. For example, the Hughes–Klotz plot (an analogue of the Lineweaver–Burk plot) consists of plotting $1/L_b$ against $1/L_f$; however, this has not been favoured and it suffers from the same defects as the Lineweaver–Burk plot. The plot used most frequently is known as the Scatchard plot. It consists of plotting $L_b/(P_tL)$ against L_b/P_t (Figure 3.8) and is an analogue of the enzyme kinetics plot of v/S against v, known as the Eadie–Hofstee plot. The slope of the graph (line a) is $-1/K_d$ and the intercept on the x-axis is the number of binding sites, n.

However, the method of preference for analysing binding results is computerized fitting of the binding equation. Since this is essentially the same as

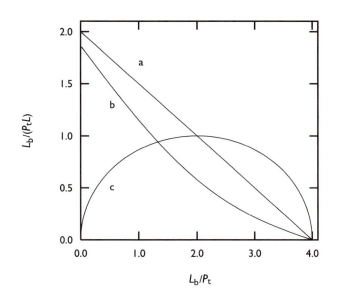

Figure 3.8 Scatchard plot
(a) Four identical independent binding sites, K_d = 2. (b) Two high-affinity sites and two low-affinity sites. (c) Four interacting, cooperative sites.

the Michaelis–Menten equation, a computer program suitable for one task may be satisfactory for the other.

3.4.2 Non–identical independent sites

Even if a protein has been purified, it is not unusual to find that it has more than one type of binding site for a particular ligand. There are a number of possible reasons for this. One is that there is a specific high–affinity site for a particular ligand, but the ligand can also bind with lower affinity and specificity to another part of the protein through hydrophobic or ionic interactions. Another possibility is that the protein sample contains a mixture of proteins of different binding affinities, either because the protein exists in a number of variant isoforms *in vivo* or because partial damage during preparation has modified the binding properties of some of the molecules.

If the different sites do not interact in any way, they behave independently and the total binding observed is just the sum of the binding at the separate sites. Thus for a protein molecule with two types of site, of which there are n_1 and n_2 per molecule, with dissociation constants $K_{d,1}$ and $K_{d,2}$, the total binding is:

$$L_b = P_t \left(\frac{n_1 L}{K_{d,1} + L} + \frac{n_2 L}{K_{d,2} + L} \right)$$

In this case, the linear graphical plots are curved (e.g. Figure 3.8, curve b). There has been a general belief that the two components can be estimated by drawing tangents to both ends of the curve on a Scatchard plot. In spite of the many instances of this continuing practice in the biochemical and physiological research literature, it has long been known that such a procedure gives grossly incorrect estimates of the two sets of parameters.[134,176] For example, no part of curve b in Figure 3.8 can be extrapolated to 2 on the x–axis — the correct value of the number of higher–affinity sites. In such cases computer fitting to the equation above can often yield the parameters of the two components.

3.4.3   Identical interacting sites
Where proteins have a number of binding sites with an initially identical binding affinity, there is the possibility that the binding of ligand at one site affects the affinity of the other sites on the protein. This is referred to as *cooperativity* in binding.

The most studied example of this phenomenon is the oxygen–binding protein haemoglobin from the blood of vertebrates. At the beginning of the 20th century, increasing accuracy in the determination of the oxygen-binding curves of blood had shown that the binding was not described by a simple binding curve for a single type of binding site. Instead of a rectangular hyperbolic binding curve, the curve was noticeably S–shaped or *sigmoid* (see Figure 3.13). At this time, the molecular mass of haemoglobin was not known, nor was it known that haemoglobin was composed of four subunits. Hill proposed that the binding curve could be explained if a haemoglobin molecule that was an aggregate of n units bound n molecules of oxygen in a single step (at least in the sense that a molecule either has zero or n oxygens bound and no intermediate number). The binding equation for the aggregates of size n in terms of the fraction of oxygen-binding sites occupied (the fractional saturation, $\overline{Y}$) is:

$$\overline{Y} = \frac{O_2^n}{K_d^n + O_2^n}$$

(3.11)

This equation does give rise to a sigmoid curve if n is greater than 1; for $n = 1$, it gives the usual hyperbolic binding equation for a single type of binding site [Eqn. (3.10)]. The values of K_d and n can be determined with a graph known as the Hill plot: if $\log[\overline{Y}/(1 - \overline{Y})]$ is plotted against $\log O_2$, the equation is converted into a linear form with slope n. When $O_2 = K_d$, $\overline{Y} = 0.5$ and $\log[\overline{Y}/(1 - \overline{Y})] = \log 1 = 0$ (Figure 3.9). The oxygen binding curve of blood generally gives a value for the slope n in the range 2.4–2.8. Hill knew the result was not a whole number, and accounted for this by assuming that the haemoglobin was a mixture of aggregates of different sizes, with 1, 2, 3 ... sites. Since the slope of the Hill plot is not therefore guaranteed to give the number of binding sites, it is usually called the Hill coefficient, h. By the 1920s, the molecular mass of haemoglobin had been measured and it was clear that it was a permanent aggregate of fixed size with four oxygen-binding sites. Adair proposed that the binding of oxygen to haemoglobin was a four-step process, *i.e.* that the intermediates $Hb(O_2)$, $Hb(O_2)_2$, $Hb(O_2)_3$ and $Hb(O_2)_4$ are formed

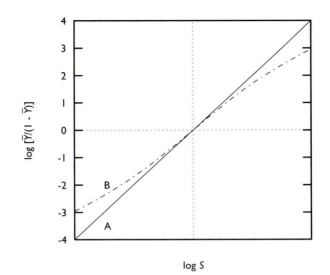

Figure 3.9 The Hill plot for cooperative binding
A linear graphical form of the Hill equation, Eqn. (3.11). Line A is the line predicted by the equation. Curve B is the form usually obtained with experimental results. The Hill coefficient, h, is the slope of the line, usually taken at the half-saturation point where the y–axis value is zero.

successively. The curve is sigmoid because after the first site has bound an oxygen, the affinity of the remaining sites becomes greater than before, and so on at each stage. This requires that the binding of oxygen at one site transmits an influence to the other sites to aid their binding; this effect is known as *cooperativity*. However, for much of the century, little was known about the molecular mechanism by which this could occur.

On the basis of energetic considerations, it was realized that the Hill equation was not a feasible description of cooperative binding, since it would require an infinite interaction energy to ensure that the affinity of all the sites increased to such an extent that they immediately filled up after the first oxygen had bound. With a finite interaction energy, the binding curve would give a sigmoid curve in the Hill plot (see Figure 3.9), having slopes of 1 at both ends (*i.e.* at very low saturations and very high saturations). This is because at very low concentrations of oxygen, only the reaction

$$Hb + O_2 \rightleftharpoons HbO_2$$

is being seen. Similarly, when the oxygen concentration is very high, the only reaction being observed is

$$Hb(O_2)_3 + O_2 \rightleftharpoons Hb(O_2)_4$$

Furthermore, the Hill coefficient could only have a maximum value equal to the number of subunits, n, for an infinite interaction energy, and with a finite interaction energy h would be less than n.

Thus the original basis of the Hill equation is no longer accepted. Nevertheless, many proteins in addition to haemoglobin exhibit cooperativity in their ligand binding, and the Hill plot is still widely used to characterize the cooperativity. This is partly because the other forms of binding curve analysis, such as the Scatchard plot, do not give linear plots for cooperative binding and cannot therefore be used to analyse the results (e.g. see Figure 3.8, curve c). The Hill plot, on the other hand, tends to have a substantial linear portion in the centre; the curvature towards a line with a slope of 1 is only observable if the extreme ends of the curve can be measured. Furthermore, the Hill coefficient, h, can be used to diagnose cooperativity even when the degree of sigmoidicity of the binding curve is difficult to detect by eye. If the value of h is greater than 1, the binding can be said to be cooperative (or even positively cooperative). A value of 1 corresponds to ordinary hyperbolic binding which should be analysable by methods such as the Scatchard plot. However, it is possible to obtain values of h of less than 1. For example, a mixture of independent binding sites of different affinity gives this result. It is also possible to conceive of the case where the first ligand to bind to a protein causes a lowering of affinity of the other sites, so they become progressively more difficult to fill. Since this is the opposite effect to the cooperativity described above for haemoglobin, it is termed *negative cooperativity*. It gives rise to non–hyperbolic binding curves and Hill coefficients of less than 1. The difficulty is that the binding experiments themselves do not distinguish between these two causes for h being less than 1. As a result there is sometimes a dispute about which explanation is appropriate in a particular case, such as with the binding of the hormone insulin by its cell surface receptor.

3.5   Allosteric enzymes

In 1956, the first two examples (threonine deaminase[250] and aspartate transcarbamylase[281]) of enzymes subject to feedback inhibition were discovered (see Chapter 7.2.1, p. 201). These enzymes were at the beginnings of metabolic pathways and were inhibited by metabolites produced further along. The significance of this is that the inhibitory metabolites by that stage do not chemically resemble the substrates or products of the enzyme, and therefore would not be expected to compete at the active site to cause inhibition. Furthermore, for these examples the inhibition was highly specific, in that analogous molecules from different metabolic pathways showed weaker or no inhibition. Following the initial discoveries, many more instances were found, and it became noticeable that these enzymes often did not give rectangular hyperbolic plots of velocity against substrate concentration, so that it was not possible to analyse their kinetics with the linear graphical methods described earlier in this chapter. Instead, these enzymes often gave a sigmoidal plot of rate against substrate concentration, like the binding curve of oxygen to haemoglobin. It is possible

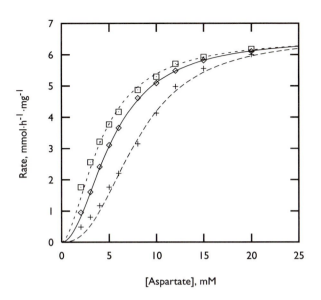

Figure 3.10 Kinetics of the allosteric enzyme aspartate transcarbamylase
The rate of reaction is shown with respect to one of its substrates, aspartate (◇). The enzyme is inhibited in a feedback manner by the pathway end product CTP (+). ATP acts as an activator (□). Based on results of Pigiet, Yang & Schachmann.[82]

to obtain a linear plot of their kinetics, at least for the results from the middle of the curve, by using the Hill plot adapted for enzyme kinetics. This consists of plotting $\log[v/(V-v)]$ against $\log S$; as with haemoglobin, the slope is the Hill coefficient, h. The intercept with the x-axis is the substrate concentration giving half the limiting rate, often designated $S_{0.5}$.

By the time Monod, Changeux and Jacob[160] reviewed the available evidence in 1963, there were sufficient examples of these enzymes to justify the following generalizations, which continue to be valid to this day.

(1) The enzymes are composed of a number of subunits, *i.e.* they are *multimeric*. The actual number varies, but tetramers (four subunits) are particularly common.

(2) The feedback inhibitor binds at a site distinct from the active site of the enzyme. Jacob and Monod named this site an *allosteric site* because the inhibitor is not a steric analogue of the substrates, and therefore the site must have a different shape. From this term, these enzymes have become known as *allosteric enzymes*. In some cases, the separation of the active site and the inhibitor site extends to their being on different subunits of the enzyme, giving *catalytic* and *regulatory* subunits.

(3) In some cases, there are activators as well as inhibitors of the enzymes. (The general term for modifiers of enzyme activity covering both activators and inhibitors is *effectors*.) The occurrence of activators makes it

even more certain that the effectors bind at sites distinct from the active site.

(4) In the majority of cases, the enzyme rate gives a sigmoid curve when plotted against the concentration of at least one of the substrates, corresponding to a Hill coefficient greater than 1. The effectors work by changing the $S_{0.5}$ of the enzyme for one of its substrates. Activators decrease the $S_{0.5}$ so that, at a given substrate concentration, the velocity is higher in the presence of the activator (Figure 3.10). On the other hand, inhibitors increase $S_{0.5}$ so that, at a given substrate concentration, the enzyme rate is lower (Figure 3.10). In both cases, the Hill coefficient is altered by the effectors. Enzymes whose activities are regulated in this way are classed as '*K systems*'. There is a minority class, the '*V systems*', where the effectors alter the rate without changing the $S_{0.5}$, and these do not necessarily exhibit sigmoid rate curves with respect to their substrates.

The characteristics of allosteric enzymes are also shared by haemoglobin in its oxygen-binding behaviour. There is also evidence that the binding of substrates and effectors to several allosteric enzymes is accompanied by substantial conformational changes of the protein detectable by a variety of physical methods. As a result, most attempts to explain how these enzymes work have assumed that the sigmoidal rate curves reflect underlying cooperativity in the substrate or effector binding. This is equivalent to making the same assumption as Michaelis and Menten that the binding of substrate is close to equilibrium because the rate of catalysis is relatively much slower. If this simplification is not applied to allosteric enzymes, explanations of their behaviour become very complicated.

There is just a handful of enzymes that show cooperative kinetics yet are monomeric and so differ from the majority. The best known example is the hexokinase IV from mammalian liver (also known as glucokinase[51]) which exhibits positive cooperativity with respect to glucose. In this case, the origin of the cooperativity is in an unusual kinetic mechanism.[50]

3.5.1   The concerted model

In 1965 Monod, Wyman and Changeux[161] proposed a structural model of allosteric enzymes to explain their cooperative binding properties and the action of effectors. They assumed that an allosteric enzyme was necessarily a protein with a number of subunits arranged in a symmetrical manner. They developed their model on the assumption that there are two structural states, or conformations of the subunits. The *tense* or T conformation is characterized by a relatively low affinity for substrate, but is well stabilized by relatively strong inter-subunit bonding. The *relaxed* or R conformation, on the other hand, shows a higher affinity for the substrate, but is less tightly bonded. Monod, Wyman and Changeux argued that the subunits in any one protein molecule

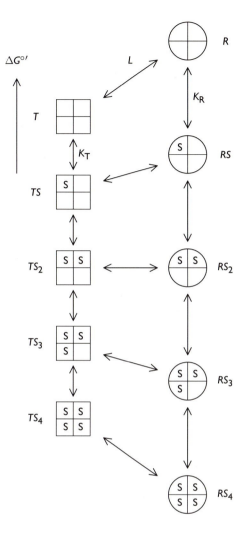

Figure 3.11 The concerted allosteric enzyme model of Monod, Wyman & Changeux
The T conformation is represented by squares and the R by circles. The different states of the protein are placed vertically according to their relative standard free energy for this specimen case. The exact relationships will vary with the values of the equilibrium constants L, K_R and K_T.

would be either all in the T state or all in the R state because symmetrical structures would be intrinsically more stable than the asymmetric ones that would result from a mixture of T and R conformations. Therefore, when the subunits change conformation, they all change simultaneously in a *concerted* manner.

Initially, in the absence of substrate, both conformations can be present, but the T state might be expected to predominate because it is more highly stabilized by the inter–subunit bonds. The R to T conversion has an equilibrium constant designated L. If the state of the protein is considered at successively higher

Box 3.1 The Monod, Wyman & Changeux equation

The equation for the fractional saturation, $\overline{Y}$, of an allosteric enzyme with n subunits that bind the ligand S according to the Monod, Wyman and Changeux model is:

$$\overline{Y} = \frac{\alpha(1 + \alpha)^{n-1} + L\alpha c(1 + \alpha c)^{n-1}}{(1 + \alpha)^n + L(1 + \alpha c)^n} \tag{3.12}$$

where L is the equilibrium constant corresponding to the T/R ratio in the absence of substrate, α is the substrate concentration relative to its dissociation constant, K_R, for an R state subunit *i.e.* $\alpha = S/K_R$, and c is the ratio of the dissociation constants for the binding of S to R and T state subunits, *i.e.* $c = K_R/K_T$. The equation may look complicated, but in fact it has a simple interpretation. The denominator is the sum of the concentrations of all the possible forms of the enzyme, $R + RS + \ldots RS_n + T + TS + \ldots TS_n$, relative to the concentration of R being arbitrarily assigned to one. If the bracketed terms in the denominator are multiplied out, there is a denominator term for each enzyme form. The numerator is the total concentration of bound substrate molecules, $RS + 2RS_2 + \ldots nRS_n + TS + 2TS_2 + \ldots nTS_n$, divided by n (again relative to $R = 1$) and again, the total number of terms in the numerator is equal to the number of liganded species. In other words, like all binding equations for the fractional saturation, the equation is merely a specific form of the general equation:

$$\overline{Y} = \frac{\text{Sum of concentrations of occupied ligand sites}}{n(\text{Sum of concentrations of enzyme species})} \tag{3.13}$$

where the denominator calculates the total concentration of ligand sites. Deriving an equation like Eqn. (3.12) can be done by taking the diagram of the model (such as Figure 3.11), assigning one of the forms the concentration one, calculating all the other concentrations relative to it by using the equilibrium constants, and inserting these concentrations into Eqn. (3.13).

The Monod, Wyman and Changeux equation [Eqn. (3.12)] therefore describes cooperative binding using three parameters, L, c and K_R; it is assumed that n is already known by other means. If $c = 1$ (corresponding to equal substrate affinity of the R and T states) or $L = 0$ (corresponding to no observable T state) the equation can be shown to reduce to an ordinary hyperbolic binding function like Eqn. (3.10):

$$\overline{Y} = \frac{\alpha}{1 + \alpha} = \frac{S}{K_R + S}$$

K_R determines the left–right positioning of the top of the curve on the Hill plot (Figure 3.9). L and c determine the shape of the Hill plot curve. It can also be shown that the maximum value of the Hill coefficient, h, depends on the values of L and c, but never exceeds the number of binding sites, n.

substrate concentrations then, at first, most of the substrate is binding with low affinity to the majority T state. However, with one molecule of substrate S bound to the protein, the equilibrium between TS and RS is somewhat more favourable for the R state because RS has stronger, more stabilizing interactions with the substrate molecule than does TS. If a second molecule of substrate

Box 3.2 The equations for inhibition and activation

In terms of the binding equation [Eqn. (3.12)], the effects of activators and inhibitors are to change the apparent value of L. For example, if an activator, B, binds exclusively to each of the n subunits of the R state with a dissociation constant $K_{R,B}$, whilst an inhibitor G binds exclusively to the n subunits of the T state with a dissociation constant $K_{T,G}$, then L in Eqn. (3.12) is replaced by L' given by

$$L' = L\frac{(1+\gamma)^n}{(1+\beta)^n}$$

where β is the relative concentration of the activator, $B/K_{R,B}$, and γ is the relative concentration of the inhibitor, $G/K_{T,G}$. If n is two or more, then this can make the substrate-binding curve of the enzyme very sensitive to the effectors in exactly the K-system manner shown by the enzyme aspartate transcarbamylase (Figure 3.10).

binds, yet more substrate–binding energy is available to stabilize the R state relative to the T state. This can be seen in Fig. 3.11 where the relative energy levels are shown for a tetrameric enzyme. At some point in the substrate–binding curve, the R state becomes more stable than the T state with the same number of substrate molecules bound. Therefore, the R state comes to be the predominant form as the substrate concentration increases. When the enzyme molecule changes from the T state conformation to the R state conformation, all the remaining unfilled substrate binding sites become high-affinity sites. This increase in affinity for the substrate after the binding of one or more substrate molecules to the enzyme gives the characteristic feature of cooperative binding.

The model also accounts for the action of allosteric effectors. An inhibitor is a molecule that binds preferentially to the T state and stabilizes it, just as the substrate stabilizes the R state. Because inhibitors stabilize the T state, they make it more difficult for the substrate to convert the molecule to the R state. An extremely effective inhibitor would stabilize the T state so much that the protein could not escape from it. The substrate would then always bind to low affinity T–state sites, and there would be no cooperativity in the substrate binding. An activator works the other way round by binding preferentially to the R state and therefore stabilizing it. This will favour the transition to the R state earlier in the substrate-binding curve. Again, a highly effective activator would stabilize the protein almost entirely in the R state, so that the binding of substrate would be to the high-affinity sites and the cooperativity in substrate binding would be lost. This explanation requires that the binding of the inhibitor and the activator both exhibit cooperativity. Indeed, the interactions between the different ligands, known as *heterotropic* effects, depend for their occurrence on the cooperativity of the substrate and/or the effector binding, the *homotropic* effects.

3.5.2   The sequential model

Koshland and his colleagues[137] developed a somewhat different theory for the action of allosteric enzymes. As in the Monod, Wyman and Changeux model, the cooperative kinetics are assumed to arise from the cooperative binding properties of a multi-subunit enzyme. Again, the conformational changes of the protein are an essential factor. However, in a link to Koshland's induced fit theory of enzyme action, the conformational change involved is specifically induced by substrate binding. The original model developed by Koshland, Nemethy and Filmer was termed the *sequential model*; later, Haber and Koshland proposed a more flexible *general model*,[93] which includes both his sequential model and the Monod, Wyman and Changeux model as special cases. However, the distinctive aspects of the Koshland models can be illustrated with the original sequential model, which is described here.

In the sequential model, the subunits of the protein are assumed to adopt two conformations, termed *A* and *B*. (*T* and *R* are not used because it is not implied that one is more stabilized by bonds than the other, as is the case with the tense and relaxed designations.) In this case, the *A* conformation is characteristic of a subunit without substrate attached. The *B* conformation is induced by the binding of substrate to the subunit; in the simple sequential model, it is assumed that the *B* conformation does not arise unless substrate binds, so there is no pre–existing equilibrium between subunits in the *A* and *B* states in the absence of substrate. In addition, the conformational change occurs one subunit at a time, in step with substrate binding, unlike the Monod, Wyman and Changeux model where all the subunits must change their conformation together. The source of the effect of the substrate binding at one site on the binding at another depends on the differences in the strengths of the interactions between subunits according to their conformations. If the interactions between a pair of adjacent subunits are considered, then the three types of interaction are *A–A*, *A–B* and *B–B*. The behaviour of the model is more complicated than that of the Monod, Wyman and Changeux model for two reasons. Firstly, it is affected by whether the *A–B* interactions are stronger or weaker relative to the *A–A* and *B–B* interactions. In particular, if *A–B* interactions are relatively weak, then the initial phases of binding where they are formed are not favoured, but the later stages of binding are promoted where the *B–B* interactions form, and the model gives positive cooperativity. However, if *A–B* interactions are strong, this assists the early stages of binding but not the later stages and the model generates negative cooperativity, which cannot be explained by the concerted model. Secondly, it is affected by the arrangement of the subunits in the protein, which determines how many subunit–subunit interactions can occur. For example, four subunits could be linked in a linear chain, in which case the two outer subunits have only one interface with another, whereas the two inner ones each have two. (However, this is thought to be an unlikely arrangement, since the protein should be able to continue growing at the ends of the line; there does not seem to be anything to stop the process at four subunits.) If

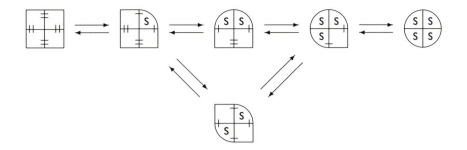

Figure 3.12 Sequential allosteric enzyme model of Koshland, Nemethy & Filmer
The A and B conformations are represented as squares and circles respectively. A tetramer with square interaction geometry is illustrated. There are two possible distinct arrangements of the tetramer with two substrates bound. Two bars at the subunit interface show an A–A interaction; one bar shows an A–B interaction; and none indicates a B–B interaction.

each subunit interacts with two neighbours, the arrangement could be schematically represented as a square composed of four smaller squares joined along two edges (without implying that the arrangement of subunits in space is geometrically square). If each subunit interacts with three others, then the four subunits would have to be arranged at the corners of a tetrahedron. The model is illustrated with the square configuration in Figure 3.12.

The action of allosteric effectors can be qualitatively explained by the sequential model. They can be thought of as inducing conformations that are more B–like for activators or more A–like for inhibitors. There is no simple way of writing activation and inhibition equations though. Thus the flexibility of the sequential model is offset by greater complexity, and since the number of parameters in the equations is fewer than the number of physically meaningful interactions that go into describing the model, effectively the values of some of the parameters are not accessible from binding experiments.

The scope for greater complexity is increased in Koshland's general model, which is like the sequential model except that it is assumed that the B conformation can exist before substrate binds. The Koshland models can be thought of as emphasizing the tertiary structural changes of a protein (*i.e.* the conformation of individual subunits) and also the linkage of the tertiary structure to the quaternary structure (*i.e.* the subunit–subunit interactions). The Monod, Wyman and Changeux model could be said to emphasize the quaternary structure, whilst the tertiary structure has less importance.

Most other models of allosteric enzymes assume that the characteristic kinetic behaviour depends on cooperativity in ligand binding and use the concepts of the two models described above, though combined in different ways. The only really different model for allosteric enzymes is the kinetic model of Rabin. Here the cooperativity in kinetic behaviour does not depend on the equilibrium binding characteristics of the enzyme, but is a consequence of the kinetic mechanism and the particular values of the rate constants for its component

Box 3.3 Equations for the Koshland models

Binding equations can be worked out using the principles described above in relation to Eqn. (3.13). However, in this case, different equations are obtained depending on the number of subunits and the interaction geometry, whereas a single equation (containing the number of subunits as a parameter) suffices for the concerted model. The original derivations considered the equilibrium constant (or free energy change) at each step in a scheme such as Figure 3.12 to be made up from a number of components: K_S, the intrinsic dissociation constant for a subunit in the B state; K_t, the equilibrium constant for the tertiary conformational change of the A subunit into a B subunit; K_{AA}, the equilibrium constant for the interaction of two adjacent A subunits (*i.e.* part of the quaternary conformational energy); K_{AB}, the equilibrium constant for the quaternary interaction between an A subunit and a B subunit, and K_{BB} the equilibrium constant for the interaction of an adjacent pair of B subunits. At each step, the change in the subunit–subunit interactions, brought about by the binding of S, has to be taken into account, and this can be different if different spatial arrangments of S on the protein subunits are possible (as in the case of two S molecules bound in Figure 3.12). Finally, it is found that in the resulting binding equation, these basic equilibrium constants always occur in certain combinations, so that they cannot be independently determined. For example, K_S and K_t always occur multiplied together, so that any pair of values that give the same product would give the same binding curve. In fact, for similar reasons, the final binding equation for a square tetramer can be expressed in terms of just two constants, formed of collections of the five constants. Unfortunately, the way the constants are collected proves to vary for different numbers of subunits and interaction geometries. Thus the assumed molecular interactions underlying the binding behaviour are not experimentally accessible from the binding curves.

steps. An occasional example of an enzyme apparently fitting the Rabin model is encountered, but it is generally believed that it is more common for allosteric behaviour to reflect binding properties, and in a number of cases there is even direct or indirect evidence to support this view.

3.5.3 Specific examples

I will now give a few examples of how the properties of certain proteins can, or cannot, be explained in terms of the allosteric models described above. They show that both of the models have some degree of success in particular cases.

3.5.3.1 Haemoglobin

Haemoglobin is an oxygen binding protein rather than an enzyme, but otherwise it has been regarded as an example of an allosteric protein. Myoglobin and haemoglobin were the two first proteins to have their three-dimensional structures determined by X–ray crystallography by Max Perutz and his colleagues at Cambridge. Myoglobin is an oxygen-storage protein that is found in partic-

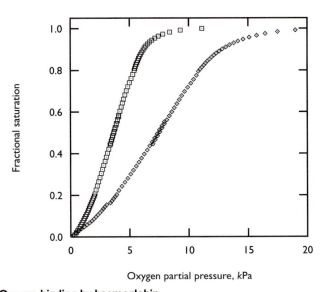

Figure 3.13 Oxygen binding by haemoglobin
The curves were measured by my student Richard Penny on human red blood cells, with an internal pH of 7.1. □, No 2,3–bisphosphoglycerate; ◇, 5 mM 2,3-bisphosphoglycerate in the cells.

ularly high levels in the muscles of diving mammals such as the sperm whale. It is relevant here because it contains a haem group and its polypeptide chain is folded in a virtually identical manner to the subunits of haemoglobin. Myoglobin, however, occurs as single subunits showing a hyperbolic binding curve for oxygen, with a much greater affinity for oxygen than has haemoglobin. The oxygen affinity of haemoglobin at the top end of its oxygen saturation curve, where the fourth oxygen is binding, is comparable to the oxygen affinity of myoglobin, so it appears that the assembly of haemoglobin into a tetrameric structure in some way inhibits the oxygen binding, as would be expected for a T–state structure in the concerted model of Monod, Wyman and Changeux.

The concept that there were two distinct conformational states of haemoglobin was supported by the crystallography studies. Crystals of deoxyhaemoglobin were grown and the protein structure was determined in this state. Significantly, if oxygen is allowed into contact with the crystals, they crack because of the conformational change on oxygen binding. Crystals of oxyhaemoglobin had to be grown separately to determine its structure; in fact, during the growth and X–ray analysis of the crystals, the iron atom in the haem group becomes oxidized, and methaemoglobin (which does not bind oxygen) is formed, but its conformation is believed to be the same as oxyhaemoglobin. The conformations of the subunits themselves scarcely differ between deoxy- and oxyhaemoglobin; the big difference was found to be the relative positioning of the subunits and the bonding between them. In accordance with the concerted model, there were more hydrogen bonding and salt linkages between the subunits in the deoxy state than in the oxy. Perutz's model of the binding of oxygen to haemoglobin assumes that there is a concerted conformational transition between the deoxy (T) state and oxy (R) state because it is as if the zig–zag surface of the interface has moved across by a complete notch, and any intermediate position would not be tenable. Nevertheless, X–ray crystallography gives a relatively static view of protein structures, which are known from other evidence to be flexible and mobile, and there is little direct evidence of the intermediate states in oxygen binding because they cannot be prepared as crystals, so the concerted transition is inferred rather than observed. However, there are well over a hundred known mutant haemoglobins that differ from normal haemoglobin by different substitutions of a single amino acid, and the effects of these on the affinity and the cooperativity of the oxygen binding can generally be interpreted in terms of the impact of the structural change on the concerted model (see question 2 at the end of this chapter).

In most mammalian red blood cells, there are high concentrations of 2,3–bisphosphoglycerate. This is normally only present in low concentrations in cells, as a cofactor for the glycolytic enzyme phosphoglycerate mutase, but in humans and many other mammals it acts as an allosteric inhibitor of oxygen binding. Its concentration is around 5 mM, comparable with the concentration of haemoglobin protein, but it varies slowly with conditions that affect the oxygenation of the blood such as the low oxygen pressure found at high altitudes. It acts as an inhibitor of oxygen binding, and is responsible for the oxygen affinity of blood being approximately half that of isolated haemoglobin, though it also slightly increases the cooperativity of binding. X–ray crystallography has shown that the binding site for 2,3–bisphosphoglycerate is in the central cavity of deoxyhaemoglobin between the four subunits; this cavity closes down in oxyhaemoglobin and would be too small to allow binding. Direct binding studies of 2,3–bisphosphoglycerate have confirmed that it binds preferentially to deoxyhaemoglobin, but they do measure weaker binding to oxyhaemoglobin, in spite of the apparent absence of the binding site in the crystal structure. The inhibitor therefore appears to behave very much as predicted in the concerted model. Proton binding, responsible for the pH–dependence of oxygen binding and the release of protons on binding of oxygen (the *Bohr effect*), does not appear to be a simple case of inhibition by preferential binding to the T state. Thus although many lines of evidence imply that haemoglobin behaves in accordance with the predictions of the concerted model, the equations of the model do not manage to describe the variation of the oxygen-binding curves at different pH and bisphosphoglycerate concentrations completely successfully, and modified versions of the theory have to be used to describe such results.[66]

3.5.3.2 Aspartate transcarbamylase

Aspartate transcarbamylase was one of the first two enzymes shown to be subject to feedback inhibition,[281] and it has been studied intensively since then.

Its reaction

carbamoyl phosphate + aspartate ⇌ carbamoyl aspartate + phosphate

is inhibited by the end product of its pathway, CTP, and is activated by ATP (Figure 3.10). The enzyme is composed of six regulatory subunits (R) that carry the binding sites for ATP and CTP and six catalytic subunits (C) with the active sites. The regulatory subunits are present as three dimers and the catalytic subunits as two trimers, so the structure is $(R_2)_3(C_3)_2$. Various chemical and denaturing treatments specifically abolish the effects of the regulatory subunits, leaving an enzyme that has hyperbolic kinetics with respect to both its substrates and that is insensitive to ATP and CTP. Some of these treatments (e.g. with mercuric compounds) cause dissociation of the catalytic trimers from the regulatory dimers. The binding curves of the substrates and effectors to the enzyme fit well with the Monod, Wyman & Changeux concerted model. The enzyme undergoes substantial changes in conformation upon binding substrates or effectors that can be readily detected by a variety of means (chemical reactivity of certain amino acid side chains, spectroscopic properties and size and shape).[82] These changes broadly fit with the expected $T \rightleftharpoons R$ transitions predicted by the concerted model. Thus aspartate transcarbamylase is probably the best established example of an enzyme that obeys the concerted model.[124]

3.5.3.3 Glyceraldehyde–3–phosphate dehydrogenase

This glycolytic enzyme is an enigma, since its properties vary greatly depending on its source for reasons that are unknown. The enzyme from yeast binds NAD^+ with positive cooperativity, and there appears to be a concerted conformational change of the enzyme in accordance with the concerted model. The enzyme from rabbit muscle, on the other hand, exhibits negative cooperativity in the binding of NAD^+, and this cannot be explained by the concerted model, though it can be by the sequential model. In fact, the negative cooperativity of this form of the enzyme is so marked that, after two molecules of NAD^+ have bound to the tetrameric enzyme, the affinities of the third and fourth sites fall substantially. It is an example of a phenomenon since found in some other multisubunit enzymes called *half of the sites reactivity*, on the basis that only a maximum of half the binding sites are occupied at any time. What remains unclear to this day is whether there is any specific function in metabolic regulation for negative cooperativity and half of the sites reactivity.

3.6   Summary

(1) The well–known Michaelis–Menten equation is not a complete description of the behaviour of single–substrate enzymes *in vivo* because of the effects of product inhibition and reversibility of the reaction.

(2) The majority of enzymes in metabolism have two substrates (and products) and catalysis can involve one of three basic mechanisms:

   • compulsory order;

   • random order;

   • double displacement.

(3) Generally, for two–substrate enzymes, the apparent K_m for one substrate will vary with the concentration of the other, so prediction of the rate at any particular set of substrate concentrations requires knowledge of the parameters of the appropriate rate equation.

(4) Many enzymes are composed of subunits. If the binding of a ligand, such as a substrate, on one subunit affects the affinity of another subunit for the same ligand, the binding is said to be cooperative and to involve homotropic interaction.

(5) Allosteric enzymes are a class of multisubunit (or multimeric) enzymes that have sites for effectors as well as the active site. As well as homotropic interactions, heterotropic interactions occur, whereby the effector can cause activation or inhibition of the enzyme by affecting substrate binding.

(6) Theories for the mechanisms of allosteric enzymes, such as the concerted and sequential models, centre around linkages between ligand binding and the conformational state of multimeric enzymes.

Further reading

Background to enzyme kinetics and allosteric enzymes: any biochemistry text such as:

Mathews, C. K. & van Holde, K. E. (1990) Biochemistry, The Benjamin/Cummings Publishing Co. Inc., Redwood City

Stryer, L. (1988) Biochemistry, 3rd edn., W. H. Freeman & Co., New York

Enzyme kinetics, general:

Cornish–Bowden, A. (1995) Fundamentals of Enzyme Kinetics, 2nd edn., Portland Press, London

Cornish–Bowden, A. & Wharton, C. W. (1988) Enzyme Kinetics, IRL Press, Oxford

Segel, I. H. (1975) Enzyme Kinetics, Wiley, New York

Computer programs

There are many programs available for fitting enzyme kinetics data. *Hyper* by John Easterby is a Windows program for fitting Michaelis–Menten kinetics, currently available as shareware on the Internet by anonymous FTP from *ftp.bio.indiana.edu* in /molbio/ibmpc/hyper.zip, or from *micros.hensa.ac.uk* in /mirrors/cica/win3/util/hyper.zip.

For fitting inhibition and two-substrate kinetics, the program *Leonora* for IBM PC-compatible microcomputers by Athel Cornish–Bowden is distributed with his book explaining the theory behind the fitting procedures: *Analysis of Enzyme Kinetic Data*, Oxford University Press, Oxford (1995).

Problems

(1) A Ca^{2+}–binding protein from bovine brain has a relative molecular mass of 17 000. Its Ca^{2+}–binding properties were investigated by an equilibrium dialysis experiment, in which the protein solution (2 mg·cm^{-3}) was placed in dialysis sacs that retain the protein and allowed to come to equilibrium with outer solutions containing various amounts of Ca^{2+} (in addition to buffer and salts). At equilibrium, the Ca^{2+} concentration is higher in the sacs than the outer solution since both contain free Ca^{2+} at the same concentration, but the sacs also contain protein–bound Ca^{2+}. The Ca^{2+} concentrations at equilibrium were measured by atomic absorption spectrophotometry, giving the results in the table below. Determine the number of binding sites on the protein for Ca^{2+} and their dissociation constant.

[Ca^{2+}], (μM)	
Outer solution	Sac fluid
0.9	47
2.1	94
4.3	152
7.7	206
18.2	284
35.0	336

(2) The following table contains data for the mid–regions of the oxygen binding curves of three haemoglobins measured in solution under identical conditions. The oxygen concentration is reported as the partial pressure of oxygen, pO_2, and the degree of oxygen binding by the fractional saturation, Y. The three haemoglobins are A (normal adult human), Hiroshima (His 146 $\beta \rightarrow$ Asp) and Kansas (Asp 102 $\beta \rightarrow$ Thr).

Plot a graph to determine the Hill coefficient, h, of each haemoglobin, and speculate on how the effects on the cooperativity and oxygen affinity could be interpreted in terms of the concerted model, given that the mutations are at the subunit interfaces rather than the oxygen-binding sites.

A		Hiroshima		Kansas	
pO_2	Y	pO_2	Y	pO_2	Y
0.67	0.044	0.133	0.045	1.33	0.193
1.33	0.243	0.267	0.179	2.67	0.371
2.00	0.500	0.667	0.620	4.00	0.500
2.67	0.691	1.33	0.822	5.33	0.592
4.00	0.874	2.00	0.948	6.67	0.660

(3) Isocitrate dehydrogenase from a slime mould catalyses the reaction:

$$\text{isocitrate} + NAD^+ \rightarrow \text{2-oxoglutarate} + CO_2 + NADH$$

The following rates of product formation (as $\mu mol \cdot s^{-1} \cdot mg^{-1}$) were measured on the enzyme for the indicated NAD^+ concentrations (mM):

	NAD^+ (mM)			
	0.2	0.4	0.8	2.0
Isocitrate (mM)	Enzyme rate			
0.05	8.5	10.1	11.2	11.9
0.15	12.6	16.6	19.6	22.1
0.25	14.0	19.0	23.1	26.6
0.50	15.2	21.3	26.7	31.5

Use the primary and secondary plot system to estimate V and the other kinetic parameters of the two-substrate rate equation. Can you deduce anything about the possible mechanism of this enzyme?

4

Traditional approaches to metabolic regulation

Until recently, biochemists tackled the problems of metabolic regulation and control either by attempting to identify the molecular details of the underlying mechanisms or by trying to formulate qualitative descriptions of the system's behaviour (see Chapter 1.2). There was general agreement that the explanations would centre around key regulatory, or rate–limiting, enzymes (Chapter 1.4.3, p. 17). I also mentioned in Chapter 1 that this conceptual framework was ultimately unsatisfactory and that the purpose of this book is to show why and to explain an alternative theory. Before I do that, I want to describe the experimental approaches that were used to identify regulatory enzymes, partly because the language and concepts are still in current use and partly to provide the context for the different approach of Metabolic Control Analysis.

The most coherent descriptions of the lines of evidence used in the traditional approaches were written by Hales[95] and by Eric Newsholme and his colleagues in Oxford (including Gevers,[169] Underwood[172] and Rolleston[201]). The plan of this chapter draws on their work and the influential textbook arising from it, *Regulation in Metabolism* by Newsholme & Start.[171] (Later, Newsholme and Bernard Crabtree were to develop their own form of quantitative systems theory.[55–57]) The following sections describe the lines of evidence that were taken to point to regulatory enzymes.

4.1 The teleological approach

Teleological arguments assume that the system has the properties necessary to fulfil its function; in other words, they assume the design is appropriate to the purpose. This can be made more biologically respectable by arguing that evolution will have favoured the adoption of efficient solutions to the problems of control and regulation. Of course, this assumes that we are able to identify

correctly the problems of constructing an efficient metabolism. The argument
applied in the search for regulatory enzymes is that it would be wasteful to have
'unnecessary' metabolism, and if pathways were controlled near their output
ends, when they were slowed down, metabolites would still continue to flow
in at the input, causing an accumulation of metabolic intermediates. Not only
might this cause the expenditure of unnecessary metabolic energy, it could
also cause osmotic problems for the cell. Therefore, it would be much better
if a controlling enzyme were to be placed at the beginning of a pathway, as
suggested by Sir Hans Krebs.[141]

The argument seems seductively reasonable, and there are many apparent
examples in its favour. This is no doubt because the argument has been influenced by the discovery of many enzymes with regulatory properties at the
points where a metabolic pathway branches off from the rest of metabolism, as
will be described later (Chapter 7.2). The problem is that there are examples
where the first enzyme in the pathway is not a regulatory enzyme (e.g. mammalian serine metabolism, see Chapter 6.3.4.2, p. 187, in which the regulatory
enzyme is the last one in a three-step pathway). In these cases, it is explained
that the regulatory enzyme is the first 'committed step'. That is the problem
with teleological arguments: when they work, they seem reasonable; when they
don't work, the story is changed slightly, and it's now reasonable that things
should be different for this particular case.

A variant on this concept foreshadowed later developments: Rolleston[201]
argued that the group of enzymes at the beginning of a pathway, including the
first non–equilibrium enzyme, could form a rate–limiting system, interacting
through substrate and coenzyme concentrations to form a functional unit.

4.2   Non–equilibrium enzymes

As discussed in Chapter 1.4.2, p.12, there was an expectation that the flux
through a pathway was not likely to be affected by changing the activity of
an enzyme catalysing a reaction that was near equilibrium, but changing the
activity of an enzyme catalysing a reaction displaced from equilibrium might
affect the flux. Of course, this principle does not explain which enzymes at non–
equilibrium steps can affect a metabolic flux, but it does suggest that the field
of candidates can be narrowed down by eliminating all the near–equilibrium
reactions.

A useful measure of the closeness of a reaction to equilibrium was defined
in Chapter 1.4.2 as the disequilibrium ratio ρ, which is the mass action ratio
relative to the equilibrium constant, Γ/K_{eq}, as defined in Eqn. (1.6). When
ρ is equal to 1, a reaction is at equilibrium, and reactions at steady state in a
metabolic pathway through which there is flow must have values less than 1.
The problem is to decide where the boundary lies between near–equilibrium
and non–equilibrium reactions. Rolleston suggested that the lowest value of ρ

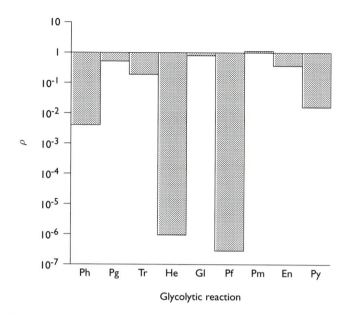

Figure 4.1   Displacement of reactions from equilibrium in glycolysis in working rat heart
The measurements were of metabolites in working perfused heart supplied with glucose but no insulin.
Both external glucose and endogenous glycogen were being used as fuels. Equilibrium constants were
corrected to measured intracellular conditions. Key: Ph, phosphorylase; Pg, phosphoglucomutase; Tr,
glucose transport; He, hexokinase; Gl, glucose–6–phosphate isomerase; Pf, phosphofructokinase; Pm,
phosphoglycerate mutase; En, enolase; Py, pyruvate kinase. Data from Kashiwaya et al.[125]

for a reaction to be classed as near–equilibrium could be as high as 0.2 or as low
as 0.05.[201] Even if 0.05 is taken as the boundary between near–equilibrium and
non–equilibrium reactions, this often leaves a significant number of reactions
in the pathway that are non–equilibrium and therefore potential candidates for
being regulatory enzymes, since reactions with ρ between 0.01 and 0.0001 are
relatively common.

Measurement of the disequilibrium ratio can pose a number of difficulties.
It depends upon measurements of metabolite concentrations, which are subject
to the problems referred to in Chapter 2.3. In addition, the equilibrium constant of the reaction must be known from *in vitro* experiments. It is possible for
the constant to have been measured inaccurately or not to have been adjusted
appropriately for intracellular conditions. Equilibrium constants of biochemical reactions may vary with pH, temperature and ionic conditions, particularly
where the reactants have weakly ionizable groups or groups that bind metal
ions such as K^+ or Mg^{2+}. Phosphorylated metabolites exhibit both properties.
(See the article by Kwack & Veech cited at the end of this chapter for examples
of how equilibrium constants can be adjusted to intracellular conditions.)

Some typical results are shown in Figure 4.1 for the glycolytic pathway in
perfused working rat heart, taken from experiments performed recently in the
laboratory of Veech and Passonneau in the United States.[125] This study was

undertaken to examine the proposal that, in the absence of the hormone insulin, transport of glucose into the heart muscle cells is the rate–limiting step for glycolysis.[162] Since insulin stimulates the movement of the glucose transporter molecules from the endoplasmic reticulum to the plasma membrane, it had also been held in the past that transport ceases to be 'rate–limiting' in the presence of insulin.[170] The design of these recent experiments included a quantitative analysis of the distribution of control by Metabolic Control Analysis. Later in this book (Chapter 5.5.1), I will return to the results of that analysis and how they relate to the disequilibrium ratios. My reason for choosing this set of results as an illustration, even though they were not used to find a rate–limiting step, is that they were undertaken with unusual thoroughness. Thus all the equilibrium constants used in the calcuations have been corrected to intracellular conditions, such as pH and the free cytoplasmic phosphate (which had been measured by ^{31}P NMR) and the free Mg^{2+} (which had been calculated from its effect on the citrate/isocitrate ratio).

The results show that three reactions, phosphorylase, hexokinase and phosphofructokinase, are very far from equilibrium, as is also pyruvate kinase, though to a lesser degree. Phosphoglucomutase, glucose–6–phosphate isomerase and phosphoglycerate mutase are close to equilibrium; indeed, the measured disequilibrium ratio for the latter is greater than 1, though not significantly so given the errors in the metabolite ratios. Glucose transport and enolase are on the boundary between the two groups. (The enzymes between aldolase and phosphoglycerate kinase could not have their disequilibrium ratios measured. This is partly because aldolase binds sufficient glyceraldehyde–3–phosphate to distort the results and also because 1,3–bisphosphoglycerate is both difficult to measure and subject to binding by enzymes.)

In the past, some researchers attributed significance to differences in the disequilibrium ratio at a step in different metabolic states. However, it is not easy to draw any conclusions from such results, and the separate changes in substrate and product concentrations were often thought to be more informative, as will be discussed in a later section of this chapter (4.6).

4.3 Isotopic measurement of flux

Another method of distinguishing between a near–equilibrium reaction (forward and reverse fluxes larger than net pathway flux) and a non–equilibrium reaction (forward flux comparable with net flux) is to measure the component forward and reverse reaction rates. This is possible because at near–equilibrium steps, an isotopically labelled substrate is converted into the product faster than would be expected from the net pathway flux. (At the start of such experiments, although the pathway is at steady state with respect to the concentrations of intermediates, it is not at isotopic equilibrium.) This can be seen in the computer–simulated examples shown in Figure 4.2. In the example where

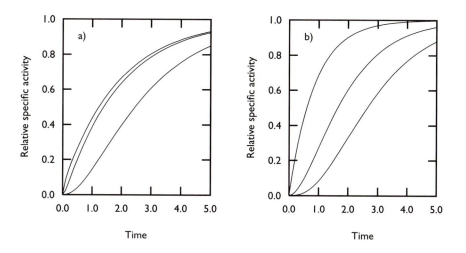

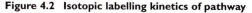

Figure 4.2 Isotopic labelling kinetics of pathway
The results have been produced by computer simulation of a pathway, and show the spread of the isotope into the first three intermediates of the pathway after its addition in the pathway source at time 0. Intermediates become isotopically labelled successively, so the leftmost curve is the first intermediate and so on. (a) The step between the first and second intermediates is near–equilibrium, with $\rho = 0.86$, corresponding to the forward rate being 7.2 times faster than the net pathway flux. The other steps are irreversible non–equilibrium steps. (b) The step between the first and second intermediates is now an irreversible non–equilibrium step, but the kinetics of the pathway have been adjusted to ensure that the pathway flux and intermediate concentrations are the same as in (a).

the first and second intermediates are linked by a near–equilibrium enzyme, the isotope is slower to accumulate in the first intermediate because of the high rate of transfer to the second intermediate. The amount of isotope in the second intermediate closely follows the amount in the first, and isotope accumulates in this intermediate faster than it does when the reaction is irreversible and non–equilibrium, as in the other example (Figure 4.2b). Computer fitting of results (such as those in Figure 4.2a) allows the forward and reverse reaction rates at the equilibrium step to be determined, as well as the pathway flux.

Many investigators have used such techniques to measure the fluxes through near–equilibrium reactions, particularly those in the tricarboxylic acid cycle and the glycolytic and gluconeogenic pathways in a wide range of cells and tissues.[10,19,58,130,192] In a study of the oxidation of [1–^{14}C]acetate by perfused rat heart, Sir Philip Randle and colleagues in Bristol found[192] that the specific radioactivities (relative to the acetate) of successive tricarboxylic acid cycle intermediates after 60 s labelling were: acetyl-CoA, 63%; citrate (in the two carbons derived from acetate), 43%; 2–oxoglutarate, 23%; malate, 13.5%; and oxaloacetate (from the four carbons contained in citrate), 4.7%. This illustrates the progressive spread of label through the intermediates in a similar manner to the example shown in Figure 4.2. The radioactivities in glutamate and aspartate were 20% and 6%, showing that these two intermediates were near-equilibrium with 2–oxoglutarate and oxaloacetate respectively (as in Figure 4.2a) through

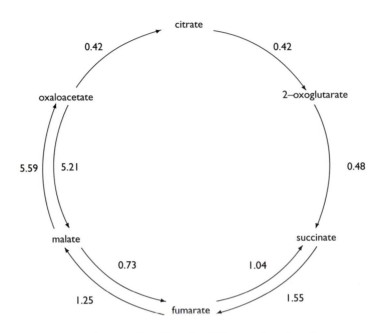

Figure 4.3 Fluxes in the tricarboxylic acid cycle of *Dictyostelium discoideum*
Only part of the metabolic network that is used in the computer fit to the experimental pattern of radioactive labelling is shown. The fluxes, in mM/min, are not perfectly balanced because of fitting errors and minor fluxes that are not shown.

the action of transaminases. These conclusions were confirmed by computer modelling of the results and estimation of the rates of the individual steps.

Figure 4.3 shows the relative rates of the non–equilibrium steps and the forward and reverse reactions of the near–equilibrium reactions of the tricarboxylic acid cycle in the slime mould *Dictyostelium discoideum* as determined by Barbara Wright's group[130] from fitting experimental results on the spread of ^{14}C.

4.4   Maximal enzyme activities

The maximal catalytic activities of enzymes (as limiting rate values) are often in considerable excess over the rates of metabolic flux; values of 100 to 10 000 times higher are not unusual. Some enzymes do not appear to be present in such 'excessive' amounts, and it is presumed that these are more likely to be regulatory. Making suitable measurements to carry out the comparison, though, raises the problems referred to in a previous Chapter (2.4). For my example in Figure 4.4, I have again drawn on the recent studies of glycolysis in working rat heart carried out by Veech, Passonneau and their colleagues[125] and used above to illustrate the displacement from equilibrium in a pathway. Their measurements were not taken to identify rate–limiting enzymes by their low activity, but they show the typical range of values observed in pathways,

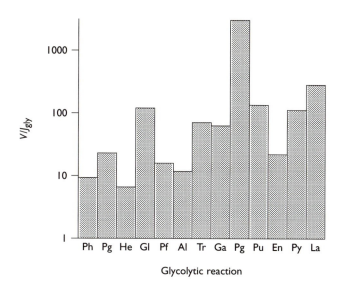

Figure 4.4   Relative enzyme activities in glycolysis in working rat heart
The limiting rates (V) were all measured at pH 7.2 in the presence of 150 mM K^+ and 5 mM Mg^{2+}. They are given relative to the glycolytic flux, J_{gly}, measured for working rat hearts using glucose as a fuel. Key: Ph, phosphorylase; Pg, phosphoglucomutase; He, hexokinase; Gl, glucose–6–P isomerase; Pf, phosphofructokinase; Al, aldolase; Tr, triose phosphate isomerase; Ga, glyceraldehyde–3–phosphate dehydrogenase; Pg, phosphoglycerate kinase; Pu, phosphoglycerate mutase; En, enolase; Py, pyruvate kinase; La, lactate dehydrogenase. Data from Kashiwaya et al.[125]

and they have the advantage that the whole set was measured in the same experiments and in constant assay conditions resembling the *in vivo* state (pH 7.2, 38 °C, 150 mM K^+ and 5 mM Mg^{2+}). The lowest activities are those of hexokinase, phosphorylase and aldolase, followed by phosphofructokinase and enolase. Apart from a lower activity of triose phosphate isomerase and higher activity of phosphoglycerate kinase than usual, the activities of the enzymes relative to one another are similar to those that have been reported previously for mammalian tissues. (See, for example, Table 3.4 in *Regulation in Metabolism* by Newsholme & Start.[171]) The consistently low measured activities of aldolase and enolase seem at variance with the usual finding that their reactions are not very far from equilibrium; this might point to a systematic measurement problem though, if so, its nature is uncertain.

Further evidence for a problem in measuring aldolase activities has recently come from Fraenkel's laboratory at Harvard. He and his colleagues inserted plasmids into *E. coli* to increase the expression of aldolase as much as 20- or 30-fold[9] and measured glycolytic flux, metabolite levels and some isotopic fluxes. Their results could only be explained quantitatively by assuming that the enzyme in the cells was 7.5 times more active than indicated by the *in vitro* assay. The same laboratory reached a similar conclusion about underestimation of the activity of glucose-6-phosphate isomerase in yeast.[14] Barbara Wright and Kathy Albe in Montana have encountered similar problems in constructing computer simulation models of metabolism of the slime mould *Dictyostelium discoideum*; the models can only be made consistent with the extensive experimental evidence (collected over many years by Wright's group) if many of the values for limiting rates measured *in vitro* misrepresent the maximal *in vivo* activities by factors of 100 or more.[278,279] (The problems of computer simulation of metabolism will be revisited later in this book, in Chapter 6.2.)

Examination of the maximal enzyme activities was often extended to measuring whether there were particular enzymes whose activities changed significantly when changes in the metabolic fluxes were caused by longer-term changes in dietary or environmental conditions or drug or hormonal treatments. In the catabolism of the amino acid tryptophan by rat liver, various hormonal and dietary treatments that increase its rate (e.g. administration of glucocorticoids[73]) specifically increase the amount of tryptophan 2,3–dioxygenase by activating its synthesis. This was interpreted as indicating a possible role for the enzyme in the control of tryptophan catabolism. Later we shall see that there has been some confirmation of this view from quantitative measurements of the influence of this enzyme on the tryptophan breakdown flux (Chapter 6.1.2, p. 148).

In many other cases, the pattern of variation of enzyme activities is not obviously informative about the potential of individual enzymes to control metabolic flux. In the case of the enzymes of carbohydrate metabolism in rat liver, three groups can be identified by their response to dietary and hormonal treatments. These are the enzymes exclusive to the gluconeogenic pathway, those exclusive to the glycolytic pathway, and those that are shared by the two pathways. The gluconeogenic group consists of pyruvate carboxylase, phosphoenolpyruvate carboxykinase, fructose–1,6–bisphosphatase and glucose–6–phosphatase (see Figure 6.17) and their amounts vary in parallel.[268] There is good evidence, though, from more recent experiments (to be described later, Chapter 6.3) that the enzymes in the group differ greatly in their degree of control over the gluconeogenic flux. Nevertheless, this and other cases where many of the enzymes of a pathway change in activity together to cause a change in metabolic flux almost certainly carry a message about metabolic control, though not one envisaged in this traditional view (see Chapter 8.1).

4.5   Addition of intermediates

If a pathway is controlled by reactions near its beginning, it would seem reasonable to expect that higher flux rates might be observed if intermediates could be fed into the pathway below this point. For example, the synthesis of cholesterol from 2–carbon precursors (acetyl-CoA) leads first to 5–carbon intermediates, which are condensed to 15–carbon intermediates, which are in turn dimerized to give the 30–carbon steroid skeleton. Higher rates of cholesterol synthesis are observed from the 5–carbon intermediate mevalonate than from 2–carbon acetate, and this has been taken as evidence for regulation of the rate of synthesis early in the pathway (at the hydroxymethylglutarylCoA reductase step). The same result is found in whole tissues and cell–free extracts, so the difference is not related to differential permeability.

Another example is the comparison of the rate of gluconeogenesis in rat kidney slices using pyruvate as a substrate with the rates measured using tricarboxylic acid cycle intermediates fumarate and 2–oxoglutarate that readily give rise to the gluconeogenic intermediate oxaloacetate (see Figure 6.17 for the pathway). Sir Hans Krebs reported[142] that the rates of glucose formation were very similar from all three compounds, and that therefore it was unlikely that the formation of oxaloacetate from pyruvate by pyruvate carboxylase is the 'pacemaker' (as he termed a rate–limiting step). However, experiments on gluconeogenesis in rat hepatocytes to be described later (Chapter 6.3) show that this enzyme has a larger influence over the rate of the pathway than any other.

The problem with such experiments on the relative rates with different intermediates is that there can be other equally reasonable explanations. If a pathway intermediate is used as a starting point, it must of necessity be supplied at higher concentrations than are normally found. The pathway would therefore be expected to operate faster merely because of this factor. On the other hand, if the pathway failed to show an increased flux, this might be because the intermediate is poorly permeable and does not reach the site of its metabolism. Therefore this method has not been regarded as reliable. Indeed, in Krebs' experiments, poor rates of gluconeogenesis were obtained from glutamate and aspartate (even though these might be expected to be efficient sources of oxaloactetate) but he discounted these results and chose to attach greater significance to the results with 2–oxoglutarate and fumarate.

4.6   The cross–over theorem

In the 1950s, Britton Chance and his colleagues in Philadelphia were studying the electron transport chain and oxidative phosphorylation in mitochondria. They measured the degrees of reduction and oxidation of various electron carriers in the mitochondria by spectrophotometric measurements on working mitochondria. In the course of these experiments, they had noted that when electron transport was partially inhibited, the carriers towards the NADH end of the chain became more reduced relative to normal (*i.e.* there was a build-up of 'substrates' of the chain) whereas the carriers from the site of inhibition towards oxygen became more oxidized (*i.e.* there was a reduction in the 'substrate').[34] They then used this phenomenon of a *cross-over* in the state of oxidation at the inhibition site to determine the sites of coupling of electron transport to oxidative phosphorylation by comparing State 3 respiration (*i.e.* phosphorylating respiration in the presence of ADP, see Chapter 6.5, p. 191) to State 4 respiration, which is inhibited by the lack of ADP for phosphorylation. They formulated a number of cross-over theorems to guide the interpretation

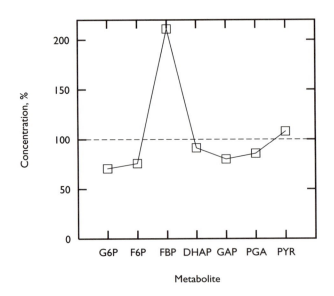

Figure 4.5 Cross–over plot of the glycolytic pathway in yeast
The metabolite levels in anaerobic conditions, when glycolysis is stimulated, are shown as percentages of their aerobic concentrations.[144] Abbreviations: G6P, glucose 6–phosphate; F6P, fructose 6–phosphate; FBP, fructose 1,6–bisphosphate; DHAP, dihydroxyacetone phosphate; GAP, glyceraldehyde–3–phosphate; PGA, 3–phosphoglycerate; PYR, pyruvate.

of these experiments[35] and they validated these theorems[33] by computer simulations. The principal theorem was that a cross–over from increased substrate (relatively more reduced carriers) to decreased substrate concentration (relatively more oxidized carriers) when the pathway flux had decreased indicated the site of an inhibition. Subsidiary theorems indicated that cross–overs in the opposite direction upon inhibition were not significant, and dealt with identification of multiple sites of inhibition (as obtained with the three coupling sites of electron transport upon limitation of the phosphorylation rate).

Other investigators then applied the principal cross–over theorem to identifying the sites of action of regulatory signals, both inhibitors and activators, on metabolic pathways. A typical example is shown in Figure 4.5 from a study[144] on the increase in rate of glycolysis that occurs when yeast that has been catabolizing glucose aerobically is transferred to anaerobic conditions (an effect known as the Pasteur effect, after the pioneering French microbiologist Louis Pasteur). The 80% increase in flux is accompanied by a fall in the levels of fructose 6–phosphate and all the preceding glycolytic intermediates, but a 220% increase in fructose 1,6–bisphosphate; the cross–over is therefore at phosphofructokinase. The subsequent crossings of the 100% line are not statistically significant because of the errors in the metabolite measurements. (In any case, one of the cross–over theorems[33] states that such reverse cross–overs should not be taken as evidence of an interaction site.) The experiments were interpreted as

showing the stimulation of phosphofructokinase by an effector; of the metabolites known to affect the yeast enzyme (including fructose 2,6–bisphosphate),
only changes in phosphate concentrations correlated systematically with the
occurrence of the Pasteur effect and this cross–over.

The applicability of the cross–over theorem to its original domain — the
electron-transport chain — has not been questioned. Indeed, it is possible to
prove that the occurrence of a cross–over must involve an inhibition at that
point on the chain. Rolleston[201] pointed out that the proof did not necessarily
validate application of the theorem to other pathways, for the proof depended
on particular properties of electron transport. In particular, the typical reaction
in the chain is:

$$A_{red} + B_{ox} \rightleftharpoons A_{ox} + B_{red}$$

where A and B are successive carriers and *red* indicates the reduced state and
ox the oxidized state. The proof depends on the *conservation* of A and B,
that is, that their total concentrations remain fixed, introducing an obligatory
coupling between the substrate and product concentrations and ensuring that
they must change in opposite directions. This is not the case in a pathway
such as glycolysis, where the total concentration of intermediates is not fixed
when glucose and phosphate are freely available, so an increase in substrate
concentration does not necessarily force a decrease in product concentration
(or *vice versa*). Furthermore, the cross-over criterion is difficult to apply for
the very common case of two-substrate two-product enzymes, since in this
case there is again nothing to force a correlation between the concentration
changes of the two substrates, which could feasibly change in opposite directions.

Now, Reinhart Heinrich & Tom Rapoport (who reappear in later chapters
as two of the founders of Metabolic Control Analysis) managed to show, using Metabolic Control Analysis arguments,[100] that in a simple linear pathway,
the cross–over theorem could be proved to be applicable. However, they also
showed that it could not be guaranteed to work in a variety of other circumstances. These included pathways where the effector causing the changes acts
on more than one site in the pathway, and pathways containing more than
one feedback loop, in which the cross–over could feasibly occur at the wrong
enzyme.

Thus the cross–over plot cannot be regarded as reliable for metabolic pathways in general. In particular, the failure to observe a cross–over when there
has been a change in metabolic flux cannot be taken as proof that an effector did
not act on an enzyme's kinetics. Even when a cross–over has been observed,
as in the yeast glycolysis example above, the significance of the finding needs
careful thought. We shall see later in Chapter 4.8, that it cannot be taken as
proof that glycolysis has been accelerated by an activation of phosphofructokinase alone, since experiments to increase that enzyme's activity specifically and
substantially have not resulted in any change in glycolytic flux.

Sir Hans Krebs suggested in 1957[141] that a site of regulatory action might be identified by the observation of anomalous changes in the substrate concentration of a non–equilibrium enzyme when comparing two metabolic states with different fluxes. That is, if the flux through the enzyme had decreased, whereas its substrate concentration had increased (which would usually be expected to cause an increase in the flux), then presumably the enzyme must have been inhibited by some other factor. (Changes in product concentration were rather summarily dismissed as a factor that could account for the change in rate of a non–equilibrium enzyme on the grounds that its reverse reaction rate is negligible; the inhibitory effect that a product can have even on an irreversible enzyme reaction was, as usual, discounted.) This is effectively a simplified version of the cross-over theorem and therefore shares some of its limitations.

4.7   Enzyme properties

A non–equilibrium enzyme might be assumed to be regulatory if:

- kinetic studies reveal that it is inhibited or activated by pathway metabolites other than the substrate [e.g. allosteric enzymes (Chapter 3.5), involved in feedback or feed–forward loops (Chapter 7.2)], or

- the enzyme is found to be subject to activity change by reversible modification reactions (Chapter 7.4).

The thinking behind this assumption is that such mechanisms are not accidental and must serve some function. This may well be true, though covalent modification of enzymes by phosphorylation seems very widespread in eukaryotic cells, and it is not known in every case what effect this has on the target enzyme — phosphofructokinase is an example of a glycolytic enzyme that undergoes phosphorylation in many mammalian tissues, but in some of these it is unclear what difference the phosphorylation makes to its properties. Furthermore, even if the molecular mechanism is brought into play in some metabolic circumstances, this does not prove that the effect has had a significant role in the situations under study. If an enzyme has its activity changed by an effector, then the proof that this interaction is of regulatory significance would have to include demonstration that the effector changes in concentration in a manner consistent with the changes in metabolic rate, that the effector concentration in the cells is in the range that affects the enzyme activity, and that changes in the activity of that enzyme can affect the overall metabolic rate. All this would involve studies at the level of the metabolic system and could not be inferred from the molecular properties of the enzyme in isolation.

In other words, the characteristics of the enzyme may contribute to an understanding of the mechanisms of regulation and control, but they cannot stand alone; there must be other supporting evidence. Furthermore, I shall present arguments later in the book to show why enzymes that are not 'rate–limiting' must even so be controlled by mechanisms such as covalent modification when the pathway flux is controlled (Chapter 8.1).

4.8 Metabolic mutants

It is arguable whether the use of mutants should be listed as a traditional technique for investigating metabolic regulation, since it is only the recent rise in molecular genetics that has made this a much more feasible experimental approach. Mutants can now more easily be isolated or made with altered regulatory properties in a specific enzyme. The gene for an enzyme in one organism can be replaced by one with different characteristics taken from another organism. The amount of a selected enzyme can be specifically varied by increasing the number of copies of its gene or changing its promoter. Some of these experiments have been carried out recently as part of quantitative investigations in Metabolic Control Analysis (Chapters 6.1.1.1–6.1.1.5), but similar techniques have been used in qualitative investigations of the role of particular enzymes in metabolic regulation. Traditional techniques have been used to isolate mutants in the regulatory properties of key enzymes in the amino acid biosynthesis pathways of bacteria, and the properties of the mutants have often been consistent with expectations.[251] On the other hand, the common view that phosphofructokinase is the rate–limiting enzyme of glycolysis has been undermined because: (a) mutants with different forms of the enzyme in *E. coli* generally show little difference in their metabolism,[76] and (b) changing the amount of the enzyme expressed in yeast makes no difference to the glycolytic flux.[96]

Thus in principle, mutant studies can be used to examine traditional concepts of metabolic control; in practice, the results obtained in this way are actually contributing to the undermining of the theory.

4.9 Conclusion

None of the lines of evidence described above has a single unambiguous meaning. In the search for regulatory enzymes and 'rate–limiting steps', it was usual to seek corroboration from several different approaches. Unfortunately, that did not always lead to a single uncontested answer, and there were many cases where groups in different laboratories produced incompatible theories about the mode of regulation of a particular metabolic pathway. The cartoon in Figure 4.6 makes fun of this. How some of these arguments have been resolved will be explained in the remainder of the book.

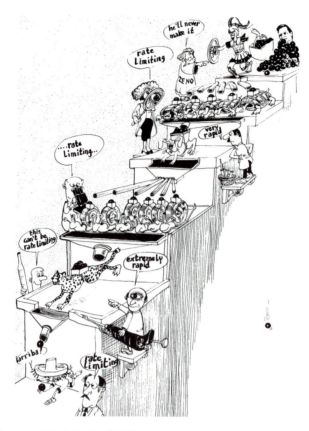

Figure 4.6 The quest for the rate–limiting step
Reproduced with permission from A. B. Tulp (1986) Trends Biochem. Sci. 11, 13

4.10   Summary

(1) For most of the second half of the 20th century, the main aim in the study of metabolic control was to find the 'rate–limiting' enzyme of a pathway. Candidate enzymes should show one or more of the following characteristics.

(2) The *teleological* argument is that there should be a rate–limiting enzyme at the first unique step of a pathway.

(3) The rate–limiting step should be a *non–equilibrium* enzyme, since otherwise it could not have a significant role in metabolic control. Candidates should be identifiable by comparing the mass action ratio with the equilibrium constant. Alternatively, isotopic measurements of forward and reverse fluxes should distinguish between near–equilibrium and non–equilibrium enzymes.

(4) A 'rate–limiting' enzyme is expected to have less capacity to work faster than other enzymes, so should show a relatively low limiting rate value in assays.

(5) The pathway flux would be expected to be higher from intermediates added after the rate–limiting step.

(6) A cross-over in relative metabolite levels between two metabolic states could indicate where a regulatory signal had acted on a rate–limiting enzyme to change the flux.

(7) Regulatory enzymes should show changes in activity in response to metabolites other than their own substrates.

(8) Alteration of the activity or regulatory properties of a rate–limiting enzyme should directly affect the metabolic flux.

(9) The results of such investigations are not always consistent. Conflicts can then arise that cannot be readily resolved within the framework of the rate–limiting step.

Further reading

Denton, R. M. & Pogson, C. I. (1976) Metabolic Regulation, Chapman & Hall, London

Hales, C. N. (1967) *Some actions of hormones in the regulation of glucose metabolism.* In Essays in Biochemistry (Campbell, P. N. & Greville, G. D., eds.), vol. **3**, pp. 73–104, Academic Press, London

Newsholme, E. A. & Start, C. (1973) Regulation in Metabolism, Wiley & Sons, London

Newsholme, E. A. & Gevers, W. (1973) *Control of glycolysis and gluconeogenesis in liver and kidney cortex.* Vitam. Horm. **25**, 1–87

Rolleston, F. S. (1972) *A theoretical background to the use of measured concentrations of intermediates in the study of the control of intermediary metabolism.* Curr. Top. Cell. Regul. **5**, 47–75

Kwack, H. & Veech R. L. (1992) *Citrate: its relation to free magnesium concentration and cellular energy.* Curr. Top. Cell. Reg. **33**, 185–207

Fraenkel, D. G. (1992) *Genetics and intermediary metabolism.* Annu. Rev. Genet. **26**, 159–177

5

Metabolic Control Analysis

5.1   The problems of the traditional approaches

Biochemists have used the investigative methods described in Chapter 4 extensively for the identification of regulatory enzymes in metabolic pathways. In many cases, several such enzymes were found in one pathway and this led to arguments between different groups of researchers who all agreed that there could only be one rate–limiting step (see p. 17), but could not agree which one it was. Is alcohol dehydrogenase the rate–limiting enzyme of human ethanol metabolism? Is the adenine nucleotide transporter the rate–limiting step in mitochondrial oxidative phosphorylation? These are just two examples of long–running disputes. It was of course possible that no group was completely right, but that some of them were partially right, because there was no single rate–limiting step. But if the control of rate was spread over a number of steps, how could their relative contributions be compared? The experiments described up to now cannot answer this question because they do not generate any quantitative measure of the degree of control of an enzyme over the rate, or *flux*, of a metabolic pathway. Apart from this practical difficulty in applying the concept of rate limitation usefully, there are theoretical difficulties.

(1) The definition states that the rate–limiting step is the slowest step in a pathway, but how is this to be interpreted? In a metabolic steady state (p. 10) all the steps along a linear pathway are going at the same rate. If 'slowest step' is interpreted as the one least able to go faster, the types of observation described in Chapter 4 do not appear to measure this inability.

(2) By the 1930s, it was known that the rate of a sequence of simple chemical reactions could depend to varying degrees on the rate constants of all the reactions. In 1964, Stephen Waley[260] showed that the rate of a sequence of unsaturated enzymes (*i.e.* enzymes for which all the metabolite concentrations are below their K_m values) depended non–linearly on the

kinetic parameters of all the enzymes. Thus in these cases, even though they are certainly simpler than a metabolic pathway *in vivo*, there is no theoretical basis for expecting that a unique rate–limiting step inevitably exists.

(3) If a rate–limiting step exists in a pathway, then varying the activity of that step alone will change the flux in the pathway, and varying any other activity will have no effect whatsoever. There are few definitive experimental observations of such a phenomenon, but many (examples of which will be discussed in the next chapter) of pathways affected by the activities of several of the steps. Furthermore, there have been attempts to increase the rate of a pathway by using gene cloning techniques to increase the amount of the supposed rate–limiting enzyme. For example, when this was applied to phosphofructokinase in yeast (the enzyme many biochemistry books cite as the rate–limiting enzyme of glycolysis), a 3.5–fold increase in the amount of enzyme had no significant effect on the anaerobic glycolytic flux.[96]

If the concept of the rate–limiting step must be replaced because it is inadequate both experimentally and theoretically, what characteristics would an alternative have to possess? It would have to allow that several enzymes might affect the flux in a pathway, and ideally it would suggest a basis for quantitatively comparing the effects that these enzymes have on the flux. Similar problems in other branches of science, and economics, have been tackled with *sensitivity analysis*. This involves the assessment of how strongly a variable (such as a pathway flux) responds to a change in any one of the factors that might conceivably affect it. Just such an approach has been introduced into metabolic biochemistry by a number of different researchers, beginning in the 1960s with Joseph Higgins.[104] In 1969, Michael Savageau started developing the sensitivity analysis that eventually became part of his Biochemical Systems Theory.[217] In the early 1970s, Henrik Kacser & Jim Burns in Edinburgh[119] and Reinhart Heinrich & Tom Rapoport in Berlin[99,100] independently made developments of Higgins' work that were eventually amalgamated into Metabolic Control Analysis (or Metabolic Control Theory). Biochemical Systems Theory and Metabolic Control Analysis are rather different in approach, though they are basically compatible where they overlap. In Biochemical Systems Theory, sensitivity analysis is just one part of a mathematical method for modelling and simulation of metabolic and physiological systems at a high level of generality. Metabolic Control Analysis is not intended to be a complete approach to the modelling of metabolism; its principal concern is with sensitivity analysis, and it maintains a closer link to the individual underlying enzymic reactions than does Biochemical Systems Theory. Since the early 1980s, a larger body of experimental work has accumulated related to Metabolic Control Analysis than to Biochemical Systems Theory. For this reason, in the rest of this book

a) The specimen pathway:

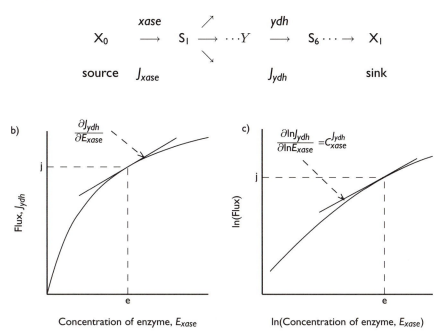

Figure 5.1   The flux control coefficient
(a) A hypothetical specimen pathway. (b) Typical variation of the pathway flux measured at a step *ydh*, J_{ydh}, with the amount of an enzyme, *xase*. The flux control coefficient at *e,j* is the slope of the tangent to the curve $\partial J_{ydh}/\partial E_{xase}$ times the scaling factor *e/j*. (c) On a double-logarithmic plot of the same curve, the flux control coefficient is the slope of the tangent to the curve.

I will use the approach of Metabolic Control Analysis, though occasionally I will mention concepts that were derived within Biochemical Systems Theory.

5.2   Flux control coefficients

The fundamental difference between the rate–limiting step concept and Metabolic Control Analysis is highlighted if we consider the question we are asking in the two cases concerning the relationship between the flux through a metabolic pathway and the activity of a particular enzyme. In the former we ask 'Is this enzyme rate–limiting?', and our answer is supposed to be 'Yes' or 'No'. In the latter we ask 'How does the metabolic flux vary as the enzyme activity is changed?'. This obviously invites a more detailed answer and allows all possibilities between 'Not at all' to 'Greatly'. Furthermore, it can be posed as a quantitative question: 'How *much* does the metabolic flux vary …?'. At the time of the rise of Metabolic Control Analysis, there were hardly any relevant experimental studies, which seems surprising since answering the question only requires measurements of flux and enzyme activity, which are standard techniques in metabolic biochemistry. There were theoretical grounds, such as Waley's equation cited earlier, for expecting the relationship between flux and enzyme activity to appear convex or hyperbolic as shown in Figure 5.1(b). The few experimental studies available at the time were consistent with this sort of relationship, and it has since been found in other investigations, some of which are referred to later in this book. In addition, the increasing availability of computers had made possible the first attempts at simulating the behaviour of sequences of enzymes, allowing theoretical investigation of their behaviour.

The important feature of the dependence of flux on the concentration of one particular enzyme (Figure 5.1b) is that the response to a change in the amount of enzyme will vary depending on the position of the starting point of the change on the x-axis. Near the origin, there could be an almost proportional increase in metabolic flux as the enzyme amount is increased; at this point, there might be some justification for terming the enzyme 'rate–limiting'. If the starting point for increasing the enzyme is part way along the x-axis, then the response of the flux to an increase in enzyme is noticeable, but weaker than before. If the starting point is far to the right on the x-axis, then an increase in the enzyme has a small or negligible effect on the flux. There is continuous variation of the response of the flux to the amount of enzyme between these extremes. Unless some suitable measurements have already been made, we do not know where the content of a chosen enzyme in a given cell type will map on this curve. Metabolic Control Analysis begins by defining a coefficient that quantifies this variable response and then finds means of measuring and using it.

5.2.1   Definition

In the pathway shown in Figure 5.1(a), suppose that a small change, δE_{xase}, is made in the amount of enzyme E_{xase}, and that this produces a small change, δJ_{ydh}, in the steady state pathway flux, J, measured at the step catalysed by ydh. If the change is made small enough, then the ratio $\delta J_{ydh}/\delta E_{xase}$ becomes equal to the slope of the tangent to the curve of J_{ydh} against E_{xase} as shown in Figure 5.1(b). In mathematical notation this tangent is represented as $\partial J_{ydh}/\partial E_{xase}$. Obviously this represents the steepness of the response of the flux to the amount of enzyme, but has the disadvantage that its numerical value and its units will depend on the units used to measure the flux and the enzyme. This problem can be avoided if we compare the fractional changes in the enzyme and flux, *i.e.* $\delta E_{xase}/E_{xase}$ and $\delta J_{ydh}/J_{ydh}$; since the numerator and denominator of each fraction are measured in the same units, the result is dimensionless. (If multiplied by 100, each of these fractional changes can be regarded as percentage changes.) The *flux control coefficient* $C_{xase}^{J_{ydh}}$ is given by the ratio of these fractional changes as $\delta E_{xase}/E_{xase}$ tends to zero:

$$C_{xase}^{J_{ydh}} \approx \frac{\delta J_{ydh}}{J_{ydh}} \bigg/ \frac{\delta E_{xase}}{E_{xase}} \qquad (5.1)$$

Box 5.1 Other definitions

The definition of the flux control coefficient given above has the advantages both of simplicity and of relevance to cellular events that change the amount of active enzyme in a cell. There are, though, more precise ways of defining it. In many circumstances, the different definitions would lead to the same answer, but in a few instances, the results could differ. In these cases, the more technical definitions should be preferred because they lead to greater consistency of interpretation, whereas the simple definition in terms of enzyme concentration would be less well-behaved. The reasons for this are given in Appendix 1, *More about flux control coefficients* (Chapter 5.7, p. 128). However, the simpler definition, as used initially by Kacser & Burns, works appropriately with the experimental results described in this book and will be retained here in order to avoid terminological differences with the research papers describing the results.

This can be rearranged so that the flux control coefficient is expressed as the tangent to a curve such as that in Figure 5.1(b) times a scaling factor E_{xase}/J_{ydh}:

$$C^{J_{ydh}}_{xase} = \frac{\partial J_{ydh}}{\partial E_{xase}} \cdot \frac{E_{xase}}{J_{ydh}} \tag{5.2}$$

In turn, this is mathematically identical to the following definition, which is useful because it shows that the flux control coefficient is the slope of the tangent on a plot of the logarithm of flux against the logarithm of the enzyme amount, as in Figure 5.1(c):

$$C^{J_{ydh}}_{xase} = \frac{\partial \ln J_{ydh}}{\partial \ln E_{xase}} \tag{5.3}$$

(Whether logarithms to base 10 or natural logarithms are used does not matter as long as the same type is used for both axes.)

5.2.2 Interpretation

What values might we expect flux control coefficients to have, and what do they signify? For the pathway shown in Figure 5.1, typical values are shown in Figure 5.2. If the curve had flattened out so that flux could no longer be increased by further addition of enzyme, as would have been seen if the graph had been extended further to the right, the flux control coefficient would be 0. It therefore seems that the values can range between 0 and 1. A value of 1 would correspond to a proportional relationship between the pathway flux and the amount of enzyme. [This can most easily be seen from Eqn. (5.1), which shows that, in this case, a given fractional change in enzyme amount produces an equal fractional change in the flux.]

It is also possible for a flux control coefficient to have a negative value. For example, in a branched pathway where one metabolite can go to two different

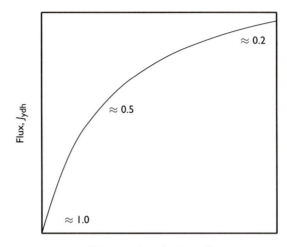

Figure 5.2 Values of the flux control coefficient
The values shown are approximately correct for the curve shown in Figure 5.1(b).

end products, an increase in the activity of an enzyme in one branch might increase the flux of the metabolite down its own branch, and thereby decrease the amount available to flow down the other branch. Therefore the enzyme could have a negative flux control coefficient on the flux in the other branch.

There is also a theoretical possibility that a flux control coefficient could have a value greater than 1 in certain control structures found in metabolism (*e.g.* Chapter 7, pp. 219 and 243). No experimental measurements have yet demonstrated that such values can be found in metabolism but there is an important piece of evidence from the genetics of diploid organisms that shows that many enzymes have small flux control coefficients. Diploids generally have two functioning copies in each cell of the gene for an enzyme, but if this copy number is changed, the amount of enzyme is usually proportional to the gene dose. In addition, there are many known examples of mutations in genes for enzymes, both naturally occurring and artificially induced, that result in the production of enzymically inactive protein. However, the important finding is that these mutations are almost invariably recessive, that is, in heterozygotes that contain one normal and one mutant copy of the gene, the organism's properties (or phenotype) appear normal. The normal gene is said to be dominant to the mutant form. For example, in 1928, the geneticist R. A. Fisher reported that 94% of mutations in the fruit fly *Drosophila melanogaster* were recessive, 6% were semi–dominant, and none was dominant. Since enzymes affect the phenotype through the flux in metabolic pathways, the observation that the wild–type is dominant effectively means that there has been no discernible change in flux in the heterozygote, even though it contains only half the enzyme present in the wild–type homozygote. In a number of cases, it has indeed been confirmed by direct measurement that the metabolic flux is only marginally reduced in heterozygotes. This is only possible if the content of the enzyme in the normal homozygote is high enough for the flux–enzyme curve to have flattened out (*cf.* Figure 5.2) to such an extent that halving the enzyme content has little effect on flux, which is equivalent to the flux control coefficient being much less than 1 and close to zero. Since it is so common for mutations in enzymes to be recessive, the implication is that most enzymes have small flux control coefficients. Furthermore, Kacser & Burns[121] also pointed out that the phenomenon of dominance has a simple explanation in terms of the systems behaviour of biochemical pathways. Previously, dominance had been difficult to explain, and mechanisms such as the one Fisher proposed assumed that it had been selected during the evolution of the control mechanisms of the pathways. Recent experiments on artificial diploids created from a normally haploid organism, the alga *Chlamydomonas reinhardtii*, showed that these new diploids also exhibited dominance of the wild–type genes over mutants in 90% of cases.[177] Since the recessive nature of mutants in the diploid could not have been subject to evolution in this haploid organism, the experiments are consistent with the interpretation devised by Kacser & Burns, but not with the earlier idea that dominance was an evolved property.

In the following subsection on the summation theorem, we shall see that there are some further restrictions on the values that the flux control coefficients can have.

If the value of a flux control coefficient is known, approximate predictions can be made about how the metabolic flux will change if the amount of enzyme is changed. Such changes might be brought about by changes in genetic expression or by covalent modification of inactive enzyme (Chapter 7.4, p. 225). (Other methods of changing enzyme activity involve changing the catalytic activity whilst the amount of enzyme is unchanged; the flux control coefficient is also involved in predicting the response to these perturbations, as will be explained in the section on the response coefficient, p. 121.) If the enzyme concentration changes from $E_{xase,1}$ to $E_{xase,2}$, by an amount small enough for $C_{xase}^{J_{ydh}}$ to be effectively constant, Eqn. (5.2) can be integrated to give:

$$\Delta \ln J_{ydh} = C_{xase}^{J_{ydh}} \Delta \ln E_{xase} \qquad (5.4)$$

where $\Delta \ln E_{xase} = \ln E_{xase,2} - \ln E_{xase,1}$. That is, the change in the logarithm of the flux is equal to the flux control coefficient times the change in the logarithm of the amount of enzyme. As pointed out by Higgins,[104] this corresponds to the power law form:

$$J = aE^C \qquad (5.5)$$

where, for simplicity, subscripts and superscripts have been omitted, so that $J = J_{ydh}$, $E = E_{xase}$, $C = C_{xase}^{J_{ydh}}$, and where a is a constant that takes the value needed to make the equation exactly true at the enzyme and flux values for which the control coefficient was measured. Eqns. (5.4) and (5.5) both describe

the tangent in Figure 5.1c), so any prediction made with the flux control coefficient of the metabolic flux at other enzyme concentrations becomes less and less
accurate the further away the new enzyme content is from the one at which the
tangent was measured. What is less obvious is that the tangent in Figure 5.1(c)
is generally a curve on the linear scales of Figure 5.1(b), that lies between the
tangent shown on that graph and the true curve. Thus Eqns. (5.4) and (5.5) are
always a better approximation to the flux–enzyme relationship than the following linear equation [based on Eqn. (5.1)], which has often been advocated:

$$\frac{\Delta J_{ydh}}{J_{ydh}} = C_{xase}^{J_{ydh}} \frac{\Delta E_{xase}}{E_{xase}} \tag{5.6}$$

Although the equations above have limited predictive power for large changes
in enzyme content, in 1993 Rankin Small & Henrik Kacser[233] devised a surprisingly simple but improved predictor. Strictly, their result only applies in cases
where the flux–enzyme relationship, such as Figure 5.1(b), is rectangular hyperbolic (as seen in Michaelis–Menten enzyme kinetics; Chapter 3, p. 47). That is to
say, the flux and enzyme amount have to be related by an equation of the form:

$$J_{ydh} = \frac{AE_{xase}}{B + E_{xase}}$$

where A and B are constants; if this is the case, a plot of $1/J_{ydh}$ versus $1/E_{xase}$
will be linear. As it happens, a number of experimentally determined results
appear to obey this relationship, although there can be no guarantee that this
will always be true. Nevertheless, when it is true in a linear metabolic pathway, measurement of the two values of the flux J_{ydh}, J_1 and J_2, at two widely
separated levels of the enzyme E_{xase}, E_1 and E_2, allows calculation of the flux
control coefficient at enzyme level E_1 as:

$$C_E^J = \frac{(J_2 - J_1)E_2}{(E_2 - E_1)J_2} \tag{5.7}$$

This differs from the small change approximation to the flux control coefficient
given earlier as Eqn. (5.6) in that the weighting factor is E_2/J_2, and not E_1/J_1.
Oddly, if E_1/J_1 is used as the weighting factor, the resulting control coefficient
is that at enzyme level E_2! This equation had also been derived by Mark Stitt
in experiments on the control of photosynthesis which are described later in
this book.

Rankin Small and Henrik Kacser also noticed that, with these equations,
the flux control coefficient measured at one point allows prediction of the flux
at a markedly different enzyme concentration with good accuracy. Suppose it
is possible to increase the enzyme amount r times; the pathway flux will be
higher by a factor f given by the equation:

$$f = \frac{1}{1 - \frac{r-1}{r}C_{xase}^{J_{ydh}}} \tag{5.8}$$

This function is plotted in Figure 5.3. What this shows is that by changing
the amount of a single enzyme, the effects on the pathway flux can be quite
limited, unless the flux control coefficient is greater than 0.5 to start with. The
maximum change in flux that can be obtained by a very considerable increase
in enzyme, when $r \gg 1$ (so that $r \approx r - 1$), is:

$$f = \frac{1}{1 - C_{xase}^{J_{ydh}}} \tag{5.9}$$

Thus if $C_{xase}^{J_{ydh}} = 0.5$, the maximum flux that can be obtained is a factor of 2.0
times greater. Only if $C_{xase}^{J_{ydh}}$ is near to 1.0 are very large changes in flux possible,
but as mentioned previously, few measurements have been made of enzymes
with such large values for their flux control coefficients. This result is very
disappointing since it implies that biotechnologists who might have hoped to
increase significantly the flux through a chosen metabolic pathway by engineering an increase in a single target enzyme will rarely find it possible. This limitation only applies, however, to increasing the metabolic flux; the same restriction
does not apply for a decrease in flux caused by a reduction in the amount of
active enzyme (*i.e.* $r < 1$), since this can always lead to a substantial drop in flux.

Equation (5.8) and Figure 5.3 also have important consequences for how
cells can control metabolic rate, and these will be discussed later (Chapter 8.1).

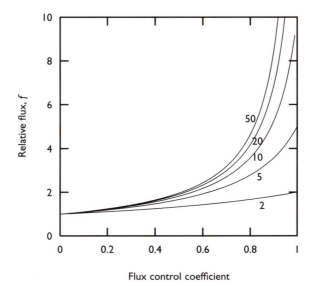

Figure 5.3   The relative change of flux for large changes in enzyme amount
The increases in flux predicted by Eqn. (5.8) against the value of the flux control coefficient. The degree
of amplification, *r*, of the enzyme amount is shown on each curve. The graph can be used in reverse
to give a quick estimate of the control coefficient if the relative change in flux has been measured for a
known change in enzyme amount.

5.2.3   The summation theorem

When Kacser & Burns first developed Metabolic Control Analysis,[119] they found that, if all the enzymes that can affect a particular metabolic flux in a cell or a metabolic system are taken and the values of their control coefficients on that flux added up, the sum comes to 1. Thus if we number all the enzymes involved from 1 to n, then:

$$C_1^J + C_2^J \ldots + C_n^J = 1 \qquad (5.10)$$

This relationship is known as the *summation theorem* for flux control coefficients, and in mathematical notation is expressed as:

$$\boxed{\sum_{i=1}^{n} C_i^J = 1} \qquad (5.11)$$

where $\sum_{i=1}^{n}$ is the mathematical symbol for summing the n items indicated by the following term. There are several ways of proving this theorem; an example is given in Appendix 1, *More about flux control coefficients*, p. 128.

The summation theorem shows that the enzymes of the pathway can share the control of flux. In a linear pathway consisting of enzymes with normal kinetics (*i.e.* where substrates stimulate and products inhibit the reaction rate), all the flux control coefficients must be zero or positive, so the maximum value any enzyme's coefficient could have is 1, when all the other enzymes would necessarily have flux control coefficients of zero. In this case, this one enzyme could be said to be 'rate–limiting', since a flux control coefficient of 1 corresponds to a proportional relationship between the activity of an enzyme and the pathway flux. The summation theorem shows that this is not a necessary feature of the pathway, as it is also possible for some or all of the enzymes to have values greater than zero but less than 1. Note that the definition states that the sum is for the flux control coefficients of *all* the enzymes in the metabolic system; for example, this potentially implies the whole cell. In practice, we would expect a pathway flux to be influenced mainly by enzymes in that pathway, and perhaps by a few closely connected pathways, and that distantly connected enzymes would have little influence at all. In other words, the flux control coefficients of hundreds, even thousands, of enzymes in a cell on our chosen flux will be zero, so even though the control of flux is shared, it is not shared evenly.

However, another consequence of the highly branched and interconnected nature of metabolism is that, for any particular pathway, there will be other pathways that could draw material or energy away from it causing its flux to decrease, so that enzymes in these pathways could have negative flux control coefficients on the flux of interest. Although this does not invalidate the summation theorem, nor the concept that control of flux is shared, it does mean that it is not possible to state definitively that the values of individual flux control

coefficients can never exceed 1. This is because if there are negative flux control coefficients, one or more flux control coefficients could have values greater
than 1. On the other hand, although negative flux control coefficients have
been measured experimentally, there are virtually no examples of an enzyme
with a flux control coefficient exceeding 1. One exception occurs in mitochondrial oxidative phosphorylation at high respiration rates, and will be described
later (see Chapter 6, p. 180).

The summation theorem also shows that the flux control coefficient of an
enzyme is a system property. This can be seen when a flux control coefficient
varies with the amount of enzyme, as shown previously in Figure 5.2. Since
the flux control coefficient decreases with an increase in the amount of the
enzyme, the summation theorem requires that the flux control coefficients of
some other enzymes must be increasing at the same time to maintain the sum
of all flux control coefficients constant at one. In addition, this must work the
other way round: the flux control coefficient of the enzyme we are considering
will be altered if the activity of some other enzyme is changed sufficiently to
affect its own flux control coefficient. This shows that an enzyme's flux control coefficient is not an intrinsic property of the enzyme itself; it is a property
of the whole system. Therefore, the value of a flux control coefficient cannot
be determined by considering the properties of the enzyme in isolation; the
characteristics and amounts of the other enzymes in the metabolic system will
affect the result. Furthermore, since the values of the flux control coefficients
can redistribute between enzymes according to circumstances, any particular
measured values apply only to the metabolic state in which they were determined. Examples showing the change in the pattern of control in different
metabolic states will be presented in the next chapter (e.g. Figure 6.15, p. 159).

5.3   Elasticities

Although the last section has demonstrated the important conclusion that the
flux control coefficient of an enzyme is a system property that cannot be related
solely to the enzyme's properties in isolation, there must of course be links
between the enzyme's kinetic properties and its potential for flux control. This
can be illustrated by considering what happens in a pathway if an enzyme
activity is changed. For example, in the pathway:

$$X_0 \quad \overset{xase}{\longrightarrow} \quad Y \quad \overset{ydh}{\longrightarrow} \quad Z \quad \overset{zase}{\longrightarrow} \quad X_1 \qquad \text{(Scheme 5.1)}$$

suppose that an extra amount of ydh is added, to increase the rate of the second
step. What is the effect on the pathway? The increased amount of ydh tends
to lower the concentration of Y.

The lower Y will:

- increase the rate of *xase* because of reduced product inhibition;

- decrease the rate of *ydh* because of lower substrate concentration.

The increased amount of *ydh* also tends to raise the concentration of Z. The increased Z will:

- decrease the rate of *ydh* because of increased product inhibition;

- increase the rate of *zase* because of higher substrate concentration.

In conclusion:

- the effects of the increased amount of *ydh* involve the relative sizes of the responses of the enzymes to the pathway metabolites;

- the effects on the metabolites could tend to counteract the change in the amount of enzyme;

- the effects on the metabolites could tend to change the rates of neighbouring enzymes to match the change in *ydh*.

This explanation has shown that the flux control coefficient of an enzyme is likely to be linked to its kinetic responses to changed metabolite concentrations, as well as its ability to influence the concentrations of metabolites in the pathway, a linkage that was shown first by Heinrich & Rapoport.[99] To be more specific about how the kinetics of enzymes relate to the flux control coefficients, we need a means of describing their kinetic responses in a manner that is compatible with the control coefficients. This measure is provided by the *elasticity coefficient*.

5.3.1 Definition and examples

Unlike control coefficients, *elasticities* are properties of individual enzymes and not of the metabolic system, even though we shall see that they are defined in a very similar way. The elasticity of an enzyme to a metabolite is related to the slope of the curve of the enzyme's rate plotted against metabolite concentration, taken at the metabolite concentrations found in the pathway in the metabolic state of interest. Again, because the value of this slope would depend upon the units of measurement, it is scaled to give a dimensionless measure (Figure 5.4a). It can be obtained directly as the slope of the logarithm of the rate plotted against the logarithm of the metabolite concentration (Figure 5.4b).

The mathematical form of the definition is just like that of the flux control coefficients given in Eqn. (5.2). For example, the elasticity coefficient for the effect of metabolite S on the velocity v of enzyme *xase* is the fractional change in rate of the isolated enzyme for a fractional change in substrate S, with all other

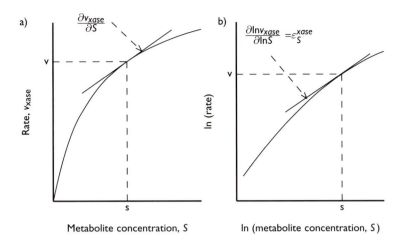

Figure 5.4 The elasticity coefficient
(a) Typical variation of the rate of enzyme $xase$, v_{xase}, with the concentration of metabolite S. The elasticity coefficient, ε_S^{xase}, at s,v is the slope of the tangent to the curve $\partial v_{xase}/\partial S$ times the scaling factor s/v. (b) On a double-logarithmic plot of the same curve, the elasticity coefficient is the slope of the tangent to the curve.

effectors of the enzyme held constant at the values they have in the metabolic pathway:

$$
\begin{aligned}
\varepsilon_S^{xase} &= \frac{\partial v_{xase}}{\partial S} \cdot \frac{S}{v_{xase}} \\
&= \frac{\partial \ln|v_{xase}|}{\partial \ln S}
\end{aligned}
\tag{5.12}
$$

(The term $\ln|v_{xase}|$ in this equation means that the logarithm of the absolute value of v_{xase} is used. That is, if v_{xase} is negative, as will be seen in Figure 5.8, its positive value is used because it is not possible to take the logarithm of a negative number.) Elasticities have positive values for metabolites that stimulate the rate of a reaction (substrates, activators) and negative values for those, like products and inhibitors, that slow the reaction. Obviously, there must be some link to the results from enzyme kinetics described in Chapter 3. In fact, the typical range of values that elasticities have can be illustrated by examining some common equations from enzyme kinetics.

For example, suppose we want the elasticity with respect to substrate of an enzyme that obeys the Michaelis–Menten equation [Eqn. (3.1)]:

$$
v = \frac{SV}{S + K_{\mathrm{m}}}
$$

If the substrate concentration at which the elasticity is required is 0.5 mM, with the $K_{\mathrm{m}} = 0.75$ mM and $V = 100\ \mu\mathrm{mol} \cdot \mathrm{min}^{-1}$, we can calculate the rate at

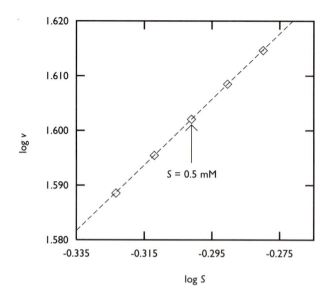

Figure 5.5 Graphical estimation of an elasticity from an enzyme rate law
The rate of reaction has been calculated for the Michaelis–Menten equation with K_m = 0.75 mM and
V = 100 μmol·min^{-1} for substrate concentrations from 95% to 105% of the required value of 0.5 mM. The
elasticity is 0.60, the slope of the tangent at S = 0.5 mM. The curve of rate against substrate concentration
has not been drawn because the curvature is so slight it barely separates from the tangent.

95%, 97.5%, 100%, 102.5% and 105% of the substrate concentration. When
the logarithms of these rate values are plotted against the logs of the substrate
concentrations, the elasticity is the slope of the graph at 100% of S = 0.5 mM
(Figure 5.5). If you know the properties of logarithms, you may be able to
spot that the limiting rate, V, moves the curve up and down the y-axis but
does not change its slope. (This is because V is a constant multiplying factor
in the calculation for v, and thus becomes a constant additive term in log v.)
Thus it does not matter what value of V is used for the calculation; an arbitrary
value of 1 suffices. Apart from the arithmetic convenience, this helps with the
biochemistry because it is not necessary to know the amount or activity of an
enzyme in a cell to know its elasticity. Elasticity values can also be obtained
from a rate equation by use of differential calculus; if you are familiar with
this, you will find more details, including the result for the Michaelis–Menten
equation, in Appendix 3 *More about elasticities* (p. 131).

Examples of the elasticity values obtained for some simple enzyme mechanisms are shown in the next few figures. Figure 5.6 shows how the substrate
elasticity of an irreversible Michaelis–Menten enzyme varies with substrate concentration; its value goes from 1 at substrate concentrations much below K_m to
0 as the enzyme approaches its maximal velocity. Note that the values have been
calculated for the presence of a fixed concentration of product, which binds at
the active site even if there is no appreciable reverse reaction. This inhibitory

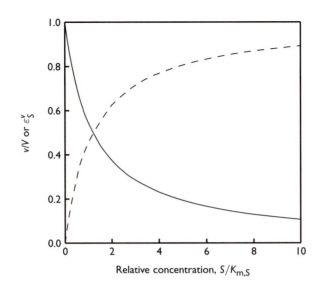

Figure 5.6 Elasticity of an irreversible enzyme with respect to its substrate at various substrate concentrations

The enzyme is an irreversible single–substrate enzyme operating in the presence of its product, according to the equation $v = V(S/K_{m,S})/(1 + S/K_{m,S} + P/K_{m,P})$, i.e. Eqn. (3.4) with $K_{eq} = \infty$ and $P/K_{m,P} = 0.2$. ———, ε_S^v. — — — — , fractional velocity, v/V.

effect of a product, even with an irreversible enzyme, means that the enzyme has an elasticity with respect to the product, as illustrated in Figure 5.7. The value is negative, going as low as -1 when the enzyme is strongly inhibited, because increasing the product concentration reduces the rate.

For enzyme reactions that are near to equilibrium, the elasticities with respect to substrate and product are mostly determined by the degree of displacement of the reaction from equilibrium rather than by the kinetic details of the reaction, and this can lead to much larger elasticity values than we have seen so far (as was first pointed out by Kacser and Burns,[119] and later developed in more detail by Bert Groen and his colleagues[90,273]). For example, consider the reversible Michaelis–Menten equation for the conversion of S to P, [Eqn. (3.4)] where v is the net rate (positive for formation of P). Algebraic calculation of the elasticity with respect to substrate by differentiation and scaling of this equation gives:

$$
\begin{aligned}
\varepsilon_S^v &= \frac{1}{1-\rho} - \frac{S/K_{m,S}}{1 + S/K_{m,S} + P/K_{m,P}} \\
&= \frac{1}{1-\rho} - \frac{v_f}{V_f}
\end{aligned}
\tag{5.13}
$$

where ρ is the disequilibrium ratio [Eqn. (1.6)] and v_f the total forward rate. The first term on the right-hand side depends on the degree of displacement from equilibrium, going from 1 in the absence of product to infinity at equilib-

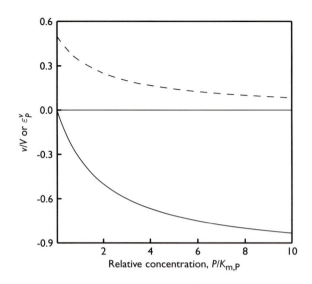

Figure 5.7 Elasticity of an irreversible enzyme with respect to its product at various product concentrations
The enzyme is an irreversible single-substrate enzyme operating in the presence of its product, according to the equation $v = V(S/K_{m,S})/(1 + S/K_{m,S} + P/K_{m,P})$, i.e. Eqn. (3.4) with $K_{eq} = \infty$ and $S/K_{m,S} = 1$. ——— , ε_P^v. – – – – – , fractional velocity, v/V.

rium, and the second term represents the fractional saturation of the enzyme with S, going from 0 in the absence of S to a maximum value of 1, giving the overall result illustrated in Figure 5.8. (Note that $S \gg K_{m,S}$ is not, in this case, a sufficient condition for the saturation term to reach 1, because the value of P counts, particularly if $P \gg K_{m,P}$; 'saturated' can be a vague concept with a near–equilibrium reaction.) In many practical cases, the elasticity of a near–equilibrium reaction will be given with sufficient accuracy by the term $1/(1-\rho)$, which generates very large values as ρ approaches 1. The product elasticity is given similarly by:

$$\varepsilon_P^v = \frac{-\rho}{1-\rho} - \frac{P/K_{m,P}}{1 + S/K_{m,S} + P/K_{m,P}}$$

$$= \frac{-\rho}{1-\rho} - \frac{v_r}{V_r} \tag{5.14}$$

Where the saturation terms are negligible, it follows that the two elasticities are related as:

$$\varepsilon_S^v + \varepsilon_P^v = 1 \tag{5.15}$$

Groen and colleagues[90] also showed that similar results can be obtained with multisubstrate rate equations having numerators of similar form to that of Eqn. (3.4).

Large elasticity values can also be obtained with allosteric enzymes, even when (as is often the case) their reactions are not close to equilibrium. With an

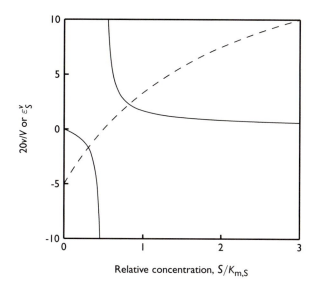

Figure 5.8 Elasticity of a reversible Michaelis–Menten enzyme with respect to its substrate at various substrate concentrations

The enzyme is a reversible single–substrate enzyme operating in the presence of its product, according to Eqn. (3.4) with $K_{m,S} = 1$; $P = 5$; $K_{m,P} = 5$; $K_{eq} = 10$. The elasticity is undefined at equilibrium ($S = 0.5$). ——, ε_S^v. – – – – – , $20 \times$ fractional velocity, v/V.

allosteric enzyme that has cooperative kinetics with respect to a substrate, the elasticity can be greater than 1, although it must be less than the Hill coefficient [see Eqn. (3.11)]. In fact, Herbert Sauro showed when he was a research student with me that, if the enzyme is an irreversible enzyme whose rate of reaction is proportional to its fractional saturation, $\overline{Y}$, with the substrate S, then:

$$\varepsilon_S^v = (1 - \overline{Y})h \tag{5.16}$$

In other words, the elasticity is similar to the Hill coefficient at low degrees of fractional saturation, when $\overline{Y}$ is near zero, but becomes progressively smaller as the degree of saturation increases. Since the Hill coefficient for an enzyme showing positive cooperativity is 1 at low saturation, becomes perhaps as high as 2–3 at mid–saturation, and then decreases to 1 again at high saturation, the elasticity in the same range will start at 1, perhaps rise above 1 and then fall away to zero (Figure 5.9). Of course, if the Hill coefficient is greater than 1, the enzyme will have a higher elasticity than it would if it were non–cooperative at an equivalent degree of saturation. (For an irreversible Michaelis–Menten enzyme, $h = 1$, and the equation above gives the same result for the elasticity as Figure 5.6 and Eqn. (5.34) in Appendix 3.)

These examples have shown how elasticity values can be obtained from equations for enzyme kinetics. However, this can only be done for an enzyme in a cell if:

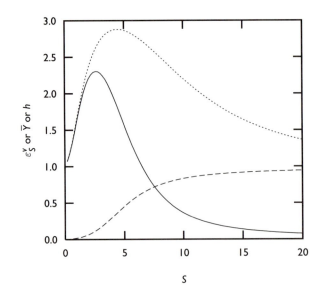

Figure 5.9 The substrate elasticity of an allosteric enzyme
The enzyme obeys the Monod, Wyman & Changeux model, Eqn. (3.12), with $n = 4$, $L = 1000$, $c = 0.01$ and $K_T = 1$ so that $S = \alpha$. ———, ε_S^v; – – – – – , fractional saturation, $\bar{Y}$; $\cdots$, the Hill coefficient, h.

- a complete kinetic equation is available that incorporates *all* the reactants and effectors that occur in the cell and affect the enzyme;

- the intracellular concentrations of all these metabolites in the compartment where the enzyme occurs are known;

- all the kinetic parameters are known under intracellular conditions.

This is quite a demanding set of requirements, often difficult to satisfy because of the patchy nature of the published results on enzymes. For instance, any particular enzyme is likely only to have been studied in a few organisms, and not necessarily in the one under study. Also, enzyme kinetics experiments often do not report the right type of results. This is partly for reasons considered in more detail in Appendix 3 *More about elasticities* (p. 131). There are also undiscovered reasons, examples of which have been given previously (Chapter 4.4, p. 91). As an alternative to determination from kinetics, there are methods for direct determination of elasticities *in vivo* (see Chapter 6.3, p. 165).

5.3.2 Use and interpretation

The function of elasticities in Metabolic Control Analysis is as a quantitative replacement for the vague concepts of responsiveness of an enzyme to a metabolite that are used in qualitative explanations of metabolic regulation, such as:

> The substrate S controls the rate of reaction because its concentration in the cell is well below the K_m of the enzyme for S ...

or

> The rate of the enzyme will be relatively unresponsive to variations
> in the concentration of S because it is well above the K_m ...

The values of elasticities are much more useful than such statements because
they are determined with the concentrations of other substrates, products and
effectors at their levels in the cell in the metabolic state being analysed. In spite
of biochemists' attachment to simple Michaelis–Menten kinetics, the rectangular hyperbola of the single–substrate enzyme in the absence of products is a
poor guide to the behaviour of enzymes *in vivo*, where the majority have more
than one substrate, are in the presence of appreciable concentrations of products, and may be catalysing a significant flux in both directions. An elasticity,
however, reflects the results of all these influences, and so it would be a useful
advance if biochemists agreed to use it as an indication of the sensitivity of an
enzyme to a metabolite, even in circumstances where they had no intention of
going any further into Metabolic Control Analysis.

5.3.3   The connectivity theorem

Now that we have defined how metabolites affect the activity of enzymes, we
can return to the question of how the flux control coefficients of enzymes can
be related to the kinetic properties of the enzymes. This link is provided by
the *connectivity theorem*[119] derived by Kacser & Burns in 1973. Suppose we
choose one pathway metabolite S and find all the enzymes in our metabolic
system whose rates respond to it; further suppose that we find there are three
and let us label these enzymes i, j and k. The connectivity theorem states
that, for each of these enzymes, if we form a term by taking its flux control
coefficient on a particular flux J and multiplying by its elasticity with respect
to S, then the sum of the terms is zero, *i.e.* :

$$C_i^J \varepsilon_S^i + C_j^J \varepsilon_S^j + C_k^J \varepsilon_S^k = 0 \qquad (5.17)$$

The mathematical statement of this theorem is:

$$\boxed{\sum_{i=1}^{n} C_i^J \varepsilon_S^i = 0} \qquad (5.18)$$

This is equivalent to the previous equation, even though the sum is now formed
of all the n enzymes in our system; this is because the enzymes that are not
affected by S will have elasticities of zero and will therefore not contribute to
the sum; perhaps only the enzyme that produces the metabolite and the one that
consumes it will have non–zero elasticities. To see how this works in practice,
consider a short section of glycolysis:

$$\ldots \xrightarrow{\text{enolase}} \text{PEP} \xrightarrow{\text{pyruvate kinase}} \ldots \qquad \text{(Scheme 5.2)}$$

Box 5.2 More complicated connectivity relationships

There is a complication in the connectivity theorem when the metabolite is one of a pair such as NAD^+ and NADH, whose ratio can vary even though the total of NAD units in the cell is effectively constant.[69] A similar problem can arise with larger 'moiety–conserved' groups, such as ATP, ADP and AMP. In essence, the right-hand side of Eqn. (5.18) for a single one of these metabolites is no longer zero, but the equations can be combined in pairs to give a zero result, with the side effect that the number of connectivity equations is reduced by one.[69] This technical complication does not invalidate the general properties and uses of the connectivity theorem.

The specific connectivity theorem involving phosphoenolpyruvate (PEP) is obtained by writing a term for every enzyme that has a non–zero elasticity for PEP; in this case, we assume this involves only enolase (denoted *eno*) and pyruvate kinase (*pk*), giving:

$$C^J_{eno}\varepsilon^{eno}_{PEP} + C^J_{pk}\varepsilon^{pk}_{PEP} = 0 \tag{5.19}$$

or

$$\frac{C^J_{eno}}{C^J_{pk}} = -\frac{\varepsilon^{pk}_{PEP}}{\varepsilon^{eno}_{PEP}} \tag{5.20}$$

Without knowing anything more about the rest of the pathway, we cannot tell the magnitude of either flux control coefficient, but we can see that the relative values of two successive flux control coefficients depend on the elasticity representing the product inhibition (*i.e.* PEP on enolase) and the substrate activation (*i.e.* PEP on pyruvate kinase) by the intermediate metabolite. For example, in working rat heart, supplied with glucose but no insulin, these two elasticities have been estimated as about -0.69 and 0.86, implying that C^J_{eno} is ≈ 1.25 times C^J_{pk}. This ratio form of the connectivity theorem [Eqn. (5.20)] shows the tendency of large elasticities (e.g. for enzymes catalysing reactions near equilibrium) to be associated with small flux control coefficients, and *vice versa*.

Since we can choose any of the pathway metabolites to form a connectivity equation, there are as many of them as there are variable metabolites in the pathway. Do we gain any advantage from having all these different equations involving control coefficients? The answer is 'yes' because the summation theorem and the set of connectivity theorems for all the metabolites of a linear pathway provide exactly the number of simultaneous equations needed to solve for the flux control coefficients of all the enzymes in terms of the elasticities. For example, we can consider a two–enzyme pathway with one pathway intermediate, Y:

$$X_0 \xrightarrow{\ xase\ } Y \xrightarrow{\ ydh\ } X_1 \tag{Scheme 5.3}$$

This pathway has a summation theorem:

$$C_{xase}^{J} + C_{ydh}^{J} = 1$$

and a connectivity theorem:

$$C_{xase}^{J}\varepsilon_{Y}^{xase} + C_{ydh}^{J}\varepsilon_{Y}^{ydh} = 0$$

If the elasticities are known, these equations form a pair of simultaneous equations in the two unknown flux control coefficients. In this case, the exact solutions are:

$$C_{xase}^{J} = \frac{\varepsilon_{Y}^{ydh}}{\varepsilon_{Y}^{ydh} - \varepsilon_{Y}^{xase}}$$

$$C_{ydh}^{J} = \frac{-\varepsilon_{Y}^{xase}}{\varepsilon_{Y}^{ydh} - \varepsilon_{Y}^{xase}}$$

Thus we have shown that although the flux control coefficients are system properties of the pathway, they are nevertheless explicable in terms of the kinetic properties of the constituent enzymes.

This is not a special result for a simple pathway; for a three–enzyme linear pathway there will be two intermediates, so the one summation theorem and two connectivity theorems will give the three equations needed to express the three flux control coefficients in terms of the elasticities. Whatever the length of a linear pathway, the procedure will work, though this is not the case for branched pathways or pathways containing certain types of cycle (such as substrate cycles). For these pathways, my student Herbert Sauro and I[69] proposed additional equations relating the flux control coefficients and the relative fluxes through different parts of the system. These equations, known as the branch–point and substrate cycle theorems, make the flux control coefficients expressible in terms of the elasticities and the flux distribution in the system. Since then, detailed mathematical analysis by other researchers (in particular Christine Reder in Bordeaux) has shown that it is always possible to write a soluble set of equations for any pathway, provided that the pathway can reach a proper steady state. The branch–point equations will not be described any further for the moment, but their use will be illustrated later in an experimental study of oxidative phosphorylation in Chapter 6.3.3.1, p. 180.

5.4   Response coefficients

There are many control mechanisms that operate on metabolic pathways, and some of these operate on the catalytically active amount of an enzyme, others do not. In the former category are mechanisms for the induction and repression of enzyme synthesis in response to hormonal and environmental stimuli, the activation or inactivation of existing enzyme protein by covalent modification reactions, and probably targeted protein degradation. In the latter category are mechanisms that change the kinetic characteristics of the enzymes, such as allosteric effectors changing the cooperativity or affinity of an enzyme for its substrate, or physiological control mechanisms that alter the concentration of the source metabolite for a pathway, or of an effector that is external to the pathway. Some biochemists have therefore been concerned that flux control coefficients seem only to relate to the first group of control mechanisms and that they are not obviously relevant to describing the second, very important, group. Later (Chapter 8.1) we will consider the possibility that the functions of this second group are not primarily flux control, in spite of what is usually claimed. For the moment, let us assume that the conventional view of the second group is correct. In this case, the argument for maintaining that flux control coefficients are still significant in spite of the criticism of their relevance has two stages: firstly, it is accepted that it is useful to define control coefficients for the response of metabolic fluxes or concentrations to factors (parameters) other than enzyme concentration, but secondly it is shown that the control coefficients we have already considered always have an influence on these other types of coefficient.

Let us consider the first stage. Why not define a coefficient for the action of some parameter P other than enzyme concentration on a metabolic flux? There is no problem at all, provided that the *parameter* is just that: a factor that influences the behaviour of the system, but that can be held constant after it has been altered while the system reaches a new steady state. On this basis, a metabolite that is synthesized and degraded by the system is not a parameter, but a *variable*, because if some alteration is made to its concentration, this alteration will fade away as the system returns to its original steady state. The strength of the effect of the parameter P on, say, the flux J_{ydh} is defined in the same way as the control coefficient, except that it is generally referred to as a response coefficient, $R_P^{J_{ydh}}$, as originally named by Kacser and Burns:[119]

$$R_P^{J_{ydh}} = \frac{\partial J_{ydh}}{\partial P} \cdot \frac{P}{J_{ydh}}$$ (5.21)

This equation for the response coefficient can also be re-expressed in the same ways as those for the flux control coefficients [Eqns. (5.3–5.5)] and has the same graphical interpretation as shown in Figure 5.1.

For the second stage of the argument, Kacser & Burns pointed out that, if an external, constant metabolite P acts on the flux J_{ydh} through being an effector of the pathway enzyme *xase*, the response coefficient for the effect of P is composed of the flux control coefficient with respect to *xase* and the elasticity of *xase* with respect to P:

$$R_P^{J_{ydh}} = C_{xase}^{J_{ydh}} \varepsilon_P^{xase}$$ (5.22)

This equation has been proved in a number of ways but, in essence, it is a

> **Box 5.3 Other definitions**
> An equivalent to the response coefficient was defined by Crabtree and Newsholme[55] (as a *net sensitivity*) and by Michael Savageau[214] (as a *logarithmic sensitivity*). The difference of emphasis between these latter authors and the adherents of Metabolic Control Analysis comes in the second step in the argument, originally made by Kacser & Burns[119] and described in the main text.

mathematical necessity given the definitions of the terms. Its importance is that it shows that *the response of a pathway to an effector depends on two factors*:

- the sensitivity of the pathway to the activity of the enzyme that is the target for the effector (given by the enzyme's flux control coefficient);

- the strength of the effect of P on that enzyme (given by its elasticity).

It is necessary for both components to be non–zero for P to be able to affect the pathway. Further, if there were a number of effectors that could act on a pathway at a particular enzyme, their response coefficients would all contain the same flux control coefficient as a component term. Thus the reason that the flux control coefficient is valuable is that it can indicate whether an enzyme has the potential to be a site at which a pathway is controlled (*i.e.* its *regulatory capacity*[106]) because the flux control coefficient is defined without reference to the existence of any particular mechanism by which the activity can be controlled. An effector cannot act on a pathway by changing the activity of an enzyme with a near–zero flux control coefficient. (The exception to this statement is when a very large increase occurs in an inhibitor of a pathway; even if the inhibited enzyme had a flux control coefficient near zero originally, it will increase as the inhibition builds up, so the response coefficient to the inhibitor may start small, but will eventually rise. Inhibitor titrations are considered in more detail in Chapter 6.1.4, p. 151.)

Another useful property of Eqn. (5.22) is that it is true regardless of the mechanism by which the effector P acts on the enzyme *xase*. For example, *P* might actually be a K–system allosteric inhibitor that exerts its effect by raising the $S_{0.5}$ of *xase* for its substrate (see Chapter 3.5, p. 70). The response coefficient equation still applies in this case because the elasticity of *xase* with respect to P takes into account that the change in activity of the enzyme occurs at constant concentration of its substrate. On the other hand, if P did directly affect the limiting rate of the enzyme, the equation would be equally applicable; it would just be that the elasticity of the enzyme with respect to P would be implemented by a different mechanism. If it seems surprising that Metabolic Control Analysis can characterize the response of metabolism to an effector without its being important how the effect is implemented at the molecular level,

---

Box 5.4 Response to a kinetic parameter
There is no particular restriction on the factors for which a response coefficient can be defined. For example, suppose we wanted to know how a metabolic pathway would respond to a change in one of the kinetic parameters of enzyme *xase*, even though we had not yet found a means of making this change. The response coefficient is once again the flux control coefficient times the elasticity of the enzyme with respect to the kinetic parameter. Elasticities can be defined with respect to a kinetic parameter in exactly the same way as to a metabolite concentration[274] and can be calculated from the enzyme rate law. In many cases, if the kinetic parameter K is a K_m or K_i value for a substrate, product or effector molecule S, then ε_K^{xase} will equal $-\varepsilon_S^{xase}$. In fact, in Appendix 1 (Section 5.7), it is shown that the combination of the response coefficient to a kinetic parameter and the elasticity to that same parameter leads to a more general definition of the flux control coefficient, compared with the definition given earlier solely in terms of enzyme concentration [Eqn. (5.2)].

---

remember that Control Analysis is intended to be a systems theory of metabolic control that aims to explain the general aspects of metabolic behaviour without being dependent on the full details of molecular mechanism.

What happens if an effector P acts on more than one enzyme in a metabolic pathway? In this case, the total response will be the sum of the individual responses from each enzyme affected.[106] (This is only true for very small changes in P, because the response coefficient, like the other coefficients, is defined as a first order approximation, true for very small changes. For a large change in P, the total effect will not be the sum of the effects on each enzyme because of the non–linear nature of the kinetics of metabolic systems.) As with the connectivity relationship [Eqn. (5.18)], we can define the overall, multisite response obtained from the n enzymes of the system as:

$$R_P^J = \sum_{i=1}^{n} C_i^J \varepsilon_P^i \qquad (5.23)$$

Contributions to the sum only come from the enzymes for which ε_P^i is not zero. This equation for the multisite response coefficient does show the potential value of control mechanisms in which an effector acts on more than one site. In the case where the effector acts only on one enzyme, then it would be rare for that enzyme to have a flux control coefficient as large as 1; the elasticity of the effector on the enzyme might be around 1, so, overall, the response coefficient is most likely to be less than 1, *i.e.* there will be less than a 1% change in flux for a 1% change in the effector concentration. If the effector acts on several of the enzymes of the pathway that together account for most of the flux control (*i.e.* their flux control coefficients add up nearly to 1), and each of the elasticities is near 1, then the response coefficient can be close to 1. (If the effector acts cooperatively on allosteric enzymes, then the elasticity terms could be greater than 1 in both cases considered.) Furthermore, there is likely to be a further, hidden advantage in the multisite response mode for the activation of a metabolic pathway. Activating a metabolic pathway via an effect on a single enzyme usually proves to be rapidly self–limiting, since even if the enzyme has a relatively large flux control coefficient to start with, it decreases, with control transferring to other enzymes, as the target enzyme is activated. This was illustrated previously in connection with large changes in enzyme amount in Figure 5.3. At the other extreme, if an effector acted equally on every enzyme in a pathway, the flux would continue to increase even for large stimulations of activity without any changes in intermediate metabolite concentrations or redistribution of control. (See the derivation of the summation theorem in Appendix 1, p. 129, for a justification of this claim, and Chapter 8.1, p. 257, for further consideration of its implications for metabolic control.) An effector acting on several enzymes, each with a moderate flux control coefficient spaced along the pathway could be an adequate approximation to this extreme case. Pure examples of this effect are difficult to give because there are usually other control mechanisms that come into play as well. However, to the extent that the nucleotide AMP can be considered an *external* effector of glycogen catabolism in muscle, it activates phosphorylase *b* and phosphofructokinase. In the longer of the synthetic pathways for amino acids, there are cases where the product amino acid (again, if it is appropriate to regard this as an external metabolite) inhibits at more than one point along the sequence (see Chapter 7.2.3, p. 206).

This equation for the multisite response coefficient, Eqn. (5.23), shows why we do not usually define response coefficients to metabolites that occur in the metabolic pathway under consideration. If P is in the pathway, the equation contains the same terms as the connectivity relationship for P, Eqn. (5.18), which proves that the response coefficient in this case, R_P^J, is zero. The physical interpretation of this result is that if we attempt to change the rate of the metabolic pathway by adding extra P, a metabolite in the pathway, this extra material will flow away through the pathway, which will return eventually to the steady state that existed before the addition, *i.e.* there are no long–term consequences of adding a pathway metabolite. (The exception to this is the case where the metabolite contains a conserved moiety that cannot be metabolized away, but in this case the connectivity relationship is not equal to zero, but has a value that indicates the response to changing the amount of the conserved material.)

5.5   Control Analysis and traditional approaches

The validity of some of the measures proposed for the identification of rate–limiting steps (described in Chapter 4) can be examined using the concepts developed in Metabolic Control Analysis. To do this, we will relax the interpretation of a 'rate–limiting step' and seek to find out whether the proposed criteria would discriminate between pathway enzymes with high and low flux control coefficients. Two particular properties are worth special consideration because they can be measured: displacement from equilibrium (Chapters 1.4.2 and 4.2) and relative limiting rates (Chapter 4.4). The only slight difficulty in carrying out such investigations is that we are no longer dealing solely with the general properties of every metabolic system (like the summation theorem) that are true irrespective of the details of the enzyme kinetics; now the equilibrium constants of the reactions, the kinetic equations of the enzymes and the values of their kinetic parameters will all enter the result. It is therefore too difficult to derive completely general algebraic solutions to these problems. For this reason, Henrik Kacser and Jim Burns examined a particularly simple case where it is possible to derive expressions for the values of control coefficients in terms of factors such as displacement from equilibrium and relative limiting rates:[119] this was a linear pathway of single substrate enzymes, all obeying the reversible Michaelis–Menten equation [Eqn. (3.4)], and with steady state metabolite concentrations all lower than the K_m values. Under these circumstances, the expressions for the elasticities of the enzymes become much simpler, and allow relative values of the flux control coefficients to be calculated *via* the connectivity theorem.

5.5.1   Displacement from equilibrium

For their simple linear metabolic pathway, Kacser & Burns determined that the relative values of the flux control coefficients of successive enzymes in the chain would be:

$$C_1^J : C_2^J : C_3^J : \ldots \equiv 1 - \rho_1 : \rho_1(1 - \rho_2) : \rho_1\rho_2(1 - \rho_3) : \ldots \qquad (5.24)$$

By considering particular sets of values of the disequilibrium ratios, it is possible to use this equation to show the following.

- Relative values of the disequilibrium ratios, ρ_i, do not themselves show the relative contributions of the enzymes to the control of flux, but the terms in Eqn. (5.24) do.

- If any step i is at equilibrium ($\rho_i = 1$), then its flux control coefficient becomes zero, because of the term $(1 - \rho_i)$. This justifies the view that control cannot be exerted by an equilibrium reaction, though only so far as for enzymes *at* equilibrium, which is not strictly possible for a reaction carrying a net pathway flux.

- It is easy to create examples where the step nearest to equilibrium is not the step with the smallest flux control coefficient.

- It is also possible to create examples where the step furthest from equilibrium is not the one with the largest flux control coefficient.

- There is a tendency, in the case of this linear pathway, for the flux control coefficients to be largest near the beginning of the pathway and to decrease with the distance along it. This is not invariant because it is affected by the specific values of the disequilibrium ratios, but the multiplication of an increasing number of terms, each of which is less than 1, has this effect.

If the disequilibrium ratios cannot be relied upon to indicate the relative influences of enzymes on the flux in such a simple pathway, there is no reason to expect them to work better in more complex cases. Additional support for this conclusion comes from Reinhart Heinrich & Tom Rapoport,[99] who used a less restrictive derivation but also found that values of disequilibrium ratios were not a reliable guide. Also, in the case of rat heart glycolysis, for which the disequilibrium ratios are shown in Figure 4.1, the relative flux control coefficients of several of the enzymes have been determined,[125] but in this real example the disequilibrium ratios alone do not rank the enzymes correctly. The equation given above, Eqn. (5.24), does rank the enzymes in the right order, though the numerical match is not very good.

5.5.2 Maximal enzyme activities

Kacser & Burns'[119] equation for the relative values of the flux control coefficients of a linear pathway was:

$$C_1^J : C_2^J : C_3^J : \ldots \equiv \frac{K_{m,1}}{V_1} : \frac{K_{m,2}}{V_2 K_{eq,1}} : \frac{K_{m,3}}{V_3 K_{eq,1} K_{eq,2}} \ldots \qquad (5.25)$$

Thus there is a tendency for the enzymes with the largest limiting rate to have the smallest flux control coefficients and *vice versa* but, again, this cannot be relied on to rank the enzymes according to their effects on the flux because K_m values and equilibrium constants enter the expressions. The equation has not been applied in any real cases because these are always more complicated (involving two substrate enzymes, for example), so it has no practical value beyond demonstrating the unsuitability of this traditional criterion.

5.6 Summary

(1) The qualitative categories of 'rate–limiting' and 'not rate–limiting' are replaced in Metabolic Control Analysis by a quantitative scale for the influence of an enzyme on a metabolic flux: the flux control coefficient.

(2) The flux control coefficient of an enzyme is a system property of a metabolic pathway since its value can be affected by any or all of the other enzymes. This is particularly apparent in the summation theorem, a system constraint that requires the control coefficients of all the enzymes on a particular flux to add up to 1.

(3) The influences of metabolites on enzymes are measured in terms of the elasticity coefficients. These are related to the kinetic properties of the enzymes, but are defined specifically for the conditions in the metabolic pathway at steady state.

(4) The connectivity theorem shows that the flux control coefficients of the enzymes in a pathway have links to the elasticities, *i.e.* the system control properties can be related to the individual kinetic characteristics of the enzymes.

(5) The action of external effectors on a pathway flux can be measured as a response coefficient, which can be shown to be the product of the flux control coefficient of the affected enzyme and the elasticity of that enzyme with respect to the effector. Both factors must be non–zero for an effector to be able to influence a flux.

(6) Metabolic Control Analysis shows that neither the degree of displacement of a reaction from equilibrium nor the relative value of the limiting rate of an enzyme is a reliable guide to the degree of control an enzyme can exert on a flux, even though these factors have been used for that purpose in the past.

5.7 Appendix 1: More about flux control coefficients

The definitions given earlier for the flux control coefficient, Eqns. (5.2) and (5.3), correspond to those originally used by Kacser & Burns (though at the time they called them *sensitivities*), and have the advantage that they directly reflect the effects of changes in enzyme amounts caused by genetic or environmental factors. However, there are occasions where subtly modified definitions are preferable.

(1) It is sometimes necessary to assign a metabolic flux a negative value, for example if it is a reversible pathway flowing in the opposite direction to that originally defined. In this case, Eqn. (5.3) cannot be used as it is because it is not possible to have the logarithm of a negative number. (Negative logarithms represent numbers between 0 and 1.) This turns out not to matter because the following modified version works just as well:

$$C_{xase}^{J_{ydh}} = \frac{\partial \ln |J_{ydh}|}{\partial \ln E_{xase}}$$

where $|J_{ydh}|$ signifies that the *absolute value* of J_{ydh} is used, *i.e.* any negative sign is ignored.

(2) The logarithms in Figure 5.1(c) and Eqn. (5.3) are the *natural logarithms*, but logarithms to base 10 can be used without any alteration to the equations.

(3) The flux control coefficient has been shown here as defined relative to the concentration or amount of an enzyme, as mentioned above. However there is the potential for complications in cases where the activity of the enzyme does not relate directly to its concentration. Such conditions are not thought to be particularly common, but the difficulties can be avoided by a variation of the definition that was proposed by Reinhart Heinrich and his colleagues, in which the coefficient is defined with respect to some parameter of the enzyme that acts on the enzyme's activity. Suppose this parameter is k; then we define the flux control coefficient as the ratio of the response of the flux to k relative to the effect of k on the enzyme activity, *i.e.* :

$$C_{xase}^{J_{ydh}} = \frac{k \partial J_{ydh}}{J_{ydh} \partial k} \bigg/ \frac{k \partial v_{xase}}{v_{xase} \partial k} \tag{5.26}$$

This equation is identical to the response coefficient relationship that was described in Eqn. (5.22) and used in determining flux control coefficients from inhibitor titrations [Eqns. (6.2) and (6.3)]:

$$C_k^{J_{ydh}} = \frac{R_k^{J_{ydh}}}{\varepsilon_k^{xase}} \tag{5.27}$$

If the rate of enzyme *xase* depends proportionally on the parameter k, then ε_k^{xase} will be 1 and the flux control coefficient will be equal to the response coefficient to k. Generally, enzyme activities are expected to be proportional to enzyme concentration, so a possible choice for k is E_{xase} and the flux control coefficient will be equal to the response of the flux to the enzyme concentration. This has been the implicit assumption in this book and the justification for the simple definition used in this Chapter. There are possible exceptions, however, such as when the enzyme concerned forms enzyme–enzyme complexes; then ε_k^{xase} need not necessarily equal 1 and the intrinsic flux control coefficient of the step catalysed by *xase* is not equal to the response coefficient of the flux to the concentration of *xase*. In such cases, the definition in Eqn. (5.26) above is preferable.

The summation theorem for flux control coefficients has been proved in a number of different ways. The simplest to understand is probably the argument originally used by Kacser & Burns. Again, we have reverted to the simple definition of the flux control coefficient relative to the amount of enzyme, Eqn. (5.2), on the assumption that for any enzyme *xase*, $\varepsilon_{E_{xase}}^{xase} = 1$. Suppose that one of the enzymes in the pathway, say the first, E_1, has its amount increased by a small fraction $\alpha = \delta E_1 / E_1$. Then according to Eqn. (5.1), the change in flux is given by:

$$\frac{\delta J}{J} = C_{E_1}^{J} \frac{\delta E_1}{E_1} = C_{E_1}^{J} \alpha$$

However, if all the enzyme amounts could be simultaneously increased by this same amount α, then all the rates would increase by this fraction α because the rates are proportional to enzyme amount. If all the rates change simultaneously by the same amount, the only change in the pathway will be that the fluxes have increased by the fraction α. There will be no changes in any metabolite concentrations because, for every metabolite, the rate of synthesis has increased by the same amount as the rate of degradation. Now the total fractional change in flux (α) is given by the sum of all the individual changes as predicted by the equation above for each of the n enzymes, *i.e.* :

$$C_{E_1}^J \alpha + C_{E_2}^J \alpha + \ldots + C_{E_n}^J \alpha = \alpha$$

Dividing through by α gives:

$$C_{E_1}^J + C_{E_2}^J + \ldots + C_{E_n}^J = 1$$

which is the summation theorem, Eqn. (5.10).

5.8   Appendix 2: Concentration control coefficients

As well as flux control coefficients, there are other control coefficients defined in the same way, such as the *concentration control coefficients* where the variable affected by the chosen parameter, such as the enzyme *xase*, is a metabolite concentration, say S:

$$C_{xase}^S = \frac{\partial S}{\partial E_{xase}} \cdot \frac{E_{xase}}{S} = \frac{\partial \ln S}{\partial \ln E_{xase}} \tag{5.28}$$

Being defined in the same way, they can be interpreted in the same way.

5.8.1   Theorems for concentration control coefficients
A set of theorems exist for the concentration control coefficients corresponding to those for the flux control coefficients. Thus there is a summation theorem:[99]

$$\sum_{i=1}^{n} C_i^{S_j} = 0 \tag{5.29}$$

where S_j represents any one of the variable metabolites of the pathway. This reflects the result mentioned in Appendix 1 on the flux control coefficients: simultaneously changing all the enzyme activities by the same small fractional amount α has no effect on any metabolite concentration.

The connectivity relationship for concentration control coefficients is more complex than for flux control coefficients[272] in that it has one form when the metabolite whose concentration is the subject of the control coefficients (say A) is different from the one in the elasticities (say B):

$$\sum_{i=1}^{n} C_i^A \varepsilon_B^i = 0 \tag{5.30}$$

but the following form when they are the same:

$$\sum_{i=1}^{n} C_i^A \varepsilon_A^i = -1 \tag{5.31}$$

As with the flux control coefficients, the form of the equation changes when metabolites in conserved cycles are involved.[213]

Generally, less attention has been given to concentration control coefficients. However, in Reinhart Heinrich & Tom Rapoport's original work[99] on control analysis, they were called *elements of the control matrix* and used to derive expressions for the flux control coefficients by means of the relationships:

$$
\begin{aligned}
C_i^{J_i} &= 1 + \sum_{j=1}^{m} \varepsilon_{S_j}^i C_i^{S_j} \\
C_i^{J_k} &= \sum_{j=1}^{m} \varepsilon_{S_j}^k C_i^{S_j}
\end{aligned}
\tag{5.32}
$$

These equations actually show how the systemic response of the flux to a modulation of an enzyme can be broken into its components. Thus, the first one shows that the response of the flux through step i to modulation of enzyme i is composed of a proportional change from the change in the amount of enzyme (the '1'), on which are superimposed the changes in activity of the enzyme because of the changes in the concentrations of each of the metabolites S_j, with each of these effects calculated from the concentration control coefficient of enzyme i on substrate S_j (to show how much the steady state concentration changes) and the elasticity coefficient for the effect a change in S_j has on the activity of enzyme i. In the second equation, because the effect of a change in enzyme i on the flux at k is sought, there is no term for a direct effect of the change in the amount of enzyme.

5.9 Appendix 3: More about elasticities

5.9.1 Elasticities and enzyme kinetics

In the main text, it was mentioned that it was possible to calculate elasticities from enzyme kinetics equations. This raises the question of why it is thought necessary to define elasticities at all if the information is available from the results of traditional enzyme kinetics? In fact, a number of points of contrast exist between the purposes for which enzyme kinetic information is usually collected and the requirements for elasticities.

(1) The equation used in enzyme kinetics is related to the presumed mechanism of action of the enzyme, and it is important that it fits the observed rates across the range of metabolite concentrations used. For the purposes

of control analysis, it is not necessary that the function used for the kinetics is soundly based mechanistically; it only has to describe the enzyme's responses to metabolites near their physiological concentrations.

(2) Because the enzyme kinetic equations provide information about mechanism, the experiments simplify the problem by using the minimum number of metabolites, for example, the substrates but not the products. The values of the elasticities must be obtained in the presence of all cellular metabolites that affect the enzyme, but such measurements are not usually taken in enzyme kinetics. The effects of products on enzymes, expressed as the product elasticities, are particularly important in Metabolic Control Analysis, even when they correspond to apparently weak product inhibition.

(3) If an enzyme responds to more than a very few metabolites, it becomes virtually impossible to carry out an experiment in which they are all varied and the results fitted to a single equation that, because it contains parameters that account for how each metabolite affects the enzyme's response to all of the others, can describe the rate under any circumstances. Such detailed information is not required for elasticities because they describe the enzyme's response to each metabolite when all the others are held constant.

(4) Enzyme kinetics experiments are performed under conditions that are convenient for obtaining the required results. Analysis of the enzyme's mechanism does not necessarily require that the measurements are taken at physiological conditions of pH, temperature and ionic composition. On the other hand, the values of the elasticities must be valid for the conditions in the metabolic system under study.

For these reasons, although enzyme kinetics could in principle supply the information required as elasticities, the published information is frequently not appropriate.

5.9.2 Algebraic evaluation of elasticities

Where a suitable rate function for an enzyme has been determined, then its elasticities can be derived by analytical partial differentiation with respect to each of the metabolites in accordance with Eqn. (5.12). Although differentiation of these functions is often tedious by hand, the wide availability of symbolic algebra programs for computers has removed the need for a high order of mathematical skill. For example, for the Michaelis–Menten equation analysed graphically in the main text we have:

$$\varepsilon_S^v = \frac{S}{v} \frac{\partial \left(\dfrac{SV}{S + K_\mathrm{m}} \right)}{\partial S} \tag{5.33}$$

The result is surprisingly simple:

$$\boxed{\varepsilon_S^v = \frac{K_\mathrm{m}}{K_\mathrm{m} + S}} \tag{5.34}$$

The final stage in the calculation of the required elasticity value is to insert numerical values for the parameters in the equation, in this case only $K_\mathrm{m} = 0.75$ mM, and the value for the concentration of the metabolite (0.5 mM), to give 0.60 as obtained previously from the graph shown in Figure 5.5.

The reason the results for most elasticities turn out to be simpler than might be expected from the complexity of the functions to be differentiated is because of the cancellations between numerator and denominator terms with the scaling factor. It is possible to define an 'elasticity calculus' that simplifies the problem of determining elasticities by avoiding generating terms that will subsequently cancel. Most enzyme rate functions, F, have the form $F = N/D$, where both N and D are functions of the metabolite concentration, S, for which we want the elasticity.

$$\begin{aligned}
\varepsilon_S^F &= \frac{S}{F}\frac{\partial F}{\partial S} \\[2mm]
&= \frac{SD}{N}\frac{\partial(\frac{N}{D})}{\partial S} \\[2mm]
&= \frac{SD}{N}\left(\frac{\partial N/\partial S}{D} - \frac{N\partial D/\partial S}{D^2}\right) \\[2mm]
&= S\left(\frac{\partial N/\partial S}{N} - \frac{\partial D/\partial S}{D}\right)
\end{aligned}$$

Even when using computer algebra packages to perform the differentiation, it is worth using the above result because many of them do not otherwise manage to simplify the results fully.

Further reading

Kacser, H. and Burns, J. A. (1973) *The control of flux.* Symp. Soc. Exp. Biol. **27**, 65–104; reprinted with modern notation and terminology as Kacser, H., Burns, J. A. & Fell, D. A. (1995) *The control of flux.* Biochem. Soc. Trans. **23**, 341–366

Kacser, H. and Porteous, J. W. (1987) *Control of metabolism: what do we have to measure?* Trends Biochem. Sci. **12**, 5–14

Kell, D. and Westerhoff, H. (1986) *Metabolic Control Theory: its role in microbiology and biotechnology.* FEMS Microbiol. Rev. **39**, 305–320

Kacser, H. (1987) *Control of metabolism.* In The Biochemistry of Plants, (Davies, D. D., ed.), Vol. 11, pp. 39–67, Academic Press, New York

Fell, D. A. (1992) *Metabolic Control Analysis: a survey of its theoretical and experimental development.* Biochem. J. **286**, 313–330

Problems

(1) Suppose an enzyme in a pathway follows Michaelis–Menten kinetics with $V = 100$ units and $K_m = 0.05$ mM:

$$v = \frac{SV}{S + K_m}$$

What is the elasticity of the enzyme with respect to its substrate (a) at a substrate concentration of 0.03 mM and (b) at a substrate concentration of 0.25 mM? (Hint: try graphical estimation, as in Figure 5.5.)

(2) The effect of a competitive inhibitor, I, on a Michaelis–Menten enzyme can be described by the equation:

$$v = \frac{SV}{S + K_m(1 + I/K_i)}$$

Suppose $V = 1$, $K_m = 1$ and $K_i = 1$ (this means the values of v, S and I have been 'scaled' so we can use dimensionless values for them). What is the elasticity of the enzyme with respect to the inhibitor at $I = 1$ for $S = 0.5$ and $S = 5$? (Hint: the solution is like that of the previous question, except that for a graphical solution, it is now $\ln v$ against $\ln I$ that is plotted.)

(3) The enzyme fumarase catalyses the reaction:

$$\text{fumarate} \rightleftharpoons \text{malate}$$

Its rate of reaction is described by the reversible Michaelis–Menten equation:

$$v = \frac{V\left(fum - \dfrac{mal}{K_{eq}}\right)}{K_{fum} + fum + \dfrac{K_{fum}mal}{K_{mal}}}$$

where $V = 20$ μmol·min^{-1}, $K_{fum} = 0.9$ mM, $K_{mal} = 1.2$ mM and $K_{eq} = 11$. What are the elasticities of the enzyme with respect to fumarate and malate at $fum = 0.4$ mM and $mal = 0.5$ mM?

(4) Consider the glycolytic pathway, particularly the successive enzymes phosphofructokinase and aldolase:

$$\cdots \text{Fru}6P \xrightarrow{PFK} \text{Fru}1,6P_2 \xrightarrow{Ald} \text{DHAP} + \text{GAP} \cdots$$

The elasticity of phosphofructokinase (PFK) with respect to fructose 1,6-bisphosphate (Fru1,6P_2), ε_{FBP}^{PFK}, is -0.01, whilst that of aldolase (Ald) to the same metabolite ε_{FBP}^{ald}, is 2.5 in a particular cell. What is the ratio of the flux control coefficients of these two enzymes on glycolysis? What is the flux control coefficient of aldolase if ε_{FBP}^{PFK} is 0? (DHAP is dihydroxyacetone phosphate; GAP is glyceraldehyde 3-phosphate.)

6

Measuring control coefficients

The previous chapter presented the main outlines of the theory behind Metabolic Control Analysis. However, up to this point I have only shown the potential of the theory: it has defined possible quantitative measures of the effects of changes in enzyme amounts or of pathway effectors on the rates of metabolic pathways, and there is the expectation that such measurements will show that control is distributed through the pathway (although it is possible for it all to be located on one enzyme). Now comes the point where it is necessary to show that:

- Metabolic Control Analysis is not an abstract theory but can be applied to measurements on metabolism; and further,

- when these measurements are made, they support the claims made earlier.

There is no doubt that the measurements required for experiments in Metabolic Control Analysis can be challenging, even though they involve many of the same experimental procedures that were described in Chapter 2 and used in earlier studies of metabolic regulation, as discussed in Chapter 4. The body of experimental evidence only started to grow in the 1980s, ten years after the theory was initially developed. This growth continues to accelerate as the value of the approach becomes more widely appreciated. The experiments that have been carried out involve a variety of pathways occurring in a range of different organisms. This means that there is little coherence in an account organized chronologically, or by pathway, and I shall therefore group the experiments according to the experimental approaches. The disadvantage of this is that some of the scientific groups involved have quite rightly used several different approaches to the same problem, either to obtain some complementary information, or to validate their experiments by making the same measurement in different ways. My method of presenting the experiments will in these cases separate the parts of what was originally a coherent set of experiments.

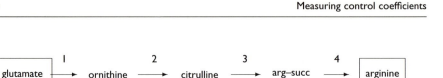

Figure 6.1 Arginine synthesis pathway of *Neurospora crassa*
The four steps of the pathway studied in the experiments by Kacser's group were: 1, the four-enzyme ornithine synthesis cycle, in which a mutant of the enzyme acetylornithine aminotransferase was used; 2, ornithine carbamoyltransferase; 3, argininosuccinate synthase; 4, argininosuccinate lyase. Arg–succ has been used as an abbreviation for argininosuccinate. The details of ornithine synthesis and the co-substrates of the pathway have not been shown.

I will concentrate on experimental methods to measure flux control co-efficients, and these I will divide initially into direct methods, which involve observation of the effects of making an alteration of an enzyme activity, and indirect methods, which involve calculation of control coefficients from other information, in particular elasticities. Obviously, looking at the indirect methods raises the question of how the elasticities can be measured.

6.1 Manipulation of enzyme activity

Since a control coefficient expresses the effect that a change in the amount of an enzyme has on a system property such as metabolic flux or metabolite concentration, the only direct method of determination of its value is to make a change in the enzyme activity and observe the consequences whilst all other conditions are kept constant. There are various ways to do this, but they all share the problem that control coefficients are defined as the response to an infinitesimally small perturbation, whereas the finite precision of any experiment requires that the response is determined from changes large enough to produce a measurable effect. One possible solution is to make a series of graded changes and extrapolate the results to an infinitely small change; both increases and decreases of enzyme activity should ideally be used to avoid bias.

Some of the different methods of altering enzyme activity that have been used are:

- alteration of expressed enzyme activity by genetic means;

- alteration of expressed activity by inducers or dietary and environmental means;

- titration with purified enzyme;

- titration of enzymes by specific inhibitors.

6.1.1 Altering enzyme activity by genetic means

In the previous chapter, when discussing the implications of dominance for Metabolic Control Analysis (Chapter 5.2.2, p. 106), I mentioned that in diploid

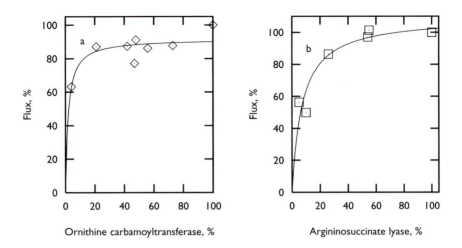

Figure 6.2 Dependence of arginine synthesis flux in *Neurospora* on enzyme levels
The results are those of Flint et al.[74] with my best–fit hyperbolic curves. Most of the points were obtained by forming heterokaryons with different ratios of wild–type and mutant nuclei. In each graph, however, the point at the lowest enzyme activity is not a heterokaryon, but a partial revertant from the mutant. (a) The dependence of the flux to arginine through argininosuccinate lyase on the activity of ornithine carbamoyltransferase, both expressed as a % of wild–type levels. (b) The dependence of the same flux on the activity of argininosuccinate lyase itself.

organisms, heterozygotes carrying a mutant allele of a gene for an enzyme will contain less enzymic activity, perhaps only 50% of the wild–type level if the mutant allele encodes an inactive enzyme. Phenotypically, these heterozygotes usually appear normal, but small differences in flux may be discernible on measurement. Nevertheless, a 50% reduction in the amount of the enzyme hardly meets our need for small increases and decreases about the wild–type level, so the results of such experiments are likely to give only an approximate value for the flux control coefficient. Fortunately there are cases where finer genetic control of enzymic activity can be obtained.

6.1.1.1 Classical genetics: gene dosage

An example of this approach is given by the experiments on arginine synthesis carried out by Henrik Kacser's group in Edinburgh during the 1970s.[74] In this case, the design of the experiment was made more favourable by their choice, instead of a diploid organism, of the fungus *Neurospora crassa*, which forms mycelia lacking cross walls between the cells so that the cells effectively have multiple nuclei surrounded by a common cytoplasm which is mixed by the continuous cytoplasmic streaming. This fungus was the one used in the 1940s by Beadle & Tatum when they formulated their *one gene, one enzyme* dictum on the basis of their genetic and biochemical analyses of mutants for the synthesis of various amino acids; as a result of this and similar work, many *Neurospora* mutants are available with known defects in particular enzymes. By mixing spores of wild–type and mutant strains, mycelia can be formed containing wild–

type and mutant nuclei in the same multinuclear cells (called *heterokaryons* in this case because the nuclei are of different types). Furthermore, a range of ratios of wild–type and mutant nuclei can be obtained by varying the ratios of spores in the mixture, whereas heterozygotes in diploid organisms only allow a 1:1 ratio. The pathway from the amino acid glutamate to arginine is shown in Figure 6.1. Null mutants, that is mutants not forming any active enzyme, were available for four of the enzymes. The results obtained by Kacser's group for the effect of two of the enzymes from this pathway on the flux through the last enzyme to arginine are shown in Figure 6.2. The hyperbolic curve I have fitted through the results for the heterokaryons of the mutants for step 2, ornithine carbamoyltransferase, gives a flux control coefficient of 0.02 at the wild–type level of enzyme, increasing to 0.31 in the mutant of this enzyme with the least activity (4%). Similarly, the hyperbolic curve I have drawn through the results for the last step, argininosuccinate lyase, corresponds to a flux control coefficient of 0.07 in the wild–type, increasing to 0.42 in the heterokaryon with 10% of the wild–type activity. Of the other two enzymes examined, in step 1 acetyl–ornithine aminotransferase also appeared to have a low flux control coefficient, around 0.06 in the wild–type organism, whereas that for argininosuccinate synthase might have been as high as 0.2, but was not very accurately determined. (Later experiments implied that this enzyme's flux control coefficient could not be so large.) Thus little of the overall control of arginine synthesis can be accounted for by these enzymes (given that the summation theorem implies that the remaining control to be found is 1 minus the sum of the four flux control coefficients in the pathway). However, the main importance of these experiments was the demonstration that, just as Kacser & Burns had predicted, the influence of an enzyme on a flux was not all or nothing, but variable depending on the activity level of the enzyme.

6.1.1.2   Classical genetics: allozymes and heterozygotes

In diploid organisms, more subtle changes in the amount of active enzyme can be generated where there are allelic forms of the enzyme, or *allozymes* with differing activity levels. The various homozygotes and heterozygotes that can be formed can give a number of different levels of enzymic activity, though interpretation of the results can become complicated if the allozymes differ in kinetic properties such as K_m as well as their limiting rates. Middleton & Kacser determined the effect of varying activities of alcohol dehydrogenase (EC 1.1.1.1) in this way on the catabolism of ethanol in the fruit fly, *Drosophila melanogaster*.[159] They used three naturally occurring alleles for the enzyme: S, F and F^d. (The letters refer to the rate of migration in electrophoresis: S for slow and F for fast. F^d is enzymically similar to F but is expressed in larger amounts.) They bred four homozygous varieties: SS, FF, F^{d}F^d and NN, where NN is the null mutant. In addition, they obtained the heterozygotes SN, FN and FS. The measurement of relative enzymic activities was complicated be-

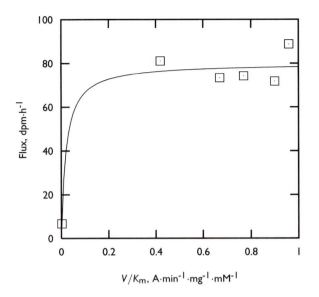

Figure 6.3 The effect of alcohol dehydrogenase activity on the flux of ethanol catabolism in
Drosophila
The genotypes giving the points are, from the left, NN, SN, FN, SS, FF and $F^d F^d$. The points on the graph
have been recalculated from the original results reported by Middleton & Kacser,[159] and a rectangular
hyperbola fitted. The result for FS is not shown as there is insufficient information to calculate its position
on the ordinate.

cause the allozymes differ in both the expressed limiting rate, V, and the K_m
for ethanol. At low fixed substrate concentration relative to the K_m values,
the activity of a two-substrate enzyme such as alcohol dehydrogenase will be
proportional to $V/(K_{ethanol} K_{i,NAD})$, as can be derived from Eqn. (3.5), p. 58.
This expression can therefore be used to compare the relative activities of the
allozymes whilst taking into account the differences in the kinetic parameters.
Accordingly, Middleton & Kacser made kinetic measurements on extracts of
the adult fruit flies and calculated $V/(K_{ethanol} K_{NAD})$ for the different genotypes. (Strictly, K_{NAD} is not the correct parameter, but there was no significant
difference in its value between the strains.) However, in order to show their
results in Figure 6.3, I have recalculated their kinetic parameters and calculated the term $V/K_{ethanol}$ as the variable reflecting the relative activity. This
does not change the basic appearance of the graph, nor their conclusion that
the enzyme's flux control coefficient is very close to zero. This is consistent
with their results on the flies' relative abilities to tolerate ethanol (which they
would naturally encounter in rotting fruit). All the enzyme–containing strains
had equal tolerance to the lethal effects of ethanol, *i.e.* they exhibited an indistinguishable phenotype; only the homozygous recessive, NN, was intolerant.
These results indicate that it is unlikely that the polymorphism at the alcohol
dehydrogenase locus is maintained through selective pressure related to alcohol
metabolism, at least in the adult fly. They are also a good demonstration of

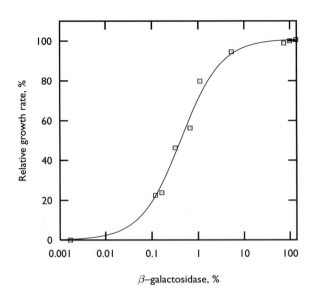

Figure 6.4 Effect of β–galactosidase on *E. coli* growth rate on lactose
The results are those obtained by Dykhuizen et al. for constitutively–expressed wild–type and mutant forms of the enzyme.[61] The enzymic activity, relative to a value of 100 for the wild–type in a constitutive mutant, has been shown on a logarithmic scale because of the wide range covered; the fitted hyperbolic curve appears sigmoidal because of this.

why mutations in alcohol dehydrogenase are recessive: although the heterozygotes do contain less enzymic activity, they have an essentially unchanged flux through the pathway.

The same technique is feasible in a haploid organism if there is a sufficient number of alleles of differing enzymic activity. Dykhuizen et al.[61] studied the effect of varying activity of the β–galactosidase (EC 3.2.1.23) of *Escherichia coli* on its rate of catabolism of lactose, which they assessed by the relative growth rates of competing strains in a chemostat, where the steady–state lactose concentration will be low enough to be restricting growth. The β–galactosidase is one of the products of the *lac* operon, which is induced by the presence of lactose in the medium. One of the other products is the lactose permease, which is the first step in the catabolic pathway because it catalyses entry of the lactose into the cell, where the galactosidase hydrolyses it to galactose and glucose which can then be catabolized. One way to vary the activity of the β–galactosidase is to vary the degree of induction of the lactose operon, but since the permease is transcribed from the same operon, its activity then varies in parallel with that of the galactosidase. To separate the effects of the two enzymes, Dykhuizen et al. used constitutive mutants of *E. coli*, *i.e.* mutants that produce the permease and galactosidase at their maximal rates regardless of the presence or absence of lactose. To get a range of strains with different β–galactosidase activities, they used revertants from a mis-sense mutant for the galactosidase gene (that is, derivatives of the mutant strain that had regained the ability to grow on lactose). These revertants contained β–galactosidases with altered kinetic properties as the result of amino acid substitutions relative to the wild–type. In addition, for the very low activity end of the range, they used strains that contained 'evolved' galactosidase activity, that is, strains that had reverted by mutation in another protein of unknown function that gave it some galactosidase activity. Because the enzymes differed in both limiting rate and K_m, relative enzymic activity was expressed as V/K_m. The results are shown in Figure 6.4, with the hyperbolic function fitted by the authors through the results. At the maximally induced or constitutive wild–type level of enzyme (100% on the graph), the flux control coefficient of the enzyme on growth rate is effectively zero, less than 0.005. The control coefficient of the permease will be referred to later (Section 6.1.2).

Mark Stitt and his colleagues, originally at the University of Bayreuth, but now at Heidelberg, have been using a variety of approaches to estimate the flux control coefficients for enzymes involved in the photosynthetic production of sucrose and starch. Their studies using heterozygotes for various enzymes are summarized in Table 6.1.1.3. Because the changes in enzyme activities in these experiments were large, the flux control coefficients were calculated from a difference equation that the authors had derived on the assumption of a hyperbolic relationship between flux and enzyme content:

$$C_{E_1}^{J_1} = \frac{\dfrac{E_2}{E_1}\left(1 - \dfrac{J_2}{J_1}\right)}{\dfrac{J_2}{J_1}\left(1 - \dfrac{E_2}{E_1}\right)} \tag{6.1}$$

where the subscript 1 signifies the flux (J) and enzyme (E) levels at the first point, and 2 those at the second. [This equation is equivalent to the 'large change' equation derived later by Small & Kacser, Eqn. (5.8), and mentioned in the previous chapter.]

6.1.1.3 Molecular genetics: gene dosage

The development of genetic engineering techniques in modern molecular biology has led to an increased number of methods for changing the amount of a target enzyme that is expressed in a cell. For a while, the pioneering experiments in this field were sufficiently difficult that achieving a change in expressed enzyme activity was virtually an end in itself. Now that the methodologies are established and becoming easier, molecular biologists are discovering, by experiment, that an ability to manipulate enzyme activities does not guarantee an ability to manipulate rates of metabolism: the need to understand the factors controlling the rate of a metabolic pathway cannot be side–stepped. However, the control of enzyme activities offered by these genetic techniques brings new opportunities for the Metabolic Control Analyst.

Table 6.1 Additional examples of the use of heterozygotes in Metabolic Control Analysis

Enzyme	Organism and organelle	Activity (% of wild type)	Flux to:	Ref.
Glucose–6–phosphate isomerase	*Clarkia xantiana* cytosol	18, 36, 64	Sucrose, starch	143
Glucose–6–phosphate isomerase	*Clarkia xantiana* chloroplast	50, 75	Sucrose, starch	143
Phosphoglucomutase	*Arabidopsis thaliana* chloroplast	0, 50	Starch	167
Glucose 1–phosphate adenylyltransferase	*Arabidopsis thaliana* chloroplast	7, 50	Starch	167

These measurements of flux control coefficients in plant photosynthesis were carried out by Mark Stitt and his colleagues.

For example, an extra copy of a gene can be inserted in a plasmid that is introduced into cells to increase the amount of enzyme expressed. This still has some problems for Control Analysis purposes. In brewer's yeast, *Saccharomyces cerevisiae*, for instance, the plasmids that are commonly used are present in multiple copies, but because of the way that yeast reproduces by budding, the number of copies received by the daughter cells is variable; as a result, the change in the amount of the enzyme carried on the plasmid can be both large and variable from cell to cell. In fact, unless the plasmid confers a specific advantage on the cells that contain it (such as conferring resistance to an antibiotic or complementing a nutritional mutation in the parent cell), it tends to be lost in culture because the cells that lose it grow faster. There is also the danger of pleiotropic effects from the expression of large amounts of one enzyme; that is, there can be phenotypic effects other than a simple change in the amount of the target enzyme. This can be simply because diverting resources into synthesizing one enzyme in unusually large amounts competes with the synthesis of other cellular components. Though this is not likely to be a problem for the small changes in enzyme amounts needed for Control Analysis, the effect has been demonstrated in extreme cases. More specifically though, the mechanisms that normally control the expression of enzymes in a metabolic pathway may be activated by the increased amount of one of the enzymes and cause a reduction in the synthesis of the others, so that any observed change in flux cannot be ascribed solely to the enzyme that has been added. Even if these problems are overcome, the experiments can still have the same difficulty as classical genetic approaches: changes in the gene dosage produce larger changes in enzyme amounts than we would normally like for determining control coefficients.

In 1986, Heinisch[96] overexpressed the allosteric glycolytic enzyme phosphofructo–1–kinase in yeast cells about 3.5–fold, but observed no effect on glycolytic flux to ethanol. This has come as rather a surprise to those who believed biochemistry textbooks that state that phosphofructokinase is the rate–limiting step of glycolysis on the basis of evidence such as that cited in Chapter 4. Similar experiments with 8 of the 11 other glycolytic enzymes have subsequently failed to show any changes in glycolytic rates either, even though hexokinase activity, for example, was increased 13.9-fold.[220] However, Davies & Brindle[59] showed in a similar experiment that although a 5–fold excess of phosphofructokinase had no effect on anaerobic glycolysis, it did stimulate anaerobic ethanol production in aerobic conditions. That is, the glycolytic rate increased slightly, but the cells nullified the effects by reducing the amount of pyruvate oxidized by the efficient aerobic route and getting rid of the excess pyruvate as ethanol. Even so, if the flux control coefficient of phosphofructokinase on glycolysis is calculated from their results using the 'large enzyme change' equation, Eqn. (5.8), it is found to be only about 0.3.

6.1.1.4   Molecular genetics: modulation of gene expression

In 1985, Walsh & Koshland[262] devised a method for getting finer control over the amount of enzyme expressed by genes carried on a plasmid. Though they had no intention of applying Metabolic Control Analysis to their results, they were studying the effects of changing the activity of citrate synthase (EC 4.1.3.7), the first enzyme of both the tricarboxylic acid and glyoxalate cycles, on the metabolism of *E. coli* growing on acetate. They placed the gene for citrate synthase on a plasmid, but they replaced the natural promoter with the synthetic *tac* promoter (a hybrid of the promoters of the tryptophan, *trp*, and lactose, *lac*, operons). The plasmid also carried the *lac* repressor so that the expression of the enzyme could be altered by varying the amounts of inducers of the *lac* operon to which the bacteria were exposed. As so often in experiments with the *lac* operon, the actual inducer used was not a metabolizable compound, such as lactose, which would interfere with the metabolism under study, but the non–metabolizable gratuitous inducer isopropyl β–D–thiogalactoside (IPTG). (The reason for using the *tac* promoter rather than just the *lac* promoter is that higher levels of enzyme synthesis can be driven by the artificial version.)

Their methodology was then adopted for Metabolic Control Analysis by Ruijter, Postma and van Dam[203] in the Netherlands in 1991. They were studying the first step in the metabolism of glucose by *E. coli*, which is its simultaneous transport across the membrane and phosphorylation to glucose 6–phosphate. As in a number of bacterial transport systems, the energy source and phosphate donor driving this linked transport and phosphorylation is the glycolytic intermediate phosphoenolpyruvate, which is converted to pyruvate in the process. This phosphoenolpyruvate–carbohydrate phosphotransferase system (PTS) consists of several components: two cytoplasmic proteins which are involved in accepting the phosphate from phosphoenolpyruvate and which are shared between the different transfer systems, and the carbohydrate–specific permeases that are located in the membrane and have one or two subunits. The glucose–specific PTS has two subunits, and the degree of control of transport on glucose metabolism was investigated by measuring the flux control coefficient of one of these, the membrane–bound permease with the elegant name enzyme II^{Glc} (EC 2.7.1.69). Ruijter et al. constructed a plasmid containing the structural gene for enzyme II^{Glc} under the control of a *tac* promoter and inserted it in an *E. coli* strain that lacked any chromosomally encoded glucose transport systems; in this way, only cells containing the plasmid could grow on glucose, and when the plasmid gene was expressed at low levels, the content of enzyme II^{Glc} was below wild type levels. On the other hand, by varying the concentration of the inducer IPTG, they could vary the level of II^{Glc} between 20 and 600% of its wild–type level with little effect on the expression of other proteins of the system. Slight variations in II^{Glc} activity near wild–type levels in the presence of excess glucose had little effect on the rates of glucose oxidation and growth, so the control coefficients were very low. At the lowest enzyme levels studied, both rates showed dependence on the enzyme content in the same sort of quasi–hyperbolic manner we have seen earlier in this chapter. Of course, one possible explanation of the low flux control coefficients at wild–type levels could have been that although transport does have some influence on glucose metabolism and growth, this control is exerted by one of the other PTS components. This was excluded by studying the flux in the transport step alone by measuring the rate of accumulation and phosphorylation of the non–metabolizable sugar methyl–α–glucoside; enzyme II^{Glc} had flux control coefficients of about 0.6 on these fluxes at wild–type levels and therefore has a larger effect than the other three components, whose flux control coefficients together cannot exceed 0.4 by the summation theorem. Of course, it should be mentioned that the measurements of the effect of the glucose permease on growth and glucose oxidation were made in just the conditions, the presence of excess glucose, that would be likely to minimize its influence on the fluxes. Lower glucose concentrations, as in chemostats at steady state, would almost certainly increase the flux control coefficients of the transport system.

A related approach that avoids the disadvantages of expressing genes from plasmids was reported in 1993 by Jensen, Westerhoff & Michelson.[113–115] They replaced the natural promoter of a chromosomal gene in *E. coli* with IPTG–inducible *lac*–type promoters (including *tac*). The enzyme they were studying was the energy–transducing proton–transporting ATP synthase (EC 3.6.1.34), which is located in the plasma membrane of the bacterium and clearly has a critical role in the transduction of energy obtained from aerobic catabolism. (See the supplementary material on oxidative phosphorylation in the Appendix, p. 191.) They determined the flux control coefficients of this enzyme by placing the *atp* operon, which codes for its subunits, under the control of the *lac*–type promoters and varying its expression from 0.15 to 4.5 times the wild–type level by altering the level of IPTG. To do this, they had to use a strain of *E. coli* that lacked the lactose permease, which catalyses the transport of IPTG into the cell, since otherwise the extent of expression of the operon was too sensitively dependent on the inducer concentration. When the bacteria were growing aerobically on succinate, the flux control coefficient of the ATP synthase at wild–type levels on growth rate was virtually zero, and on succinate consumption and respiration rate was actually slightly negative at −0.25. The results with glucose as the substrate were very similar at the same wild–type level of enzyme. It also appeared that the wild–type level of ATP synthase in *E. coli* gives a minimal dependence of growth rate on the enzyme content.

6.1.1.5 Molecular genetics: antisense RNA

Another method of varying the expression of a chromosomal gene is to insert a gene that expresses antisense RNA relative to the normal gene transcript. This results in hydrogen bonding between the two complementary strands and formation of double–stranded RNA, which tends to be translated poorly and degraded quickly. Thus the amount of active enzyme protein formed can be

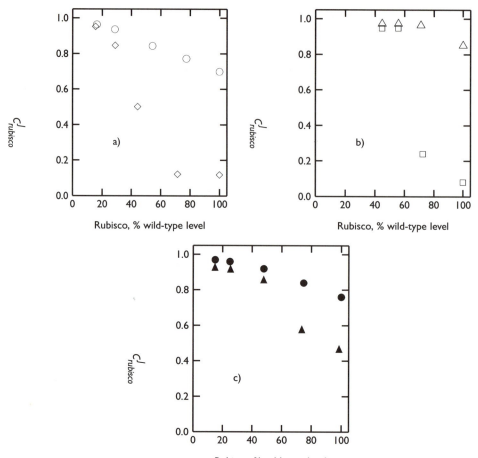

Figure 6.5 Flux control coefficients of rubisco on photosynthetic carbon assimilation in transgenic tobacco plants

The diagrams have been replotted from the results obtained by Stitt's group.[243] The amount of rubisco was reduced below wild–type levels by using transformed plants expressing antisense RNA. (a) Variation of the flux control coefficient at high (1050 μmol. quanta.m^{-2}.s^{-1}) (o) and moderate (350 μmol. quanta.m^{-2}.s^{-1}) ($\Diamond$) light intensities. Other conditions: 35 Pa. CO_2; 65% relative humidity; 22°C. (b) Variation of the flux control coefficient above (45 Pa) ($\Box$) and below (25 Pa) ($\triangle$) ambient CO_2. Other conditions: 1050 μmol·quanta·m^{-2}·s^{-1}; 65% relative humidity; 22°C. (c) Variation of the flux control coefficient at 85% (•) and 35% (▲) relative humidity. Other conditions: 1050 μmol·quanta.m^{-2}.s^{-1}; 35 Pa CO_2; 22°C.

reduced below wild–type levels. An example of the application of this technique in Metabolic Control Analysis was reported in 1991 by Mark Stitt and his co–workers,[189,243] who used it to determine the flux control coefficients of the enzyme responsible for CO_2 fixation in plant photosynthesis: ribulose–bisphosphate carboxylase (or *rubisco*, EC 4.1.1.39). Many plant biochemists seem to assume that this enzyme is 'rate–limiting' for photosynthesis, partly because it is present in an exceptionally high concentration, for an enzyme, of about 4 mM in the chloroplasts of green plants; this concentration, coupled with the large amounts of plant biomass, makes it the most abundant enzyme in the biosphere. Biochemists are also dissatisfied with it, since some 2 billion years of evolution have not eliminated its side reaction with oxygen, instead of CO_2, which leads to apparently wasteful *photorespiration*. On these grounds, plant molecular biologists had started programmes to engineer improved versions of the enzyme in the expectation that this would increase the rate of carbon fixation by plants. In fact, at the time Stitt's group started their experiments, no–one knew whether increasing the activity of rubisco in plants would change the rate of photosynthesis, because the flux control coefficient had not been measured. In the experiments, tobacco plants were transformed with an 'antisense' gene to *rbcS*, the gene for the nuclear–encoded small subunit of rubisco. The transformed plants exhibited varying degrees of reduced expression of the enzyme, with only minor changes in the contents of other photosynthetic enzymes. The flux control coefficients of the enzyme on photosynthesis in the leaves were determined by comparing the rate of carbon fixation in leaf discs cut from wild–type and transformed plants under varying conditions of light, CO_2 and humidity. In spite of rubisco's reputation as the 'rate–limiting' enzyme of photosynthesis, the experiments showed that the maximum flux control coefficient was about 0.8 for the wild–type range of enzyme contents; the highest values were only observed with strong illumination, high humidity and low CO_2, whereas they fell to about 0.1 at high levels of CO_2 or low light intensity (Figure 6.5), and were intermediate at average levels of these environmental parameters. Thus there must generally be other steps that are also contributing to the control of the rate of photosynthesis, and the influence of environmental factors is very strong. Given the values of the flux control coefficients, Figure 5.3, which shows the expected change in flux for a change in enzyme activity, reveals that very substantial improvements in rubisco activity would have to be made to produce modest changes in photosynthetic flux under most conditions, at least for tobacco plants.

6.1.2 Natural alteration of expressed activity

The responses of an organism to changes in its diet or environment generally include metabolic adaptations and, especially when the changes are sustained, these often reflect alterations in the amounts of enzymes. In some pathways, the amounts of several or even many of the enzymes change (see Chapter 8.1), but there are also cases where the number of enzymes affected may be small, even just one. Indeed, in Chapter 4.7, I mentioned that this was one of the pieces of evidence used in the qualitative identification of important regulatory enzymes, and Metabolic Control Analysis shows that this has some justification. For, as was seen in Figure 5.3, a change in the amount of a single enzyme is only likely to cause a significant change in flux if its flux control coefficient is reasonably close to 1. Moreover, where the change in metabolic flux in response to one

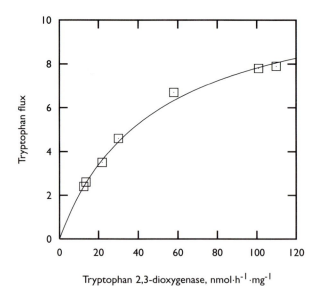

Figure 6.6 Effect of varying tryptophan 2,3–dioxygenase activity on the catabolism of tryptophan in hepatocytes
The enzyme activity was adjusted by various dietary and hormonal treatments of rats.[207] The smooth
curve is a fitted rectangular hyperbola.[233]

of these natural signals can be correlated with the change in a single enzyme, there is the possibility of going further than this qualitative conclusion and of estimating the flux control coefficient of the enzyme.

For example, Salter et al.[207,208] were interested in the factors determining the rate at which the mammalian liver broke down amino acids from the blood. Not surprisingly, this biochemical system responds to the requirements that the amount of protein in the diet and the physiological state of the mammal place upon it. Accordingly, they used a range of dietary and hormonal treatments that specifically change the degree of induction of an enzyme in the pathway for the catabolism of the amino acid tryptophan — tryptophan 2,3–dioxygenase (EC 1.13.11.11) — in the livers of rats. Tryptophan that has been brought into the cells by a transporter in the plasma membrane is converted by this enzyme into kynurenine, which is in turn further catabolized by kynureninase and other enzymes. Hepatocytes (i.e. liver cells) isolated from these treated rats retained the induced changes in enzyme amount, and the differences in their rate of breakdown of tryptophan could be measured under standardized conditions. The hyperbolic relationship between the amount of tryptophan 2,3–dioxygenase and the catabolic flux is shown in Figure 6.6. The enzyme's flux control coefficient varied from 0.75 in the rats on a normal diet (at the lower end of the range of enzyme content) to 0.25 in the maximally induced state. We shall see in a later section that they managed to identify where most of

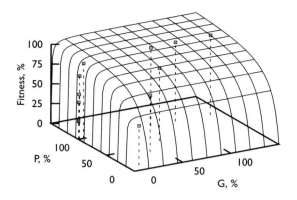

Figure 6.7 Dependence of the growth of E. coli on variation of the permease and β–galactosidase activities
The axes are expressed as percentages of metabolic flux and enzyme activities (P for permease and G for galactosidase) obtained with maximal induction of the *lac* operon. The experimental values at 100% permease activity are the same results as in Figure 6.4. The three–dimensional surface is that fitted by Dykhuizen et al.

the remaining control could be found by other means (Chapter 6.1.4.3, p. 160 and Chapter 6.3, p. 165).

I have already mentioned the experiments that estimated the control coefficient of β–galactosidase on the growth rate of *E. coli*. Dykhuizen et al.[61] also carried out further experiments in which they used variable induction of the *lac* operon by the gratuitous inducer IPTG to produce parallel changes in the activities of the lactose permease and the β–galactosidase, since the genes are in the same operon under the control of a single promoter. As in their experiments mentioned previously (p. 140), in which the activity of β–galactosidase was varied at a constant level of the permease, the rate of lactose metabolism was measured in terms of the relative growth rate in a chemostat under conditions of lactose limitation. This time, however, they were attempting to measure the flux control coefficient of the permease. Although in this case two of the pathway enzymes changed simultaneously, the contribution from the changes in β–galactosidase was known from the previous experiments. They combined the results of the two experiments and fitted them to an equation that assumed the metabolic flux depended on each enzyme in a rectangular hyperbolic manner, as shown in Figure 6.7. When the enzymes are only partly induced by the natural effect of the lactose in the chemostat, the two flux control coefficients can be calculated to be $C_{perm} = 0.53$ for the permease and $C_{\beta-gal} = 0.04$ for the β–galactosidase. (These figures differ slightly from those given by Dykhuizen et al. in their paper, but have been calculated from their fitted function.) The coefficients at the maximally induced level of expression are 0.11 and 0.004. One surprising conclusion from this numerical analysis, which is qualitatively apparent in Figure 6.7, is that the production of permease would have to be increased 30–fold to reduce its flux control coefficient to the same level as that

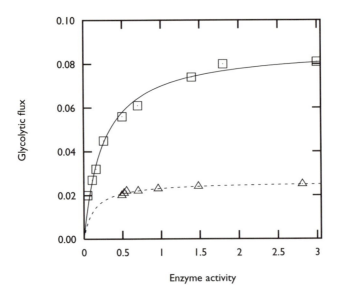

Figure 6.8 Dependence of glycolytic flux in a rat liver homogenate on added enzymes
The enzymes added were hexokinase (□) and phosphofructokinase (△). The results are those of Torres
et al.[248] with computed best–fit rectangular hyperbolas. The leftmost point on each curve represents
the original activity in the homogenate. The phosphofructokinase activity has been multiplied by a factor
of 10 for display purposes. Titration with glucose–6–phosphate isomerase gave no change in flux.

of the β–galactosidase, but the coordinate expression of the proteins in the same
operon prevents this happening. Another interesting feature is that, in these
experiments, the lactose permease had a relatively large flux control coefficient
but, in the same organism, the experiments by Ruijter et al. described above
showed the glucose PTS system had a negligible flux control coefficient[203] on
growth rate. No doubt a relevant factor is that in the lactose utilization experiments the bacteria were growing in a chemostat on limiting lactose, whereas
in the others the bacteria were growing in batch mode on excess glucose.

6.1.3 Titration with purified enzyme

The experiments described so far have used a variety of methods to force cells
to make more or less of a chosen enzyme. But many enzymes can be obtained
in purified form, and are often available commercially. Why not just take one of
these purified enzymes and add it to a metabolizing system in order to discover
the effect of increasing the enzyme content? The obvious difficulty is that the
metabolites inside cells would not get out across the plasma membrane to reach
the enzyme, and the enzyme would be too large to cross the plasma membrane
into the cell. However, biochemists do not always work on intact cells and
tissues: cell homogenates often exhibit functioning metabolic pathways even
though the permeability barriers have been removed by membrane disruption.

   Enzyme addition has been tried on rat liver homogenates, in studies of
their glycolytic activity carried out by Enrique Meléndez–Hevia's group in the

Canary Islands, starting in the mid 1980s. The experiment was designed to study the distribution of control in the upper part of the glycolytic pathway in liver. To simplify the problem, the pathway was effectively limited to the first three enzymes by adding an excess of (fructose bisphosphate) aldolase and glycerol–3–phosphate dehydrogenase.[248] This traps all the fructose 1,6–bisphosphate produced by hexokinase IV (glucokinase), glucose–6–phosphate isomerase and 6–phosphofructokinase, and converts it into glycerol. Furthermore, the rate of utilization of NADH during glycerol production can be determined spectrophotometrically and indicates the flux in the pathway. Titrating this system with various additional amounts of the more readily available yeast hexokinase (HK, for supplementing hexokinase IV) and 6–phosphofructokinase (PFK) gave hyperbolic responses of the flux (Figure 6.8), but there was virtually no response to extra glucose–6–phosphate isomerase (GPI). The flux control coefficients derived from the fitted hyperbolas for the liver homogenate without added enzymes are[233] $C_{HK} = 0.79$, $C_{GPI} = 0.0$ and $C_{PFK} = 0.21$. (Torres et al.[248] reported marginally different values calculated from parameters derived from double–reciprocal plots of their results.) Note that the results show no discrepancy from the summation theorem, as the coefficients add up to 1 (though this is somewhat fortuitous as the experimental uncertainties are of the order of 5%).

These experiments were an interesting demonstration of the potential of a simple method though their physiological relevance is doubtful. The reasons include: liver is more typically gluconeogenic than strongly glycolytic; the homogenate was more dilute than cytosol; the study was limited to just three enzymes, and the method used to shorten the pathway is likely to lower fructose 1,6–bisphosphate below *in vivo* levels. On the other hand, some very rough enzyme supplementation experiments performed by other groups on red blood cells, which are only capable of anaerobic conversion of glucose to lactate, are consistent with significant control of the glycolytic flux to lactate being shared predominantly by hexokinase and phosphofructokinase.

6.1.4   Titration of enzymes by specific inhibitors

Specific inhibitors of enzymes have long had a place in the study of metabolism, because the involvement of an enzyme in the formation of a particular metabolic product could be shown by demonstrating that large doses of the inhibitor blocked the pathway. Blocking a pathway with inhibitors was also a way of increasing the concentrations of metabolic intermediates to more readily detectable levels during the initial discovery phase of metabolic biochemistry.

In 1979 Rognstad suggested application of such inhibitors to the identification of rate–limiting steps in metabolic pathways.[200] He expected that if an inhibitor acted on the rate–limiting enzyme of a pathway, it would cause an immediate hyperbolic inhibition of pathway flux, starting at the lowest concentration that had an effect on the enzyme. For a strong non–competitive inhibitor, Rognstad proposed that the graphical appearance of the reciprocal

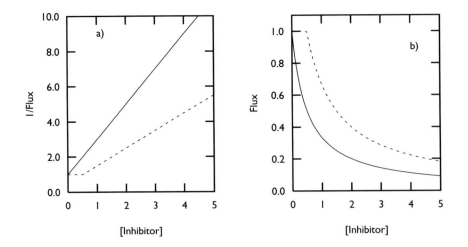

Figure 6.9 Expected effects of non–competitive inhibitors on pathway flux according to Rognstad
(a) The reciprocal of pathway flux has been plotted against inhibitor concentration because this plot is linear for an isolated enzyme. The solid line shows the result expected if the inhibitor acts on a rate–limiting enzyme, and the dashed line the biphasic response expected if it acts on one that is not. The numeric scales are arbitrary. (b) The same responses plotted as flux against inhibitor concentration.

of pathway flux against inhibitor concentration would be as shown in Figure 6.9(a), on the basis that non–competitive inhibitors give this type of linear plot with isolated enzymes. On the other hand, if the pathway flux did not initially respond to an inhibitor of an enzyme at concentrations known to affect the enzyme, but showed a stronger response at higher inhibitor concentrations, then the enzyme was originally 'non–rate–limiting' but became rate–limiting as its activity was reduced. This would give rise to the 'biphasic' line shown in Figure 6.9(a), as there is supposedly no effect on flux until the enzyme has been inhibited sufficiently to become the rate–limiting enzyme, but thereafter, the plot follows the line expected for the enzyme inhibition. Translated into a flux versus inhibitor graph (Figure 6.9b), the rate–limiting enzyme would give a hyperbolic plot, whereas the non–rate–limiting enzyme would show a biphasic plot again (or sigmoidal if the sudden transition were rounded off). A somewhat more realistic plot, typical of the curves observed in practice, is shown in Figure 6.10. Unfortunately, if these are plotted as reciprocal flux versus inhibitor, both of the cases give curved (or biphasic) lines. Rognstad illustrated his proposal with results he obtained on the gluconeogenic pathway for the formation of glucose from lactate in isolated rat hepatocytes. 3–Mercaptopicolinate, a specific inhibitor of the enzyme phosphoenolpyruvate carboxykinase (PEPCK, EC 4.1.1.32) gave the result he predicted for a rate–limiting enzyme (see Figure 6.12). On the other hand, aspartate transaminase (which is involved in the shuttle between the mitochondria and the cytoplasm during the conver-

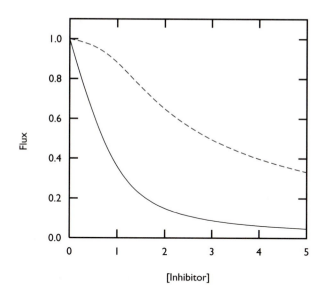

Figure 6.10 Action of an inhibitor on pathway flux
The plot shows a more realistic graph of the response of the flux to a non–competitive inhibitor than Figure 6.9(b). The solid line is for inhibition of an enzyme with a flux control coefficient of 1, whereas the dashed line is for an enzyme with a coefficient of 0.05. The curves were plotted with an approximate equation derived by Rankin Small[229] that gives curves very similar to those experimentally observed.

sion of pyruvate to phosphoenolpyruvate) gave biphasic responses with the inhibitors amino-oxyacetate and cycloserine and was therefore classed as not rate–limiting.

Readers should not by now be surprised to learn that Metabolic Control Analysts were not content with Rognstad's use of inhibitors to divide enzymes into the two classes of *rate–limiting* and *not rate–limiting*. However, perhaps just as important is the question of whether the shapes of the plots are reliable qualitative indicators for making this classification anyway.

6.1.4.1 Theory

The application of Metabolic Control Analysis to the problem was first tackled by the group of researchers at the University of Amsterdam who have given experimental and theoretical studies of Metabolic Control Analysis such a great boost from the early 1980s onwards. This group included, amongst others, Tager, van Dam, Groen, Westerhoff, Wanders and Meijer, some of whom have already had their work mentioned in this chapter. Rognstad's proposal was analysed by Bert Groen et al. in 1982,[90] both in general terms and with reference to his specific conclusion about the role of PEPCK in gluconeogenesis.

The effect of an inhibitor, I, of some enzyme *xase*, on flux is described by a response coefficient R_I^J, as defined earlier in Eqn. (5.21). As shown in Eqn. (5.22), Chapter 5.4, this response is composed of the enzyme's flux control

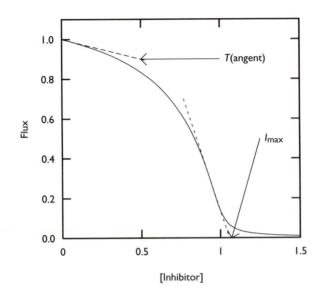

Figure 6.11 Titration with an irreversible non-competitive inhibitor
The curve is from inhibition of an enzyme with a flux control coefficient of 0.2 by an inhibitor with very high affinity. The initial slope at zero inhibitor is shown by the dashed line *T*. The linear region at the other end has been extrapolated to zero flux to give the amount of inhibitor, I_{max} needed to bind all the enzyme.

coefficient and the elasticity of the inhibitor I on *xase*, *i.e.* :

$$R_I^J = C_{xase}^J \varepsilon_I^{xase} \tag{6.2}$$

Therefore, the flux control coefficient of the enzyme can be obtained from the response of the metabolic flux to an inhibitor relative to the effect of the inhibitor on the isolated enzyme:

$$C_{xase}^J = R_I^J / \varepsilon_I^{xase} \tag{6.3}$$

This is not, though, a suitable equation for experimental implementation; it looks as though the way to evaluate it would be to measure the flux at a series of inhibitor concentrations, and use these to estimate the response coefficient. However, we want the value of the flux control coefficient in the absence of inhibitor, and the response coefficient is not easy to obtain for $I = 0$. For example, the response coefficient is the slope of a double logarithmic plot of flux versus I, but $\log 0$, for $I = 0$, cannot be plotted. The way around this devised by Groen et al.[90] is as follows. The equation above is rewritten with the response coefficient and elasticity written out in full, for the limit ($\lim_{I \to 0}$) as I approaches zero:

$$\lim_{I \to 0} C_{xase}^J = \lim_{I \to 0} \frac{\partial J}{\partial I} \frac{I}{J} \bigg/ \left(\frac{\partial v_{xase}}{\partial I} \frac{I}{v_{xase}} \right) \tag{6.4}$$

The inhibitor concentrations in the numerator and denominator cancel to give:

$$\lim_{I \to 0} C_{xase}^J = \lim_{I \to 0} \frac{\partial J}{\partial I} \frac{1}{J} \Big/ \left(\frac{\partial v_{xase}}{\partial I} \frac{1}{v_{xase}} \right) \tag{6.5}$$

The two terms of this equation are easier to evaluate. The numerator, $(\partial J/\partial I)(1/J)$, is the slope of a graph of J versus I (in the limit that $I = 0$) times $1/J_0$, where J_0 is the pathway flux in the absence of inhibitor. Let us call the value of the slope T (for tangent) as in the example in Figure 6.11; the numerator is therefore T/J_0.

The denominator term, $(\partial v_{xase}/\partial I)(1/v_{xase})$ in the limit where $I = 0$ (i.e. $\lim_{I \to 0}$), can be determined from the effect of the inhibitor on the enzyme's kinetics, but different types of inhibitor give different results. The simplest case is the very strong inhibitor that can be considered effectively irreversible because, once bound to the enzyme, it dissociates very slowly. The degree of inhibition of the enzyme is proportional to the amount of inhibitor added, up to 100% inhibition when the amount of inhibitor I_{max} is equal to the amount of enzyme sites. That is, the enzyme activity goes linearly from v_{xase} at $I = 0$ to 0 at $I = I_{max}$. The slope $\partial v_{xase}/\partial I$ is therefore $-v_{xase}/I_{max}$, so our denominator term in Eqn. (6.5), $(\partial v_{xase}/\partial I)(1/v_{xase})$ is $-1/I_{max}$. I_{max} can often be estimated from the inhibitor titration graph itself as shown in Figure 6.11. If the values for the terms are now substituted into Eqn. (6.5), the value of the flux control coefficient from a titration with an irreversible inhibitor will be:[90]

$$\boxed{C_{xase}^J = -T \frac{I_{max}}{J_0}} \tag{6.6}$$

For other types of inhibitor, the denominator term can either be evaluated experimentally by an inhibitor titration of the (isolated) enzyme activity, or by calculation from the rate law and the inhibition constant. In the first case, Douglas Kell and Hans Westerhoff pointed out that if the pathway flux and the enzyme rate were both expressed as fractions of their uninhibited values and plotted on the same graph, then Eqn. (6.5) is just the ratio of the initial slopes of the two curves.[129] Jean–Pierre Mazat and Thierry Letellier have been using this method recently in Bordeaux for the study of the control of oxidative phosphorylation in relation to diseases caused in humans by mitochondrial mutations; they used inhibitor titrations of both the flux and the isolated enzyme activity. Their application of this method will be seen later in Figure 6.16.

As an example of the method using calculation from the enzyme rate law, the denominator term for a non-competitive inhibitor can be shown to be $-1/(I + K_i)$, which when substituted with $I = 0$ into Eqn. (6.5) gives:

$$\boxed{C_{xase}^J = -T \frac{K_i}{J_0}} \tag{6.7}$$

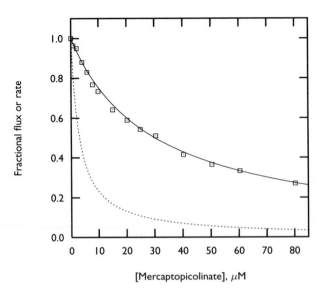

Figure 6.12   Inhibition of gluconeogenesis from lactate by mercaptopicolinate
The points are fractional rates of glucose formation by rat hepatocytes measured by Rognstad[200] and
replotted from his graph of 1/Flux against the inhibitor concentration. The solid curve through the points
is a transformation of the line Rognstad fitted on his graph. The dotted line is the fractional rate of
PEPCK against mercaptopicolinate calculated from its K_i value of $3\,\mu M$.

The conclusion from this is that the flux control coefficient of an enzyme is
related both to the initial slope of the inhibitor titration curve and the strength
of the inhibitor effect on the isolated enzyme. The shape of the titration curve
does not seem to give a reliable indication. This became apparent when Groen
et al.[90] used Rognstad's data[200] on the inhibition of gluconeogenesis by the
action of mercaptopicolinate on PEPCK and applied their equation. Whereas
Rognstad had classed the enzyme as rate–limiting because of the shape of the
inhibition curve, they calculated that the flux control coefficient was only 0.08.
We shall see later that this value was corroborated by an entirely different type
of experiment. Rognstad's results are shown in Figure 6.12. Also plotted is the
expected inhibition curve for PEPCK based on the reported inhibition constant
of $3\,\mu M$; as can be seen, the initial slope of the enzyme inhibition curve is about
10 times steeper than the flux inhibition curve, corresponding to a flux control
coefficient of about 0.1 on the basis of the Kell & Westerhoff slope ratio method.

6.1.4.2   Experimental application to oxidative phosphorylation
The study of oxidative phosphorylation has been a very fruitful area for the
application of inhibitor titrations. This is partly because there are more strong
and highly specific inhibitors known for this system than for any other. However, there was also a powerful motivation to apply Metabolic Control Analysis

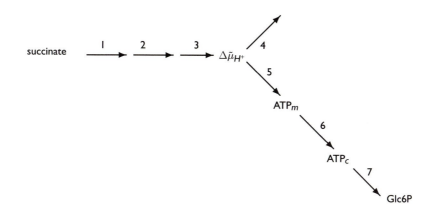

Figure 6.13 Schematic representation of mitochondrial oxidative phosphorylation system
The following steps were studied by Groen and his colleagues:[92] 1, dicarboxylate carrier for succinate transport; 2, bc_1 complex in Complex III [the succinate dehydrogenase (ubiquinone), Complex II, was not measured]; 3, cytochrome c oxidase; 4, proton leak; 5, ATP synthase (not measured in these experiments); 6, adenine nucleotide translocator; 7, hexokinase. $\Delta\tilde{\mu}_{H^+}$ is the protonmotive force.

to oxidative phosphorylation because it was a notable example of how the concept of the 'rate–limiting step' failed to achieve anything but the generation of unresolved arguments. In particular, different research groups debated in the literature about whether the 'rate–limiting' step was cytochrome c oxidase or the adenine nucleotide translocator when mitochondria were phosphorylating ADP at maximal or near–maximal rates. To understand the arguments it is necessary to have a working knowledge of mitochondrial oxidative phosphorylation. A brief summary of the major points relevant to this discussion is provided in the Appendix, p. 191.

Bert Groen and his colleagues in Amsterdam[92] applied their inhibition titration technique in the original Control Analysis study on rat liver mitochondria. The system they analysed is shown in Figure 6.13. Several of the steps were titrated with specific inhibitors. For example, the adenine nucleotide translocator was titrated with carboxyatractyloside, which is an essentially irreversible inhibitor, at different respiration rates obtained by using different amounts of hexokinase to alter the rate of ADP regeneration. Examples of the curves they obtained are shown in Figure 6.14. From the initial slopes of the curves and the I_{max} value for carboxyatractyloside, the flux control coefficient of the translocator was measured at each respiration rate. In addition, the dicarboxylate carrier (which transports the respiratory substrate succinate into the mitochondria) was titrated with the competitive inhibitor phenylsuccinate. The flux control coefficient of the hexokinase was determined by the addition of extra amounts of the enzyme, *i.e.* the enzyme titration method described previously. Finally, the flux control coefficient of the proton leak was measured by an analogue of the inhibitor titration method — an activator titration. In this, an uncoupler,

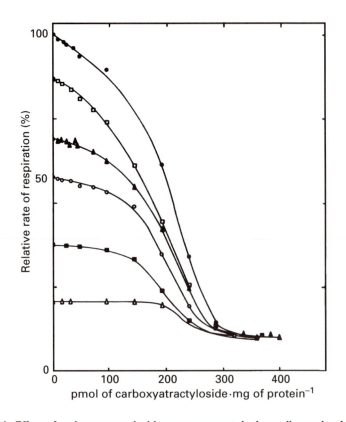

Figure 6.14 Effect of carboxyatractyloside on oxygen uptake in rat liver mitochondria
Mitochondria were incubated with succinate, ATP, glucose and varying amounts of hexokinase to give
different initial respiration rates, as measured by oxygen consumption with an oxygen electrode. At
each respiration rate, the system was titrated with increasing amounts of inhibitor. Carboxyatractyloside
does not cause complete inhibition of respiration, since the leak reaction is responsible for some oxygen
consumption when phosphorylation has been completely inhibited. The I_{max} value for the inhibitor was
estimated from the curves. This graph is reproduced with permission from Groen's Ph.D. thesis.[89]

carbonyl cyanide p-trifluoromethoxyphenylhydrazone (FCCP), was added to
stimulate respiration by increasing the the leak of protons through the membrane. The flux control coefficients of all these steps on respiration varied with
the respiration rate as shown in Figure 6.15.

A further set of measurements was made at the maximal rate of phosphorylating respiration (State 3) by titrating cytochrome c oxidase with the non–
competitive inhibitor azide and the bc_1 complex with the non–competitive inhibitor hydroxyquinoline N–oxide. The results for the six steps studied are
given in Table 6.2.

These results are a powerful example of the utility of Metabolic Control
Analysis. For a start, they show the complete futility of the previous arguments
between different research groups as to whether the cytochrome c oxidase or
the adenine nucleotide translocator was the rate–limiting step by showing that
neither of them was. Instead no step is rate–limiting because the control of

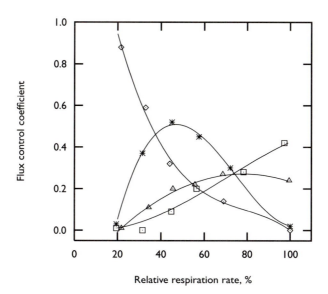

Figure 6.15 Flux control coefficients of four steps in oxidative phosphorylation as a function of respiration rate
Mitochondria were incubated and the flux control coefficients determined by various titrations,[89, 92] as in Figure 6.14. Results of inhibitor titrations are shown for the translocator (△) and the dicarboxylate carrier (□). ∗ is ATP utilization titrated with hexokinase. The control coefficient for the leak (◇) was determined with an activator titration method.

respiratory flux is shared between the different steps. In addition, the results show how that distribution changes according to the rate of phosphorylation that the mitochondria are performing. In particular, the ATP–consuming step, hexokinase, has a zero flux control coefficient at the lowest and highest respiration rates, but goes through a maximum of 0.52 at intermediate rates. The step that comes closest to being rate-limiting is the leak reaction at the lowest respiration rates, where there is no phosphorylation and all the respiration is accounted for by the leak. However, the method of calculation of this flux control coefficient from the activator titration has been criticized, and so this flux control coefficient has almost certainly been over–estimated in these experiments. Nevertheless, we shall see later that a different method of performing this experiment has produced essentially similar results. The results in Table 6.2 show that the measured flux control coefficients account for 0.86 relative to the expected summation theorem total of 1. Two steps have not been measured though: the succinate dehydrogenase (ubiquinone) (Complex II), and the proton–translocating ATP synthase. These might account for the missing control, if indeed there is any missing as opposed to some experimental error. Although Groen et al. did not measure the flux control coefficient of the ATP synthase, they believed it to be low because of the results of previous experiments on the inhibition of oxidative phosphorylation by the ATP synthase inhibitor oligomycin.

Table 6.2 Distribution of control in rat liver mitochondria in State 3 respiration

No.	Step	C_i^{resp}
1	Dicarboxylate carrier	0.33
2	bc_1 complex	0.03
3	Cytochrome c oxidase	0.17
4	Proton leak	0.04
6	Adenine nucleotide translocator	0.29
7	Hexokinase	0
	Total	0.86

The results are from Groen et al.[92] The numbers of the steps correspond to those in Figure 6.13. C_i^{resp} is the control coefficient of step i on the respiratory flux.

Some very similar experiments carried out by Thierry Letellier and Jean–Pierre Mazat in Bordeaux[148] illustrate the application of the slope ratio method. Figure 6.16 shows the inhibition curve of mitochondrial respiration with pyruvate and malate as substrate, using the Complex IV inhibitor cyanide; on the same scale is shown the inhibition of the 'isolated' Complex IV step under the same conditions. The ratio of the slopes leads to a value of the flux control coefficient for Complex IV of 0.2.

6.1.4.3   Other experimental applications

The inhibitor titration method has been applied in a range of other pathways, some examples of which are summarized in Table 6.3. The results shown there for the control coefficient of tryptophan uptake by rat hepatocytes on tryptophan catabolism complement the results cited earlier on the role of tryptophan dioxygenase in this pathway (Chapter 6.1.2, p. 148). The flux control coefficient of uptake is 0.22 when that of the dioxygenase is 0.75, and is 0.70 when that of the dioxygenase is 0.25. Thus between them, the control coefficients of these two steps sum to almost 1 and, according to the summation theorem, this leaves little scope for other steps to have a significant influence.

6.1.4.4   Problems

The versatility of the inhibitor titration as a method of determining flux control coefficients is demonstrated by the examples I have cited. Of course, the method is capitalizing on a long history in biochemistry of discovering and using inhibitors of enzymes, not least because inhibitors are potential drugs.

Table 6.3 Additional examples of the use of inhibitor titrations in Metabolic Control Analysis

Enzyme	Inhibitor	Pathway	C_E^J	Ref.
PEPCK	Mercaptopicolinate	Gluconeogenesis (hepatocytes)	0.24	198
Diacylglycerol acyltransferase	2–Bromo-octanoate	Triacylglycerol synthesis	0.76	154
Ornithine carbamoyltransferase	Norvaline	Urea cycle	< 0.02	265
Carbonic anhydrase	Acetazolamide	Urea cycle	< 0.02	265
Alcohol dehydrogenase	TMSO[a] and isobutyramide	Ethanol catabolism (rat liver)	0.5–0.7	179
Tryptophan uptake	Phenylalanine	Trp catabolism	0.22–0.70	207
Kynureninase	Amino–oxyacetate	Trp catabolism	< 0.01	239
Tyr aminotransferase	Amino–oxyacetate	Tyr catabolism	0.29–0.71	207
Glutaminase	Glutamine γ–hyrazide	Gln catabolism	0.96	151
Glyceraldehyde–3–P dehydrogenase	Iodoacetate	Yeast glycolysis	≈ 0	22
Glucose phosphotransferase system	Xylitol	Glycolysis in *Clostridium pasteurianum*	< 0.2	264
Glucose transport	6–Chloro–6–deoxyglucose	Respiration in *Agrobacterium radiobacter*	0.1–0.3	47
Glucose transport	6–Chloro–6–deoxyglucose	Exopolysaccharide synthesis *A. radiobacter*	0.1–0.3	47

Where a range of values has been given for the flux control coefficient (C_J^E), this is because the value varies with the experimental conditions.

[a] Tetramethylene sulphoxide

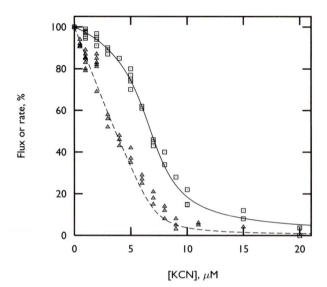

Figure 6.16 Inhibitor titration of mitochondrial respiration flux and Complex IV rate with cyanide
The substrate for oxidation was pyruvate + malate. □, Inhibition of mitochondrial respiration. The solid line is a fitted curve. △, Inhibition of Complex IV activity. The dashed line is calculated from the parameters that fitted the other points for mitochondrial respiration. Data supplied by Letellier.[148]

In spite of these successes, there is a difficulty with the inhibitor titration, connected with the need to determine the initial slope at zero inhibitor concentration of the flux against inhibitor curve. Examination of the experimental results in Figures 6.14 and 6.16 shows why this is not easy. The response of the flux is often significantly curved, so there is not necessarily an initial linear region. In any case, the experimental variance in the flux measurements makes it difficult to tell whether the initial region is a concave curve, linear or a convex curve, all of which are possible shapes. In addition, one form of the method requires an estimate of I_{max} from the graph, and another requires the initial slope of the enzyme rate against inhibitor graph. My student Rankin Small[228] found that these problems could cause bias and uncertainty in the estimates of the flux control coefficients. Both he[229] and Gellerich and his colleagues[81] proposed that it was better to use a computer fit to the curve. The difficulties of doing this are made greater because the exact equation governing the curves is generally not known, and would in most cases be very complex if it were. Instead, approximate equations have been devised, matched to the type and properties of the inhibitor, but computer simulation tests do show that this approach does work better. The titrations of oxidative phosphorylation shown in Figure 6.16 were fitted in this way; the curve drawn through the flux measurements was computer–fitted to Gellerich's equation. A measure of the success of this approach is that the fitted curve predicts the degree of inhibition of the isolated enzyme step, and this predicted inhibition curve is the one drawn through the experimentally measured enzyme rate values on that same graph. In this example, there was relatively little difference between the flux control coefficients obtained by the slope ratio method and the computer fit, but the latter is regarded as more reliable.

6.2 Control coefficients from computer models

It is impossible to look at the enzyme kinetic equations for the set of enzymes in a pathway and guess how the system will behave, but for the past thirty years it has been possible to use computers to simulate numerically what will happen. Computer simulation of metabolism was pioneered by Garfinkel,[79] Park and Chance amongst others. More recently it has played an important role in the development of Metabolic Control Analysis by allowing the rapid evaluation of the control properties of particular metabolic structures. The experiment that can be so difficult to do in the laboratory — specifically altering the activity of one enzyme whilst keeping all other conditions constant — is so much simpler in a computer model, where it generally involves no more than the alteration of a single number.

This would suggest that a simple way of finding the flux control coefficients of a metabolic pathway would be to use the experimental information about the pathway to build a computer model, and then to use the model to calculate the flux control coefficients. Unfortunately, the first stage has proved to be very difficult, and there are still relatively few computer simulations of metabolic pathways that are realistic and reliable. This is in spite of the fact that there have been successive improvements in the computer programs designed for simulating metabolism and calculating flux control coefficients, so that very little mathematical skill is needed to carry out the simulations.[52,158,209,211] The problem seems to lie elsewhere: in the amount and reliability of the experimental information and/or the assumption that the simulation can use the kinetic equation for each enzyme. (Enzyme kinetics equations are actually derived for conditions where enzyme concentrations are very low relative to substrate concentrations, and this is often not the case in cells.) It seems to be a common experience that when the experimentally determined information about the enzymes and their activities is incorporated into the metabolic model, it is rare for this to give results that match well with the experimental observations of steady state concentrations and fluxes. One particular finding is that it is only possible to make a computer model behave in a realistic and stable manner by including some degree of product inhibition on even the irreversible enzymes. (This is one of the lines of evidence for the importance of product inhibition effects in spite of their relative neglect in biochemistry. See also Chapter 6.3.4, p. 187.) Also, it is frequently necessary to change the values of some of the enzyme activities by a hundredfold or more to make the simulation match the observed results. This has been reported by Barbara Wright,[279] for example, whose research group has measured the amounts and properties of the enzymes of carbohydrate metabolism in the slime mould *Dictyostelium discoideum* with the express purpose of collecting the information needed to build a computer model. Indeed, the model has been built, has succesfully represented a number of the features of the slime mould metabolism, and has been used to calculate control coefficients.[2,278] Nevertheless, the reasons for the discrepancies in this and other examples (such as those mentioned in Chapter 4.4, p. 91) are not completely clear, but probably include the existence of many unknown weak interactions, between metabolic intermediates and enzymes, that have not been characterized. There are also the possibilities of unknown compartmentation of pathways and metabolites and of direct enzyme–enzyme interactions.

Certainly, the small number of working simulations does show how far the reductionist approach to biochemistry (building up explanations from the molecular details; see Chapter 1.2.1) has to go before it can be regarded as truly successful.

Many of the contributions from Reinhart Heinrich and his colleagues in Berlin to the theory of Metabolic Control Analysis have been linked to to the development of models of the metabolism of the human red blood cell from an initial model with just the glycolytic pathway[193] through a series of versions to one that includes the 2,3-bisphosphoglycerate bypass and, via the membrane ATPase, ion fluxes and volume changes.[97,98,194] Control coefficients for the fluxes and metabolite concentrations have been calculated. Other models of red cell metabolism, also developed in Berlin by Hermann–Georg Holzhütter's group, have included theoretical examination of the effects of inherited enzyme deficiencies[108,109] and the regulation of the hexose monophosphate shunt.[222] Of course, it is more reasonable to expect to be able to build a comprehensive model of human erythrocyte metabolism because the cells contain no nuclei or mitochondria, so there is no nucleic acid and protein synthesis, nor oxidative phosphorylation.

David Garfinkel, one of the pioneers of computer simulation of metabolism, developed large models of catabolism in muscle cells. Kohn and colleagues have applied Metabolic Control Analysis to some of these models.[135,136] However, it must be said that these models show one of the difficulties of large computer models: once they reach a certain complexity, even if they are exhibiting similar behaviour to the *in vivo* system, it can be almost as difficult to understand why the model behaves as it does as it is for the real system.

A number of models of various aspects of photosynthesis have been proposed to aid understanding of how its rate responds to environmental conditions. Some of these have been subject to one or other types of sensitivity analysis, including Metabolic Control Analysis.[86,87,182,276] Predictions made by the models differ about the dependence of the control coefficients for the photosynthetic flux on the conditions, but, like the various experimental studies reported earlier (e.g. Figure 6.5), they show that whereas the flux control coefficient for the CO_2–fixing enzyme, ribulose bisphosphate carboxylase, is high in some conditions, in others, it declines and other steps have comparable or higher coefficients.

6.3   Control coefficients from elasticities

There are three ways in which linkages with elasticities can be of use for the experimental determination of control coefficients.

(1) The connectivity theorem links the ratio of the control coefficients of adjacent enzymes to the inverse ratio of their elasticities to their common metabolite. Thus if a control coefficient of one enzyme has been determined by some means, knowledge of the elasticities of that enzyme and its neighbour would allow the calculation of the unknown control coefficient. This was used by Wanders et al. in Amsterdam[265] to estimate that the flux control coefficient of carbamoyl–phosphate synthase on the flux to citrulline synthesis (as part of the urea cycle in rat hepatocytes) was 0.96, relative to the control coefficient of the next enzyme ornithine carbamoyltransferase, which had been determined by inhibitor titration. (See Problem 1 at the end of this chapter.)

(2) The response of a flux to an external metabolite (such as the pathway source) is a relatively easy measurement to make; the response is equal to the product of the flux control coefficient of the enzyme affected by the external metabolite and the elasticity of that enzyme to the external metabolite. Thus if the elasticity value is combined with the response co-efficient, the flux control coefficient can be calculated from Eqn. (5.21). This was used by Groen et al.[91] in their study of gluconeogenesis from lactate and pyruvate in hepatocytes. The response of the flux to external pyruvate was divided by the elasticity to pyruvate to obtain an estimate of the combined flux control coefficients of a block of reactions at the start of the pathway. The result agreed well with the results they obtained by a different method (see below). The same technique was also used to determine the flux control coefficients of the aromatic amino acid transporters on catabolism of the amino acids in hepatocytes [207] by measuring the responses of the rate of catabolism to the external concentrations of tryptophan, tyrosine and phenylalanine and dividing by the elasticity of the transporter. The resulting flux control coefficients varied between 0.2 and 0.9 depending on the amino acid and the previous treatment of the hepatocytes. This formed part of the study mentioned previously in Chapter 6.1.2, Figure 6.6, Chapter 6.1.4.3 and Table 6.3.

(3) As explained in the section on the connectivity theorem (5.3.3, p. 119), all the control coefficients of a pathway are expressible in terms of elasticities, and, for certain types of pathway, relative fluxes and concentrations,

by using the summation, connectivity and, if necessary, branch point theorems. Therefore, it is in principle possible to measure the elasticities and calculate all the control coefficients of a pathway. This was first achieved by Bert Groen and his colleagues in Amsterdam in their study of the control of gluconeogenesis from lactate in rat hepatocytes,[89,91] which remains to this day the largest and most detailed experiment of this type.

Of these three methods, the most informative is the third, but the control coefficients obtained in this way are derived entirely indirectly, for the experimental observations neither directly measure changes in flux as a function of a known change in a single enzyme activity, nor relate the flux control coefficients to another known flux control coefficient (as in the first method). In addition, it involves certain assumptions, in particular:

- that all the relevant steps in the metabolic system have been identified, and that all the significant influences of the metabolites on each of these steps have been recognized. *i.e.* that all the non–zero elasticities involved in the system are known;

- that the theorems of control analysis apply to the system, *i.e.* that the metabolic system reaches a *quasi* steady state (as defined in Chapter 1.4.1) and there are no features of the pathway that would require the use of modified theorems or invalidate their application altogether. Such problems are mostly beyond the scope of this book, though a brief account of some of them is given in Chapter 8.3, p. 274.

My research group and I showed that, provided that these conditions are satisfied, it should be possible to carry out such analyses on any metabolic pathway.[69,213] Still, in order to show that the assumptions are justified, it is best if results obtained in this way are confirmed by direct measurement of one of the control coefficients to check that similar results can be obtained by a different method.

Before explaining some of the methods available to measure elasticities, I will first give an example of how flux control coefficients have been determined from them.

6.3.1   An experimental example

Groen et al.[89,91] determined the flux control coefficients for gluconeogenesis with lactate as substrate in rat hepatocytes by measuring or calculating the elasticity values. This was a new approach compared with previous studies of gluconeogenesis, which had attempted to identify the rate–limiting step. As we saw earlier, in Chapter 6.1.4, Rognstad was one of the supporters of the claims that the rate–limiting step was the enzyme PEPCK. There were other researchers who favoured pyruvate carboxylase. The position of these enzymes in the pathway can be seen in Figure 6.17. The first problem that Groen and

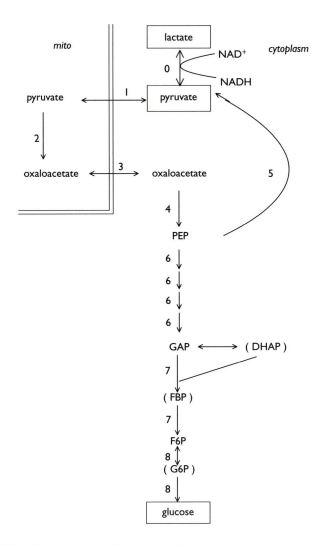

Figure 6.17 Gluconeogenesis from lactate in hepatocytes
The source and sink are shown in boxes. The numbers on the reactions refer to the groups used by
Groen et al.[91] for estimation of the flux control coefficients from the elasticities. The six metabolites
shown without parentheses or boxes are the ones used for elasticity estimates, though they were
not all directly measured (see text). The reactions are: 0, lactate dehydrogenase (assumed to be
at equilibrium); 1, pyruvate transport into the mitochondrion; 2, pyruvate carboxylase; 3, the malate
and/or aspartate shuttle systems for oxaloacetate transport; 4, PEPCK; 5, pyruvate kinase; 6, enolase,
phosphoglycerate mutase, phosphoglycerate kinase and glyceraldehyde–3–phosphate dehydrogenase; 7,
aldolase and fructose bisphosphatase; 8, glucose–6–phosphate isomerase and glucose–6–phosphatase.
Hexokinase IV (glucokinase) and phosphofructokinase were inactive under the conditions used.

his colleagues had to solve was ensuring that they could make observations in
a quasi–steady state. They solved this by *perifusing* the hepatocytes in a flowing isotonic buffer. In this way, the energy–providing substrate (the fatty acid
oleate) and the substrate for gluconeogenesis (lactate) were continually replen-
ished. Along with the lactate, it was necessary to provide sufficient pyruvate

to prevent the cytoplasmic redox balance being perturbed. (This is because lactate, pyruvate, NAD^+ and NADH are kept close to equilibrium by the action of lactate dehydrogenase; see Figure 6.17.) The build–up of glucose was prevented because it was carried away in the buffer stream, and its steady state concentration was less than the normal level in rat blood. The hepatocytes were contained in a closed stirred container and were prevented by a filter from escaping in the outflow, though samples could be removed for analysis of the internal metabolites. In the case of mitochondrial metabolites, this also involved rapid cell fractionation by the digitonin method (Chapter 2.3.3, p. 35). The perifusate was collected and analysed for lactate, pyruvate and glucose. In this way, it was possible to tell when a steady state had been reached because the glucose concentration in the perifusate would become constant (after about 20–30 min). Some change in the conditions, such as substrate concentration, could then be made and the cells allowed to reach a new steady state, so that as many as six experiments could be performed on a single sample of cells. The concentration of glucose in the perifusate also indicated the gluconeogenic flux.

Experiments were carried out in the presence of the hormone glucagon, which stimulates the liver to form glucose, and in its absence. One of the major differences between these two sets of conditions is that, in the presence of glucagon, the return loop from phosphoenolpyruvate, catalysed by the glycolytic enzyme pyruvate kinase, is suppressed by inactivation of the enzyme by phosphorylation (Chapter 7.4.3.1). In the absence of the hormone, some of the phosphoenolpyruvate is recycled to pyruvate.

The complete pathway from lactate to glucose involves about 15 steps (excluding transport of lactate and glucose into and out of the cell). To measure the elasticities of all these steps would have required measurement of all the metabolites that affected them, and this would have been an enormous amount of work. In addition, not all the metabolic intermediates are easily measurable. Groen and his colleagues therefore reduced the size of the problem by grouping some of the reactions together and treating them as a unit. This means that it is not necessary to know the metabolite concentrations inside the group. The control coefficient of a group must be the sum of the control coefficients of the component enzymes (for the summation theorem to remain valid). It is also possible to imagine that the group has elasticities to its overall substrate and overall product.[69] The relationship of these elasticities to the component elasticities of the individual steps is more complex, though it can be calculated. However, if the group elasticities are going to be measured experimentally, this does not matter. The gluconeogenesis pathway was therefore simplified to a set of seven or eight groups of steps between intracellular (cytoplasmic) pyruvate and external glucose (Figure 6.17). Seven steps are involved when glucagon is present because it suppresses the flux through pyruvate kinase. The interconversion of lactate to pyruvate was discounted since the belief is that this enzymic reaction is always close to equilibrium. The eight groups interconvert six internal metabolites, which are mitochondrial pyruvate

Table 6.4 Flux control coefficients in gluconeogenesis from lactate

		Flux control coefficient	
Step		+ Glucagon	− Glucagon
1	Pyruvate transport	0.01	0.00
2	Pyruvate carboxylase	0.83	0.51
3	Oxaloacetate transport	0.04	0.02
4	PEPCK	0.08	0.05
5	Pyruvate kinase	0.00	-0.17
6	Enolase — PGK	0.00	0.29
7	TIM — FBPase	0.03	0.27
8	PGI + G6Pase	0.00	0.02

The results are those reported by Groen et al.[91] for rat hepatocytes incubated with 5 mM lactate and 0.5 mM pyruvate, in the presence and absence of the hormone glucagon. The enzyme groups correspond to those shown in Figure 6.17, where the full enzyme names are given. The flux control coefficients inevitably add up to 1, allowing for rounding error, because the summation theorem was one of the equations used in the calculation.

and oxaloacetate, cytoplasmic oxaloacetate, phosphoenolpyruvate, glyceraldehyde 3–phosphate and fructose 6–phosphate. These metabolites were measured either directly or, as in the case of the oxaloacetate concentrations, indirectly from the malate concentrations on the assumption that the malate dehydrogenase reaction is near equilibrium. The other metabolites estimated indirectly were glyceraldehyde–3–phosphate (GAP) from dihydroxyacetone phosphate (DHAP) measurements, assuming that the triose phosphate isomerase reaction was close to equilibrium, and fructose 6–phosphate (F6P) from glucose 6–phosphate (G6P), assuming that the glucose–6–phosphate isomerase reaction was near equilibrium.

By a variety of means, some of which will be described in the following sections, the elasticities of the groups were determined from these metabolite measurements. This information was used to set up seven (or eight) simultaneous equations involving the seven (or eight) flux control coefficients (depending on whether pyruvate kinase was active or not). These equations were:

- the summation theorem;

- six connectivity theorem equations for each of the internal metabolites;

- in the absence of glucagon, a branch–point equation linking the control coefficients of the groups between phosphoenolpyruvate and pyruvate and between phosphoenolpyruvate and glucose with the relative fluxes in these two branches.

Their results for 5 mM lactate are summarized in Table 6.4; the results at 0.5 mM and 1 mM lactate gave a similar pattern but are not shown.

Their conclusions were that, in the presence of glucagon, the largest flux control coefficient was that of pyruvate carboxylase (0.83–0.89); no other enzyme (including PEPCK) had a control coefficient above 0.1. In the absence of glucagon, the largest control coefficient was still that of pyruvate carboxylase (0.51 in the presence of 5 mM lactate), but there were a number of other significant values: pyruvate kinase, −0.17; the enolase to phosphoglycerate kinase group, 0.29, and the triose phosphate isomerase to fructose bisphosphatase group, 0.27. PEPCK showed very small control coefficients under all conditions. Furthermore, independent validation of the calculations is provided by the reanalysis of the inhibitor titrations of PEPCK, quoted earlier in Chapter 6.1.4, that suggested a flux control coefficient of at most 0.1. Also, the response of the pathway to pyruvate was used as described in the previous section to calculate that the flux control coefficient of the block of reactions (groups 1–4) converting pyruvate to PEP was 0.65 in the absence of glucagon. This is in close agreement with the values in Table 6.4.

Now that the potential value of determining control coefficients from elasticities has been illustrated, I will describe some of the methods used both by Groen and his colleagues and other research groups to obtain elasticity values experimentally.

6.3.2   Experimental measurement *in vivo by modulation*

A method for measuring elasticities *in vivo*, called the *double modulation method*, was first suggested by Kacser & Burns[120] a few years after they first advocated measuring flux control coefficients. Let me illustrate their method by showing how it might be applied to the enolase (eno) reaction in glycolysis:

$$\cdots \longrightarrow 2PG \xrightarrow{\text{eno}} PEP \longrightarrow \cdots \qquad \text{(Scheme 6.1)}$$

The rate of enolase depends solely on the two glycolytic metabolites 2PG (2-phosphoglycerate) and PEP (phosphoenolpyruvate). Mathematically we state this as $v_{eno} = f(2PG, PEP)$, where $f(...)$ means *is a function of* and is used to indicate that, at this point, either we do not want to, or we cannot, be more specific about what this relationship is. At steady state, $v_{eno} = J$, where J is the glycolytic flux. In a control experiment, the flux J_c and the concentrations $2PG_c$ and PEP_c have to be measured, whilst in a parallel experiment, the rate of glycolysis is perturbed in some way by a small amount, for example by altering the input glucose level, and the new levels of flux, J_{e1}, and concentrations, $2PG_{e1}$ and PEP_{e1}, measured at steady state. Mathematical theory for approximating the change in rate ($\Delta J_1 = J_{e1} - J_c$) in terms of the changes in the metabolite concentrations gives the result:

$$\Delta J_1 \approx \frac{\partial v_{eno}}{\partial 2PG}\Delta 2PG_1 + \frac{\partial v_{eno}}{\partial PEP}\Delta PEP_1 \qquad (6.8)$$

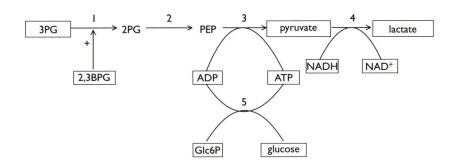

Figure 6.18 A three enzyme *in vitro* segment of glycolysis
This was the system used by Giersch[85] to measure flux control coefficients from elasticities and to compare them with the values obtained by enzyme titration. The three enzymes are: 1. phosphoglycerate mutase; 2. enolase, and 3. pyruvate kinase. In addition, 4. lactate dehydrogenase and 5. hexokinase are present in excess. Lactate dehydrogenase enables the flux to be continuously monitored by measuring the absorbance at 340 nm by NADH. Hexokinase regenerates ADP. The variable metabolites of the system are the ones not boxed, i.e. 2–phosphoglycerate (2PG) and phosphoenol pyruvate (PEP).

Scaling this equation, by dividing throughout by $J_c = v_{eno}$ and substituting the definitions of the elasticities [Eqn. (5.12)] leads to:

$$\frac{\Delta J_1}{J_c} \approx \varepsilon^{eno}_{2PG} \frac{\Delta 2PG_1}{2PG_c} + \varepsilon^{eno}_{PEP} \frac{\Delta PEP_1}{PEP_c} \tag{6.9}$$

If a second independent change can be made in the glycolytic flux, say by inhibition of an enzyme downstream from PEP, leading to another equation:

$$\frac{\Delta J_2}{J_c} \approx \varepsilon^{eno}_{2PG} \frac{\Delta 2PG_2}{2PG_c} + \varepsilon^{eno}_{PEP} \frac{\Delta PEP_2}{PEP_c} \tag{6.10}$$

then the pair of equations can in principle be solved for the two unknown elasticities. It is important for the accuracy of the method that the two imposed changes result in mathematically independent equations (*i.e.* $\Delta 2PG_1/\Delta PEP_1 \neq \Delta 2PG_2/\Delta PEP_2$), otherwise the result will be dominated by the experimental error. Theoretical analyses by Rankin Small[228] and Christoph Giersch[84] have suggested that the only viable experimental strategy is to make one change upstream of the enzyme under investigation, and one change downstream.

This was the form of the double modulation method Groen et al.[91] used in the experiment described in the previous section on the control of gluconeogenesis in hepatocytes. They determined the elasticities of the transport of oxaloacetate by the malate/aspartate shuttles between mitochondria and cytoplasm (see Figure 6.17) by changing the amount of the pathway substrate lactate and by inhibiting PEPCK with mercaptopicolinate as the two perturbations. The substrate and product concentrations, mitochondrial and cytoplasmic oxaloacetate, had to be estimated and the flux from lactate measured.

Although the double modulation equation [Eqn. (6.9)] has often been presented as shown above, the approximation formula used is not the best. Since

Box 6.1 A complete analysis of Giersch's modulation experiments

Giersch's experiment aimed to determine the flux control coefficients of an *in vitro* segment of the glycolytic pathway between 3–phosphoglycerate and pyruvate, involving the three enzymes phosphoglyceromutase (PGM), enolase (eno) and pyruvate kinase (PK). The system used is shown in Figure 6.18. The experiment had two aims:

(1) To show that flux control coefficients could be obtained from elasticities measured by modulation experiments, using a generalized version of the double modulation method devised by Giersch.[84]

(2) To validate the method by comparing the flux control coefficients obtained in this way with the flux control coefficients obtained in the same experimental system directly by the enzyme titration method.

Giersch's analysis of the modulation results is more flexible and extensive than the simple double modulation method, and I am grateful to him for providing me with his results and for giving me permission to analyse them in a different way. The first enzyme, phosphoglycerate mutase, was modulated by varying the concentration of the obligatory cofactor 2,3-bisphosphoglycerate (Figure 6.19b). For the second modulation, the third enzyme, pyruvate kinase, was subjected to variations in the concentration of its second substrate ADP (Figure 6.19a). The four lines on the figure give the coefficients in the following two equations:

$$1 = -0.182\varepsilon_{2PG}^{eno} - 0.632\varepsilon_{PEP}^{eno}$$
$$1 = 2.59\varepsilon_{2PG}^{eno} + 2.44\varepsilon_{PEP}^{eno}$$

From these, we calculate that $\varepsilon_{2PG}^{eno} = 2.58$ and $\varepsilon_{PEP}^{eno} = -2.32$.

To complete the analysis of Giersch's experiment, we need to consider a simplification of the modulation equation, Eqn. (6.11). If one term in Eqn. (6.9) is known or insignificant, only a single perturbation type is needed. Let us therefore term this variant the *single modulation method*. It could apply either because one of the elasticities is zero or because one of the metabolite concentrations does not change. For example, at the start of a pathway, the first enzyme has a pool metabolite as its substrate, and the

☞

the elasticity is given directly by the slope of a graph of the logarithm of the rate against the logarithm of the metabolite concentration, a better approximation is obtained starting from $\ln v_{eno} = f(\ln 2PG, \ln PEP)$, to give:

$$\Delta \ln J_1 \approx \varepsilon_{2PG}^{eno}\Delta \ln 2PG_1 + \varepsilon_{PEP}^{eno}\Delta \ln PEP_1 \qquad (6.11)$$

where $\Delta \ln J_1 = \ln J_{e1} - \ln J_c$. Furthermore, we can turn this into the basis of a simple graphical analysis of the results of a modulation experiment. Dividing through by $\Delta \ln J_1$ gives:

$$1 \approx \varepsilon_{2PG}^{eno}\frac{\Delta \ln 2PG_1}{\Delta \ln J_1} + \varepsilon_{PEP}^{eno}\frac{\Delta \ln PEP_1}{\Delta \ln J_1}$$

☞ **Box 6.1 (continued)**

experiment will be arranged so either this concentration does not vary significantly (so that the metabolite modulation term is zero), or the first enzyme is saturated with this source metabolite (equivalent to an elasticity of zero). A similar situation arises with the final step of the pathway, where the term involving the sink metabolite should be zero. Both of these cases apply in the three-enzyme pathway studied by Giersch. Taking the experiment shown in Figure 6.19(a), the enzyme modulated to alter the flux was pyruvate kinase. However, flux changed at all three enzymes. In the case of enolase, as we have seen, the change in flux was related to the changes in the concentrations of its substrate and product. In the case of phosphoglycerate mutase, however, only the concentration of its product, 2PG, changed, so the double modulation equation reduces to:

$$1 = \varepsilon_{2PG}^{PGM} \frac{\partial \ln 2PG}{\partial \ln J} \tag{6.12}$$

where $\partial \ln 2PG / \partial \ln J$ is the slope of the 2PG line in Figure 6.19(a), which is -0.182. It follows that the elasticity, $\varepsilon_{2PG}^{PGM} = -5.49$. Similarly, in Figure 6.19(b), where the first enzyme PGM is modulated by varying the concentration of its cofactor, the flux through pyruvate kinase varies solely because of the change in the concentration of phosphenolpyruvate. The slope of the PEP line in this Figure, 2.44, is $1/\varepsilon_{PEP}^{PK}$, giving $\varepsilon_{PEP}^{PK} = 0.411$.

The analysis of these two modulation experiments has, in this case, given all the information that is needed to determine the flux control coefficients of the three-enzyme system. There are three equations involving the flux control coefficients: a summation theorem and two connectivity theorem equations with respect to 2PG and PEP respectively:

$$
\begin{aligned}
C_{PGM}^{J} + C_{eno}^{J} + C_{PK}^{J} &= 1 \\
C_{PGM}^{J} \varepsilon_{2PG}^{PGM} + C_{eno}^{J} \varepsilon_{2PG}^{eno} &= 0 \\
C_{eno}^{J} \varepsilon_{PEP}^{eno} + C_{PK}^{J} \varepsilon_{PEP}^{PK} &= 0
\end{aligned}
$$

Subsituting the values obtained above for the four elasticities allows calculation of the three flux control coefficients as $C_{PGM}^{J} = 0.07$, $C_{eno}^{J} = 0.14$ and $C_{PK}^{J} = 0.79$.

In the limit as the change $\Delta \ln J_1$ tends to zero, the approximation becomes the equality:

$$1 = \varepsilon_{2PG}^{eno} \frac{\partial \ln 2PG}{\partial \ln J} + \varepsilon_{PEP}^{eno} \frac{\partial \ln PEP}{\partial \ln J} \tag{6.13}$$

The reason that this is particularly useful is that $\partial \ln 2PG / \partial \ln J$ is the slope of a graph of $\ln 2PG$ against $\ln J$, which can be obtained by modulating the system by a series of varying perturbations and measuring $2PG$ and J each time (e.g. Figure 6.19). In the same experiments, if PEP is measured, then the graph of $\ln PEP$ against $\ln J$ can also be plotted. The advantage of the graphical analysis is that, by using a number of different sized modulations and drawing a line or

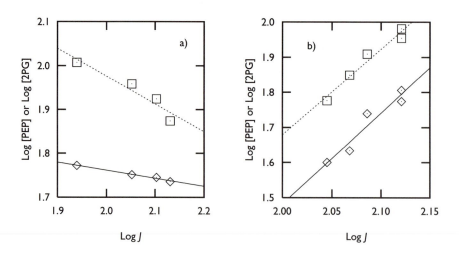

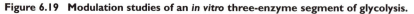

Figure 6.19 Modulation studies of an *in vitro* three-enzyme segment of glycolysis.
The system under study is shown in Figure 6.18. ◇, 2–phosphoglycerate (2PG); □, phosphoenolpyruvate (PEP). (a) Modulation of the third enzyme, pyruvate kinase, by varying the concentration of its second substrate ADP. The gradient of the regression line through the 2PG points is −0.182, and that through the PEP points is −0.632. (b) Modulation of the first enzyme, phosphoglycerate mutase, by varying the concentration of the obligatory cofactor 2,3-bisphosphoglycerate. The gradient of the regression line through the 2PG points is 2.59 and that through the PEP points is 2.44. The results have been replotted from experiments reported by Giersch.[85]

smooth curve through the results, the slopes can be more precisely determined than by taking differences between a control and a single modulated point. Thus, with an experiment of this type, the two elasticities become the only unknown terms in Eqn. (6.13) above. Repeating the experiment by applying a second type of modulation to varying degrees will give two equations in the two unknowns. This analysis was originally proposed by Rankin Small [228,230] and can be illustrated by applying it to some modulation experiments performed by Christoph Giersch in Darmstadt.[85] By perturbing the *in vitro* model of a short section of glycolysis shown in Figure 6.18, he obtained the results plotted in Figure 6.19. From the four slopes, the elasticities of enolase to 2–phosphoglycerate and phosphoenolpyruvate can be calculated as $\varepsilon_{2PG}^{eno} = 2.58$ and $\varepsilon_{PEP}^{eno} = -2.32$.

Some additional examples of the use of modulation methods for measuring elasticities are shown in Table 6.5. This is not comprehensive, because we shall see in the next section that modulation methods have been incorporated into an experimental protocol for measurement of flux control coefficients.

Table 6.5 Additional examples of the use of modulation methods for elasticity measurements in Control Analysis

Enzyme	Pathway	Type	Modulation Perturbation	Ref.
Pyruvate carboxylase	Gluconeogenesis	Single	Inhibition of PEPCK	91
Pyruvate kinase	Gluconeogenesis	Single	Lactate/pyruvate ratio	91
Ornithine carbamoyltransferase	Citrulline synthesis	Single	ATP level (via TCA cycle inhibition)	265
Carbamoyl–phosphate synthase	Citrulline synthesis	Single	Inhibition of ornithine carbamoyltransferase	265
Fructose bisphosphatase	Photosynthesis (spinach)	Double	Light input and sucrose concentration	242
Sucrose phosphate synthase	Photosynthesis (spinach)	Double	Light input and sucrose concentration	242, 166
Fructose bisphosphatase	Photosynthesis (Clarkia)	Double	Light input and GPI enzyme level	242, 165
Sucrose phosphate synthase	Photosynthesis (Clarkia)	Double	Light input and GPI enzyme level	242, 165

These examples do not include the similar 'top–down' type of experiments described in the next section. The examples above fall into two groups: those carried out on hepatocyte metabolism by members of the Amsterdam group, and the photosynthesis experiments by Mark Stitt and his co-workers. TCA, tricarboxylic acid; GPI, glucose-6-phosphate isomerase.

Box 6.2 Advanced modulation methods

If the activity of an enzyme is affected by three of the variable metabolites (for example, if the enzyme is subject to feedback inhibition), then three independent perturbations are needed, and this may be even more difficult to arrange. Giersch's generalized modulation method[84] should be consulted for the method of calculation. His method could also potentially find 'unknown' elasticities, that is, it could detect interactions between metabolites and enzymes that had previously not been expected. Another multiple modulation method that allows calculation of the elasticities in a system, again detecting them for each metabolite on every enzyme, is the co–response coefficient analysis of Cornish–Bowden & Hofmeyr,[53] which extends and generalizes the use of the slope measurements on log–log graphs of metabolite concentrations and fluxes described above.

6.3.3   Experimental measurement *in vivo*: the 'top–down' approach

A problem about the use of elasticity determination for evaluating flux control coefficients is that the amount of experimental information needed for a pathway appears daunting. In the gluconeogenesis example presented earlier, it was necessary to reduce the number of elasticities and flux control coefficients under consideration by forming groups of enzymes and transport steps, and even then it remained a large and complex experiment. If a pathway is newly under investigation, how can it be decided how many steps can feasibly be studied? Then if the conclusion implies the need to form groups of enzymes, what groups should be formed? There are no general answers to these questions; each case has to be decided on its merits, taking into account the relative difficulty of measuring different metabolite concentrations. This has almost certainly deterred researchers who have been interested in using Metabolic Control Analysis but have had difficulties devising a feasible approach.

In Cambridge (England), a group of researchers consisting of Martin Brand, Guy Brown, Patti Quant and their co-workers suggested that the solution to these problems was to look at them from the other end. Instead of starting with the components of a pathway and seeking how to group these into a small number of components (a bottom–up approach), they proposed taking the pathway and choosing a point at which it could be broken into two or three components. They called this method the *top–down approach* to emphasize that it worked in the opposite direction. For example, a linear pathway might be divided into two about a single metabolite which is the product of one block and the substrate of another, *i.e.* :

$$X_0 \xrightarrow{\text{Block 1}} S_1 \xrightarrow{\text{Block 2}} X_1 \qquad\qquad \text{(Scheme 6.2)}$$

As far as the theory of Metabolic Control Analysis is concerned, this does not raise any difficulties. We have already seen that it is legitimate to have flux

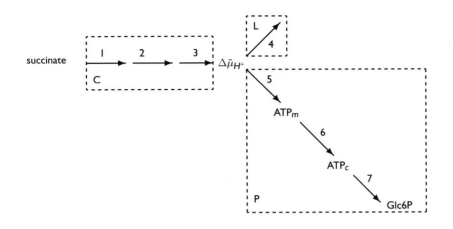

Figure 6.20 Top–down analysis of mitochondrial oxidative phosphorylation
The steps were grouped by Hafner et al.[94] into the three blocks outlined by dashed lines: C, the
respiratory chain; L, the proton leak; P, the phosphorylation system. $\Delta\tilde{\mu}_{H^+}$ is the protonmotive force.
The numbered steps correspond to the components studied by Groen et al. as described in Figure 6.13.

control coefficients of groups of reactions that must, by reason of the summation theorem, be formed of the sums of the flux control coefficients of their
component steps. There is also no difficulty about applying the definition of
the elasticity to a group of reactions rather than to a single one,[69,116,213] though
we would almost certainly have to measure its value experimentally, since we
cannot state general relationships between the kinetics of the components and
the elasticity in the same way that we can relate the kinetics of an individual
enzyme to its elasticity. In addition, it is necessary that the two blocks are
independent of one another, that is, no metabolite from one block is a substrate or effector of any of the steps in the other block apart from the single
intermediate metabolite.

One of the advantages of the top–down approach is that it simplifies the
experimental procedure enormously. If we wanted the elasticities of the two
blocks in Scheme 6.2, then only two single modulation experiments are required. Thus, to determine the elasticity of Block 1 to S_1, it would be necessary
to measure the flux in the system and the level of S_1 whilst altering the activity of Block 2 (for example by using an inhibitor of one of its enzymes) and
keeping everything else constant, particularly X_0. The slope of a plot of $\ln J$
against $\ln S_1$ is the elasticity $\varepsilon_{S_1}^{Block1}$, by reason of the definition of the elasticity
and also by analogy with Eqn. (6.12). The next step would be to determine
the elasticity of Block 2 with respect to S_1 by modulating Block 1 (perhaps
by varying the concentration of the source X_0) and measuring the flux and S_1
again. With the two elasticities, we can find the flux control coefficients of
the two blocks by solving the pair of equations formed from the summation
theorem and the connectivity theorem with respect to S_1.

Box 6.3 Experimental details

The protonmotive force, $\Delta\tilde{\mu}_{H^+}$ has two components: a membrane potential, ψ, across the inner mitochondrial membrane and a pH difference, ΔpH. In these experiments, the membrane potential was measured from the distribution of a lipophilic cation, methyltriphenylphosphonium cation (Ph_3MeP^+). A known amount was added to the mitochondrial suspension, and, because it is lipophilic, it equilibrated rapidly across the membrane with the equilibrium values of the inner and outer concentration dependent upon the membrane potential as described by the Nernst equation. The external concentration was continuously monitored by an electrode specific for the Ph_3MeP^+ ion, which allowed the matrix concentration, and hence the membrane potential, to be calculated. The pH difference could be measured by its effect on the distribution of the weak, permeant acid, [^3H]ethanoic acid between the mitochondrial matrix and the exterior but, in a number of tests where the distribution of the radioactivity from the ^3H was measured, it was found to be small and invariant relative to the membrane potential component.

There are three fluxes in the system: the formation of the protonmotive force by the respiratory chain, J_C; the dissipation of the protonmotive force by the leak of protons across the inner mitochondrial membrane, J_L, and the consumption of the protonmotive force by the ATP–synthesizing branch, J_P. These were all expressed in terms of the rate of oxygen consumption for three reasons.

(1) It was necessary for the analysis that all three fluxes were expressed on the same scale, since then $J_C = J_P + J_L$.

(2) The rate of oxygen consumption could be continuously monitored with an oxygen electrode, which was non–invasive and made it easier to ensure that flux measurements were made in a steady state.

(3) It avoids the uncertainties that would arise in converting the oxygen fluxes into proton or phosphorylation fluxes because of uncertainties in the stoichiometric ratios between these.

The experiments were performed on a series of steady states involving different rates of respiration, between the resting rate in the absence of phosphorylation and the maximal possible in a phosphorylating system (100% level), which were obtained by using different amounts of hexokinase. At each steady state, the respiratory chain

☞

Would this help? Let us imagine the possible results of the experiment. Either both blocks could have significant flux control coefficients, showing that the control is distributed, or one could be near 1, when the other would necessarily be near zero, showing that most of the control is somewhere inside one of the blocks. In both cases, the next step is to choose a different central metabolite, *i.e.* to form the blocks in a different way. In the first case, the results of the flux control coefficients for these two different blocks could be compared

☞ **Box 6.3 (continued)**

flux J_C and the protonmotive force $\Delta\tilde\mu_{H^+}$ were measured as the reference point, and a series of perturbations were made to measure the other variables.

Firstly, the phosphorylation and leak fluxes were measured as follows. In a sample of the same mitochondria, phosphorylation was suppressed with the inhibitor oligomycin, i.e. $J_P = 0$, $J_C = J_L$. This resulted in a lower respiration rate but higher protonmotive force than in the reference state. The protonmotive force and the respiration rate were then successively reduced in a titration with the respiratory chain inhibitor malonate (a competitive inhibitor of succinate dehydrogenase). A graph of these titration results was plotted, and the respiration rate that gave the same protonmotive force as in the reference state was read from the graph. This was taken to be J_L in the reference state, and the phosphorylation flux was found by difference $J_P = J_C - J_L$.

This same graph was also used to determine the elasticity of the leak block with respect to the protonmotive force. The slope of the graph is $dJ_L/d\Delta\tilde\mu_{H^+}$, and this is scaled by the values of the rate and protonmotive force at the reference state to give:

$$\varepsilon^L_{\Delta\tilde\mu_{H^+}} = \frac{dJ_L}{d\Delta\tilde\mu_{H^+}}\frac{\Delta\tilde\mu_{H^+}}{J_L}$$

A similar malonate titration experiment, except without oligomycin so that phosphorylation was active, was carried out and the respiratory chain flux plotted. The difference between the two graphs was taken as the phosphorylation flux J_P and this was in turn plotted against the protonmotive force. The gradient of this graph gave the elasticity of the phosphorylation block to the protonmotive force, i.e. :

$$\varepsilon^P_{\Delta\tilde\mu_{H^+}} = \frac{dJ_P}{d\Delta\tilde\mu_{H^+}}\frac{\Delta\tilde\mu_{H^+}}{J_P}$$

Finally, the elasticity of the respiratory chain block was measured by modulating one of the two branches and measuring J_C and the protonmotive force. Two methods were used: gradual increase of the leak flux by titration with an uncoupler, or increase of the phosphorylation flux by titration with hexokinase. As in the previous cases, the initial part of the titration gave a linear slope, and the gradient gave the elasticity:

$$\varepsilon^C_{\Delta\tilde\mu_{H^+}} = \frac{dJ_C}{d\Delta\tilde\mu_{H^+}}\frac{\Delta\tilde\mu_{H^+}}{J_C}$$

with the original set of results to allow deduction of the control coefficients for three blocks: the beginning and end blocks, and the block between the two chosen metabolites. In the second case, it might be found that the second experiment narrows down even further the section of the pathway where most of the control resides.

6.3.3.1 Experimental example: mitochondrial oxidative phosphorylation

Brand, Brown and co-workers applied this top–down methodology to the control of mitochondrial respiration and oxidative phosphorylation.[21,23,94,163] The system they studied was essentially similar to the one used by Groen et al. for the inhibitor titration studies discussed earlier in Chapter 6.1.4 in which isolated rat liver mitochondria oxidized succinate and drove an ATP-utilizing system that converted the ATP formed in phosphorylation back to ADP, thus allowing the system to attain a steady state. They chose the protonmotive force as the central metabolite, which divides the system into three blocks, as shown in Figure 6.20. It might seem odd to regard the protonmotive force as a metabolite, but it is the intermediate that is formed by respiration and is used by the proton leak and phosphorylation. Furthermore, the protonmotive force is logarithmically related to the proton concentration in the matrix, and since logarithms of concentration usually appear in elasticities, the protonmotive force itself can be used to define the elasticity. It is, of course, necessary to measure the protonmotive force. The fluxes were measured in terms of the oxygen consumption, measured for the respiration branch with an oxygen electrode. The distribution of the flux at the branch point had also to be measured, *i.e.* the relative contributions of the leak and the phosphorylating system to the consumption of the protonmotive force had to be determined. A more detailed explanation of how this was done is given in the Box 6.3.

The elasticity of any one block with respect to the protonmotive force was determined by inhibiting or stimulating one of the other blocks in order to change the value of the protonmotive force. Thus if the elasticity of the phosphorylating system was required, it was obtained from the slope of the phosphorylation-coupled component of the respiration rate as the respiratory chain block was titrated with the inhibitor malonate. Again this is covered in more detail in Box 6.3.

The results were calculated by the simultaneous solution of three equations. For example, the control coefficients on the respiratory chain flux came from solving the summation equation:

$$C_C^{J_C} + C_P^{J_C} + C_L^{J_C} = 1 \qquad (6.14)$$

the connectivity equation:

$$C_C^{J_C} \varepsilon_{\Delta\tilde{\mu}_{H^+}}^C + C_P^{J_C} \varepsilon_{\Delta\tilde{\mu}_{H^+}}^P + C_L^{J_C} \varepsilon_{\Delta\tilde{\mu}_{H^+}}^L = 0 \qquad (6.15)$$

and a branch-point equation worked out according to a set of rules devised by Herbert Sauro and myself[69]

$$\frac{C_P^{J_C}}{J_P} - \frac{C_L^{J_C}}{J_L} = 0. \qquad (6.16)$$

The results obtained in this way by Hafner, Brown & Brand[94] are shown in Figure 6.21. The range of the control coefficients on the respiration flux between the minimum and maximum respiration rates was approximately: $C_L^{J_C} =$

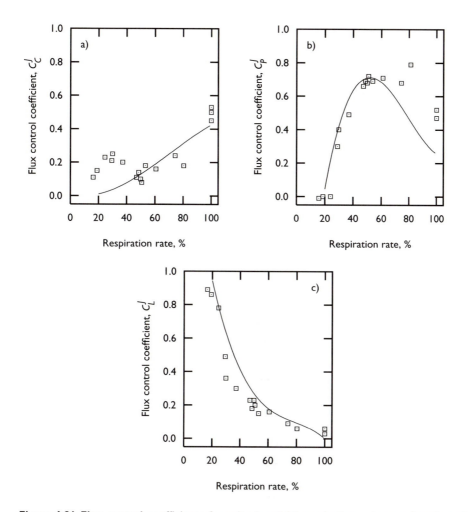

Figure 6.21 Flux control coefficients for mitochondrial respiration rate as a function of respiration rate

The results of Hafner et al.[94] are compared with the corresponding results of Groen et al.[92] (a) The flux control coefficient of the respiratory chain (block C, Figure 6.20). Points from Hafner et al. are shown with the curve of Groen et al. for the dicarboxylate carrier only (step 1 in block C, Figure 6.20) taken from Figure 6.15. (b) The flux control coefficient of the phosphorylation block (block P, Figure 6.20). Again, the experimental points are shown with the sum of the two curves through the the coefficients for the adenine nucleotide translocator and hexokinase (steps 6 and 7, block P) from Figure 6.15. (c) The flux control coefficient of the leak (block L). The experimental points are shown with the corresponding curve from Figure 6.15.

0.9–0.0; $C_P^{J_C} = 0.0$–0.7, and $C_C^{J_C} = 0.1$–0.5. The profiles between these points resembles the results Groen et al.[92] had obtained by inhibitor titrations, although to see this, it is necessary to group these latter results into the appropriate blocks. In order to do this, I used the smooth curves drawn on the graph of their results (Figure 6.15) and superimposed them on Figure 6.21. Under the circumstances, the degree of agreement between the results of the Cambridge

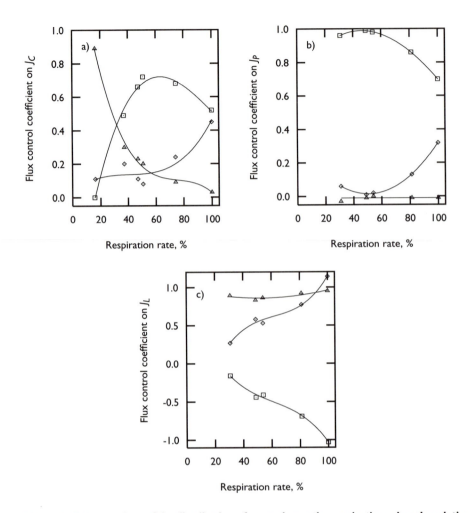

Figure 6.22 Comparison of the distribution of control over the respiration, phosphorylation and leak fluxes in mitochondrial oxidative phosphorylation
The results were derived by top–down control analysis of rat liver mitochondria.[94] (a) Control of the respiration flux, J_C. Points from a single experiment from Figure 6.21 summarized on one graph. (b) Control of the phosphorylation flux, J_P. One of the sets of results from Figure 6.21 recalculated. (c) Control of the leak flux, J_L, again recalculated from results in Figure 6.21. $\diamond$, flux control coefficients for the respiratory chain block; $\square$, flux control coefficients for the phosphorylation block; $\triangle$, flux control coefficients for the leak block. This Figure is based on one by Brand.[20]

and Amsterdam groups is remarkably good, and it can be taken as providing some independent validation of both experimental methods: the inhibitor titration method, and the top–down control analysis via block elasticities.

Once again, the results demonstrate that the distribution of the control of flux varies according to the metabolic steady state. There is also another feature of control that can be illustrated by further analysis of this system. Because there are three fluxes in this branched system, we can ask whether the distribution of control is the same for all three; we shall see that it is not.

Suppose that we wish to calculate the distribution of control over the flux in the phosphorylation branch, J_P. The flux control coefficients will be related by a summation theorem, exactly the same as Eqn. (6.14) above, except with J_P instead of J_C. The connectivity theorem equation will likewise be the same as Eqn. (6.15) above. The third equation, the branch point equation, is, however, different. It is now:

$$\frac{C_C^{J_P}}{J_C} + \frac{C_L^{J_P}}{J_L} = 0. \tag{6.17}$$

Just as Eqn. (6.16), which applied to the respiratory chain flux J_C, did not contain the control coefficient $C_C^{J_C}$, the new equation does not contain the control coefficient with respect to the phosphorylation block, $C_P^{J_P}$. The sign has also changed, because the two fluxes now involved have opposite orientations, in that J_C produces the protonmotive force and J_L uses it whereas, in the previous case, both the fluxes related to utilization of protonmotive force. The solutions of the set of three equations are consequently different, as can be seen in Figure 6.22(b). Over most of the range of respiratory rates, the majority of control of the phosphorylation flux lies in its own block. This top–down experiment cannot tell the distribution of this control between the different steps within the block. However, the share of the phosphorylation control exerted by the adenine nucleotide translocator and the ATP-utilization system should be the same as their share of respiratory control as observed by Groen et al. in Figure 6.15. (This ratio of control is not affected by the change in the reference flux.)

When the flux control coefficients are calculated for the control over the leak flux, J_L, a different pattern is seen again. Once again, the same summation and connectivity theorem equations apply, but the branch-point equation is different and does not contain J_L:

$$\frac{C_C^{J_L}}{J_C} + \frac{C_P^{J_L}}{J_P} = 0 \tag{6.18}$$

The results are shown in Figure 6.22(c). At high respiratory flux rates, the solution is remarkable for having two flux control coefficients near 1, and the third near -1. Under all circumstances, the leak itself has a high level of control over its flux, but the degree of control of the other two blocks increases with increasing rate of respiration.

6.3.3.2 Experimental example: hepatocyte energy metabolism

The studies on the control of oxidative phosphorylation in isolated mitochodria have led to a considerable advance over previous attempts to identify the rate–limiting step. Nevertheless, to what extent can these findings be applied to mitochondria working in cells? After all, in the experiments, large amounts of succinate are made available externally, whereas *in vivo*, succinate would be generated in smaller concentrations in the matrix of the mitochondria. The ATP-utilizing reactions in the cell are also more varied than the single reaction

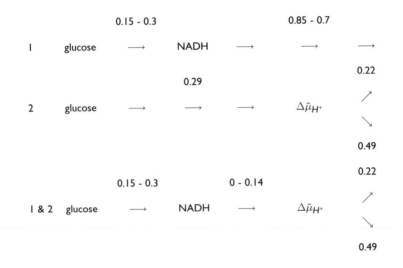

Figure 6.23 Two overlapping top–down analyses of cellular respiration
The two experiments used NADH and $\Delta\tilde{\mu}_{H^+}$ as the two central intermediates and are shown in the first two lines. At the end of the second and third lines, the upward arrow is the dissipation of protonmotive force by the leak and the downward arrow is phosphorylation and ATP utilization. The third line combines the two results to infer a flux control coefficient for the respiratory chain.

(hexokinase) used in the experiments. The Cambridge group went on to consider this by applying the top–down experimental approach to the control of respiration in isolated hepatocytes[23] supplied with glucose as an oxidizable substrate. In one set of experiments, they took the mitochondrial $NAD^+/NADH$ pair as the central metabolite, dividing the system into an NADH supply block (glycolysis and the Krebs cycle) and an NADH demand block (the respiratory chain, phosphorylation, etc). To do this, they had to measure the mitochondrial NADH by fluorescence; oxygen consumption flux was once again measured with an oxygen electrode. The flux control coefficient of the NADH producers, C_{supply}^{Jc}, was estimated to be in the range 0.15–0.3, with that of the NADH users, C_{demand}^{Jc}, 0.85–0.7.

In another set of experiments, they used the mitochondrial protonmotive force as the central 'metabolite', effectively repeating the mitochondrial experiments described above, except that this time they were using whole cells. As before, metabolism was divided into three blocks: a block generating the protonmotive force by oxidizing glucose and the leak and phosphorylation blocks consuming it. They showed that the flux control coefficient of the phosphorylation block was about 0.49, that of the generating block was 0.29, and that of the leak block was 0.22.

From the overlaps between these two sets of experiments, a more detailed picture of the control can be built up as shown in Figure 6.23. The two important conclusions are first that the pattern of control over the rate of respiration is very similar to that observed in the studies of isolated mitochondria for intermediate respiration rates (e.g. Figure 6.22a). In particular, the block containing the phosphorylation of ADP to ATP and the consumption of ATP by cellular processes is the one exerting the largest amount of control. Much less control is shared between catabolism and the respiratory chain. (This concentration of control in the lower end of the pathway is highly significant, for reasons that will be analysed later in Chapter 7.1.) Secondly, Control Analysis is shown to be applicable to the totality of cellular energy metabolism and, with two applications of the top–down approach, the section of metabolism having the largest influence on respiratory rate has been identified.

6.3.3.3 Fatty acid metabolism

Top–down analysis is also being used by Patti Quant and her colleagues in Cambridge to study the control of fatty acid utilization and ketone body formation.[153,187,188] In the case of ketogenesis, the traditional criteria for identifying rate–limiting enzymes had led some groups to favour carnitine palmitoyltransferase I and others to support hydroxymethylglutaryl-CoA synthase. The measurements of control coefficients so far show that their values vary with metabolic state, but neither of these enzymes is fully rate–limiting in any of the experiments. (Some of their results are presented in Problem 5 at the end of this chapter.)

6.3.4 Calculation of elasticities
6.3.4.1 Theory

Perhaps readers may be surprised that the calculation of elasticity values from metabolite concentrations and enzyme kinetic information was not one of the first options to be discussed as a means of deriving control coefficients from elasticities. After all, in Chapter 5.3 I introduced elasticities in terms of their relationships to known enzyme kinetic functions, and in Appendix 3 to that Chapter, *More about elasticities*, p. 131, I gave more detail about how elasticities could be calculated from any enzyme rate law. However, in that Appendix, I also mentioned some of the difficulties that arise in this approach because the enzyme kinetics experiments recorded in the biochemical literature were not made with this application in mind and therefore often do not include all the relevant measurements. Even so, a day in the library conducting a literature search sometimes yields some appropriate information, though the chances that the measurements were made on the cell type you want to study are not high unless it is *Saccharomyces cerevisiae*, *Escherichia coli* or rat liver cells.

If the kinetic rate law and its parameters are known, the next set of information required is the concentrations of all the metabolites that influence the enzyme rate, measured in the metabolic steady state of interest. This raises all the usual problems of interpretation (see Chapter 2.3, p. 30). Are the measurements of cellular metabolite concentrations representative of the actual concentrations experienced by the enzyme in the cell? That is, do they reflect the free concentrations of the metabolites or are they affected by significant amounts of bound metabolites? Are the measurements applicable to the compartment of the cell where the enzyme is located? Perhaps this list of problems seems formidable, but even so, I do not believe we should give up. None of them is unique to Metabolic Control Analysis; they apply equally to other forms of biochemical explanation, and the reductionist ethos of much biochemistry (see Chapter 1.2.1, p. 5) would be undermined if there were no confidence in the applicability of such results. Would it be sensible to believe that incorporating the available information into a logical quantitative framework such as Metabolic Control Analysis would give less reliable results than applying the same information in a set of semi–quantitative principles (see Chapter 4) which we have seen can only be partially justified and can often be misleading? For example, qualitative theories of control will often assess the potential importance of a regulatory interaction by comparison of a metabolite concentration with its K_m, K_i or K_a value for a particular enzyme on the assumption that the enzyme will respond if the two are of comparable magnitude. We have seen, in the chapter on enzyme kinetics (for example, Chapters 3.2 and 3.3) that a single kinetic parameter cannot serve to define the effect of a metabolite concentration on an enzyme rate without considering the concentrations of other relevant metabolites and their associated parameters. The elasticity, on the other hand, does reflect the interaction of all these factors. Furthermore, we know that the elasticity alone is not enough; its influence on the flux control coefficient or response coefficient of the enzyme has to be considered.

In spite of the admitted problems in getting reliable information for elasticity calculations, there is another reason why it may still be worth attempting. This is that the results of Metabolic Control Analysis are not necessarily particularly sensitive to inaccuracies in the information used in the calculations either of the elasticities or, from them, of the flux control coefficients. One reason can be seen by looking at the diagrams of elasticity values against metabolite concentration (Figures 5.6–5.9): for much of the range, the elasticities are not changing very rapidly relative to substrate concentration, so errors in the substrate concentration (or equivalently, in the corresponding K_m value) do not cause errors of corresponding size in the elasticity. Two cases where this is not so turn out to be rather different from one another. One case is for enzymes near to equilibrium, where the elasticity grows very rapidly as the metabolite concentrations tend to their equilibrium values. Inaccuracy here is of little significance because, as summarized in Chapter 5.5.1, Kacser & Burns showed[119] that the flux control coefficients of such enzymes tend to zero. The other concerns small inhibition elasticities; studies with my co-workers Rankin Small and Simon Thomas have shown that these are much more important.

In our work,[228,232,246] they devised procedures for assessing the influence that individual elasticity values have on the calculated values of the flux control coefficients. Some of our conclusions have been that:

- the values of the control coefficients are not equally sensitive to the values of all the elasticities;

- the dependence of the value of any control coefficient on the value of an elasticity follows a hyperbolic or inverse hyperbolic response, *i.e.* the value of the control coefficient changes relatively rapidly with the elasticity when the elasticity is small (much less than 1), but tends to a constant value as the elasticity increases;

- this applies particularly to elasticities of near equilibrium reactions, because the elasticities are not only large in magnitude, but appear in substrate–product pairs whose contributions tend to cancel, leading to the tendency to small control coefficients mentioned above;

- small feedback and product inhibition elasticities will tend to be particularly important, in that small changes in their values will have the largest effects on the control coefficients. (See also Section 6.2, p. 163, for evidence from computer modelling that even weak product inhibition effects are important in metabolism.)

The general conclusion is that using an approximate value for many of the elasticities will not make a significant difference to the calculated flux control coefficients, and the validity of this assumption can always be tested by the procedures devised by Small and Thomas. Simon Thomas' computer program Metacon automates the calculations.[245,246] Therefore, as previously mentioned, the elasticity values of near–equilibrium enzymes can frequently be calculated with sufficient accuracy using only the displacement from equilibrium terms in Eqns. (5.13) and (5.14). The elasticity values that will cause problems are small ones, particularly those associated with weak inhibition effects; not only is it necessary to have an accurate value for them, it is essential to know that they exist at all, and here there is a weakness in the biochemical literature, because weak inhibition effects have not been of much interest, since it is only recently that it has become apparent how important they are.

6.3.4.2 Applications

Keith Snell drew my attention to the evidence that the control of the pathway for synthesis of the amino acid serine in mammalian liver might be rather unusual. The pathway branches off from the glycolytic intermediate 3–phosphoglycerate and involves three enzymes, phosphoglycerate dehydrogenase, phosphoserine aminotransferase and phosphoserine phosphatase catalysing the sequence:

3–phosphoglycerate $\longrightarrow$ phosphohydroxypyruvate

$\longrightarrow$ phosphoserine $\longrightarrow$ serine   (Scheme 6.3)

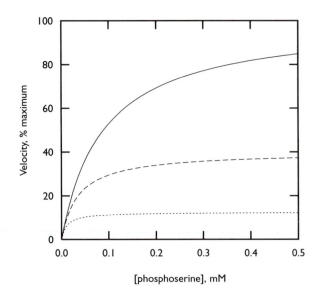

Figure 6.24 Inhibition of rat liver phosphoserine phosphatase by serine
The inhibition is of the uncompetitive type. Note that the curves are close together at low substrate concentrations and diverge at higher ones. The solid curve is in the absence of serine; the dashed one is at 1 mM, and the dotted one, 6 mM. Levels of serine in rabbit liver are typically between these values, and intracellular phosphoserine is about 0.4 mM.

The first step is an NAD–dependent oxidation, the second a transamination with glutamate as donor, and the third the hydrolysis of a phosphate group. The pathway can be regarded as starting at 3–phosphoglycerate because the flux to serine is so small relative to the glycolytic flux that the serine pathway will have little effect on the 3–phosphoglycerate levels. What appeared unusual about this pathway was first that published measurements of the metabolite levels in rabbit liver suggested that the first two steps were nearer to equilibrium than the final step, and secondly that the most obvious regulatory interaction known from previous enzyme kinetic studies was inhibition of the third step, phosphoserine phosphatase, by the end product serine.

At first sight, there seemed to be enough information to calculate the elasticities of the enzymes and thus the flux control coefficients, but as so often is the case, not all the information was quite complete. For example, phosphohydroxypyruvate concentrations in liver are too low to be readily measurable; however, since 3–phosphoglycerate and phosphoserine were nearly in equilibrium (taking into account the NAD^+, NADH, glutamate and 2–oxoglutarate levels), the first two reactions could be combined as one near–equilibrium reaction and its elasticities to 3–phosphoglycerate and phosphoserine calculated from the displacement from equilibrium. The kinetic information on the other step was also not ideal, in that the measurements had been made on chicken liver and rat liver, not rabbit liver. However, we reanalysed the measurements and showed that both sets were explained best by the serine inhibition being of the uncompetitive type (Figure 6.24). Although there were differences in the K_m values and inhibition parameters between the rat and chicken enzymes, these were not so great as to give grounds for believing that the rabbit enzyme would be very different. With the equation for uncompetitive inhibition and the parameters of the rat liver enzyme, we calculated the elasticities of phospho-serine phosphatase to its substrate phosphoserine and the pathway end product, serine.

Thus the problem we analysed had become a two step pathway with a single intermediate, phosphoserine, for which we had the elasticities. Examples of the calculation method have already been given, so it will not be shown here; Question 2 in the Problems section asks you to calculate the solution. We found[71,235] that, in normal rabbit liver where there is a relatively high biosynthetic flux, phosphoserine phosphatase has the largest flux control coefficient (0.97), whereas the first two enzymes are close to equilibrium and have negligible flux control coefficients. Phosphoserine phosphatase is inhibited by the pathway product serine, giving a calculated response coefficient of −0.63 for the effect of serine on the pathway flux. In contrast, the response coefficient of the flux to the pathway source, 3–phosphoglycerate, is about one-tenth of this value, so the flux is largely determined by the serine concentration through inhibition of the final step. This is an exception to the common pattern where the first enzyme after a pathway branches off is usually the enzyme subject to end–product inhibition. The strong control exerted by serine on the pathway flux is dependent on the strange properties of uncompetitive inhibition. In uncompetitive inhibition, the inhibitor has contradictory actions: it inhibits by reducing the apparent limiting rate (like a non–competitive inhibitor), but at the same time it reduces the K_m of the enzyme for its substrate, which would normally cause an activation. This has the result that the stimulatory and inhibitory effects are almost in balance at low substrate concentrations, but inhibition predominates as the substrate concentration increases. As can be seen from the graph of phosphoserine phosphatase kinetics (Figure 6.24), the degree of inhibition is higher at high substrate concentrations than at low ones. This is the exact opposite of competitive inhibition, but is well adapted to feedback inhibition, since the general effect of inhibiting a pathway enzyme is to increase the concentration of its substrate, which could potentially nullify the action of a competitive inhibitor. In fact, at intracellular levels of serine in rabbit liver, phosphoserine phosphatase is effectively almost saturated with its substrate.

6.3.4.3 Hybrid examples
Several research groups have adopted a hybrid strategy towards the determination of elasticity values, in that they have calculated elasticity values for steps with well-characterized kinetics or that are not likely to have a significant influence on the values of the flux control coefficients, but have measured more

critical elasticities, or those for which there is inadequate information. In fact, some of the studies mentioned previously have relied on calculation methods for some of the elasticities, for example, the study of the control of gluconeogenesis in hepatocytes by Groen et al.[89, 91] described earlier in Chapter 6.3.1.

Galazzo & Bailey[77] have used NMR to measure the concentrations of intermediates in the glycolytic pathway of yeast (*Saccharomyces cerevisiae*). They then used these concentrations in the kinetic equations of the glycolytic enzymes to calculate their elasticities and then their flux control coefficients. The results varied for the different incubation conditions they had used, though the largest control coefficients were shown by glucose entry into the cell, phosphofructokinase and ATP consumption processes. However, the conclusions depend strongly on two elasticities that are not well characterized: the feedback inhibition of glucose transport by glucose 6–phosphate and the group elasticity of ATP–utilizing processes with respect to ATP.

Salter et al. also used some calculated elasticities in their study of the control of aromatic amino acid metabolism by hepatocytes[207] (see Chapters 6.1.2 and 6.1.4.3, and Table 6.3). In particular, they calculated the elasticities of the amino acid transporters to their amino acids from the displacement from equilibrium, and combined them with the response coefficients of the catabolic fluxes to the external levels of the amino acids to calculate the flux control coefficients of the transport steps. These varied from about 0.25 for transport of tyrosine and tryptophan at basal catabolic levels to 0.93 for phenylalanine transport when catabolism was induced.

6.4   Summary

(1) There is now a large and growing body of experimental measurements of flux control coefficients in a range of different pathways and organisms. Although the experiments require a good degree of accuracy in order to obtain reasonably reliable values for flux control coefficients, they are based on familiar experimental techniques from genetics, molecular biology and biochemistry.

(2) Direct methods of measuring flux control coefficients involve measuring the change in flux when the amount or activity of an enzyme is manipulated by some means. Indirect methods, including the top–down approach, involve calculation of the control coefficients from measured elasticity values (or from calculated elasticities based on experimental measurements of metabolites and enzyme kinetic parameters).

(3) Values of flux control coefficients vary depending on the prevailing conditions.

(4) There are only a few cases where a flux control coefficient is very close to 1.0, and in some of these, in extreme rather than physiologically normal

conditions. Thus the control of a pathway by a single, rate–limiting enzyme has been experimentally proved not to be the norm.

(5) As predicted by the theory, the control of flux is distributed, with more than one step in a pathway having some measure of control. However, most flux control coefficients are found to be relatively small or zero.

6.5 Appendix: Oxidative phosphorylation revision

Oxidative phosphorylation is most commonly studied on intact mitochondria isolated from cells and consists of the steps from the oxidation of compounds such as NADH and succinate by oxygen and the associated phosphorylation of ADP by phosphate to form ATP. The rate of substrate oxidation is determined from the oxygen consumption, which is measured with an oxygen electrode. Although mitochondria would normally generate their own oxidizable materials via pathways such as the tricarboxylic acid cycle and β–oxidation, in the experiments, the oxidizable substrate is added externally. This brings minor complications. For example, succinate is normally produced internally in the matrix of the mitochondrion *in vivo*, but has to be transported across the mitochondrial membranes in the *in vitro* experiments. In addition, externally added NADH cannot be oxidized by animal mitochondria because it does not cross the mitochondrial inner membrane and the NADH oxidase is only accessible from the mitochondrial matrix. Therefore, to study the oxidation of NADH, it is necessary to supply the mitochondria with metabolites that will be transported into the mitochondrial matrix and be oxidized there by NAD^+–dependent dehydrogenases; examples of suitable compounds include β–hydroxybutyrate, pyruvate plus malate and glutamate plus malate.

The oxidation of the substrates by oxygen is carried out by the electron transport chain, which is composed of a number of complexes of electron transport components. Complex I is NADH–ubiquinone oxidoreductase (EC 1.6.5.3); Complex II is succinate dehydrogenase (ubiquinone), EC 1.3.5.1. (The supposed succinate dehydrogenase, described by many textbooks, that reacts with FAD is merely a partial reaction of the catalytic cycle of this complex.) The ubiquinol (or reduced Coenzyme Q) produced by these complexes is oxidized by Complex III, or ubiquinol–cytochrome *c* reductase (EC 1.10.2.2). Reduced cytochrome *c* is oxidized with oxygen by the cytochrome *c* oxidase complex (EC 1.9.3.1) or Complex IV. In animal mitochondria, Complexes I, III and IV are coupled to the phosphorylation of ADP, but this does not imply, as previously assumed, that oxidation of an NADH generates 3 ATP molecules whereas oxidation of a succinate generates 2.

The linkage between oxidation and phosphorylation is described by Mitchell's chemiosmotic theory. The electron transport complexes coupled to phosphorylation move protons out of the mitochondrial matrix across the inner mitochondrial membrane, thereby creating both a concentration difference

(or ΔpH) and a membrane potential difference (or $\Delta\psi$) that together consti-
tute the protonmotive force (PMF or $\Delta\tilde{\mu}_{H^+}$). The PMF is the reservoir of
energy that drives phosphorylation of ADP. This reservoir is tapped by the
H$^+$–transporting ATP synthase (EC 3.6.1.34), which allows protons back into
the mitochondrial matrix and captures their energy for the formation of ATP
from ADP and phosphate. The oxidation of NADH results in four protons
being pumped out at Complex I, two at Complex III and four at Complex IV,
giving a total of ten protons. It is thought that a total of four protons are needed
to take in ADP and phosphate from outside the mitochondria, turn them into
ATP and return the ATP outside the mitochondrion. Therefore, the P/O ratio,
that is the number of ATP molecules formed per oxygen atom used in oxidation
of NADH, is 10/4 or 2.5. Since succinate is not oxidized via Complex I, its
P/O ratio is 6/4 or 1.5.

Some of the PMF can dissipate without protons going through the ATP synthase. The principal cause of this is the 'leak' reaction, which is most significant
when phosphorylation is going slowly and least significant when phosphorylation is rapid. The 'leak' reaction can be stimulated by uncouplers, which
increase the permeability of the mitochondrial membrane to protons.

The phosphorylation process requires that ADP is transported into the mitochondrion and returned back to the outside as ATP. These two transport
steps are coupled as an exchange process catalysed by the adenine nucleotide
translocator.

There are two basic types of experiments performed on mitochondria in
the study of oxidative phosphorylation. In pulse experiments, mitochondria
are supplied with an oxidizable substrate and their rate of respiration measured. A known amount of ADP is added; this causes a noticeable stimulation
of respiration (known as State 3 respiration) until all the ADP has been converted to ATP, when the respiration rate returns close to its original rate (State
4). From the oxygen consumption profile, it is possible to calculate the amount
of oxygen used to phosphorylate the known amount of ADP. However, in this
experiment, the steady states are only transient; the mitochondria pass from
zero phosphorylation to maximal phosphorylation rate and back with relatively
brief periods in the intermediate states. This is unlikely to be similar to physiological conditions in most cell types. The alternative is to set up a steady state
phosphorylation rate. One way of doing this is to use the enzyme hexokinase
in the presence of glucose as a means of recycling the ATP back to ADP (along
with the formation of glucose 6–phosphate, which can be measured to find out
the phosphorylation rate) as shown in Figure 6.13. By varying the amount of
hexokinase, the rate of phosphorylation, and hence oxygen consumption, can
be adjusted, and the steady state lasts until the oxygen runs out.

Most of the characteristics usually described in the textbooks relate to mammalian mitochondria, or more specifically, rat liver mitochondria. Experiments,
including Control Analysis studies, have been performed on mitochondria from
other sources, for example from yeast and from various plants, even though it is

more difficult to isolate the organelles successfully from them. There are, however, some significant differences between the details of the electron transport components and coupling sites of these mitochondria from the animal ones.

Further reading

Fell, D. A. (1992) *Metabolic Control Analysis: a survey of its theoretical and experimental development.* Biochem. J. **286**, 313–330

Quant, P. A. (1993) *Experimental application of top–down Control Analysis to metabolic systems.* Trends Biochem. Sci. **18**, 26–30

Salter, M., Knowles, R. G. & Pogson, C. I. (1994) *Metabolic control.* In Essays in Biochemistry (Tipton, K. F. ed.), vol. 28, pp. 1–12, Portland Press, London

Computer programs

Several programs are available to carry out simulation and Metabolic Control Analysis of metabolic pathways. At the time of writing, the following programs for PC-compatible microcomputers are available over the Internet by 'anonymous FTP' from my laboratory at *bmsdarwin.brookes.ac.uk* in the directory *pub/software/ibmpc*:

- SCAMP, a package for carrying out simulation, steady state analysis and Metabolic Control Analysis;[209,211]

- Gepasi, a similar package to SCAMP with an interface for the Windows operating system;.[158]

- Metamodel, a package for steady state and control analysis of simple pathways;[106]

- Metacon, a package for determining the algebraic expressions relating control coefficients to the elasticities of a network and calculating the uncertainties in the control coefficients that arise from the errors in the elasticity measurements.[245,246]

Problems

(1) Citrulline is synthesized in mitochondria by the reactions:

    (a) $NH_4^+ + HCO_3^- + 2ATP \longrightarrow$ carbamoyl-phosphate $+ 2ADP + P_i$

    (b) carbamoyl phosphate $+$ ornithine $\longrightarrow$ citrulline $+ P_i$

Reaction 1a is catalysed by carbamoyl-phosphate synthase (CPS) and reaction 1b by ornithine transcarbamoylase (OTC). If the elasticities
of these two enzymes with respect to carbamoyl phosphate (cp) are
$\varepsilon_{cp}^{CPS} = -0.011$ and $\varepsilon_{cp}^{OTC} = 0.92$, what are the relative values of their
flux control coefficients C_{CPS}^J and C_{OTC}^J?

(2) In the serine biosynthesis pathway:

$$3\text{-phosphoglycerate} \xrightarrow{\ 1\ } \text{phosphoserine} \xrightarrow{\ 2\ } \text{serine}$$

the elasticity of the first step, ε_{pser}^1, is -1.43 in the liver of rabbits on
a normal low-protein diet. (The first step is actually catalysed by two
enzymes, but the elasticity is the 'combined' elasticity for them both, so
they can be treated as a single step.) The elasticity of the second step,
ε_{pser}^2, is 0.041. What are the flux control coefficients, C_1^J and C_2^J, of the
two steps?

The response coefficients for the responses of flux to changes in the pathway source, phosphoglycerate (3pg), and the product, serine (ser), are
given by the Kacser & Burns combined response equations:

$$R_{3pg}^J = C_1^J . \varepsilon_{3pg}^1 : R_{ser}^J = C_2^J . \varepsilon_{ser}^2$$

where $\varepsilon_{3pg}^1 = 2.43$ and $\varepsilon_{ser}^2 = -0.65$. ('$J$' signifies the pathway flux.) What
does this suggest to you about the regulation of this pathway?

(3) Stitt et al. determined how the rate of photosynthetic sucrose synthesis in
spinach cytosol depended on two groups of enzymes. Group 1 consists
of aldolase and fructose bisphosphatase and converts triose phosphate
(delivered by the chloroplasts) into hexose phosphate. Group 2 contains phosphoglucose isomerase, phosphoglucomutase, UDPG synthase,
sucrose phosphate synthase and sucrose phosphatase and converts hexose phosphate to sucrose. Elasticities for hexose-phosphate on the two
groups were determined as $\varepsilon_{hexose-P}^1 = -0.8$ and $\varepsilon_{hexose-P}^2 = 1.0$. What
are the flux control coefficients of the two groups, C_1^J and C_2^J, on the
flux J to sucrose?

Group 1 responds to the supply of triose phosphate from the chloroplasts
with an elasticity estimated as $\varepsilon_{triose-P}^1 = 1.6$. What is the response
coefficient, $R_{triose-P}^J$, for the effect of triose phosphate on the flux to
sucrose?

(4) Brand et al. considered the control of respiration in non–phosphorylating
mitochondria (i.e. in the absence of ADP). They argued that the system
can be considered as one in which the respiratory chain (rc) produces an
intermediate (the protonmotive force, $\Delta\mu$) which is consumed by leakage
back across the membrane. It is possible to regard $\Delta\mu$ as an intermediate

and estimate elasticities for the two reactions rc and leak, i.e.:

$$\text{oxidizable substrate} \xrightarrow{\text{rc}} \Delta\mu \xrightarrow{\text{leak}} \text{dissipation}$$

The fluxes were measured in terms of the rate of oxygen consumption, J_O, accompanying substrate oxidation. The measured elasticities were $\varepsilon_{\Delta\mu}^{rc} = -15.2$ and $\varepsilon_{\Delta\mu}^{leak} = 7.9$. What are the two flux control coefficients $C_{rc}^{J_O}$ and $C_{leak}^{J_O}$?

(5) In experiments on the top–down analysis of ketogenesis, the acetyl-CoA/CoA couple can be regarded as the central metabolite, produced by β–oxidation and utilized by ketogenesis. Both steps can be simultaneously modulated by using pyruvate to perturb the acetyl-CoA level, giving the following results:

[Pyruvate] (mM)	[Acetyl-CoA]/ [CoA]	$J_{\beta - \text{oxidation}}$ (nmol·min^{-1}·mg^{-1})	$J_{\text{ketogenesis}}$ (nmol·min^{-1}·mg^{-1})
0.0	1.25	21.1	18.9
2.5	2.23	15.8	19.2
5.0	4.75	5.3	23.9

Make two log–log plots of the fluxes against [acetyl-CoA]/[CoA] and measure the slopes to determine the elasticities. Using these elasticity measurements, determine the flux control coefficients of the acetyl-CoA-producing block and the -consuming block. (This calculation method will not give exactly the same answer as that published by Quant and colleagues using a different method of analysis.[188])

Control structures in metabolism

So far, we have considered the potential that an enzyme might have for controlling a pathway without having given particular consideration to its place in the metabolic network. However, there is further organization in metabolism beyond the serial sequences of reactions that we call metabolic pathways. In this chapter, we shall look at some of the features of these higher levels of organization and their potential roles in control, both as conventionally interpreted and in the light of Metabolic Control Analysis. Once again we will find that there are aspects of the conventional views that do not stand up to close analysis.

7.1 Supply and demand

First let us consider the most basic problem of metabolic regulation and control: how to regulate the concentration of a metabolite when controls are exerted to alter the rate of its production and consumption. The simplest structure that we can analyse in metabolism that exhibits this feature is the synthesis of some metabolite M from a source metabolite X_{source} by a *supply* pathway and its use by a *demand* pathway:

$$X_{source} \xrightarrow{\text{supply}} M \xrightarrow{\text{demand}} X_{sink} \qquad \text{(Scheme 7.1)}$$

This is just the same simplification that is used in the 'top–down' method of Metabolic Control Analysis considered in Chapter 6.3.3, p. 176 and, as in that method, the supply and demand steps can each be a composite of many individual steps without changing the essential nature of the problem. For example M might be an amino acid, in which case the supply step would be its synthetic pathway and the demand step could be protein synthesis. Alternatively,

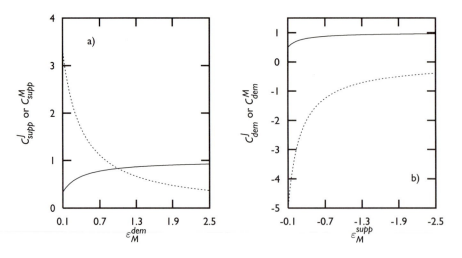

Figure 7.1   Control of flux and regulation of concentration
Relationships between the control coefficients and elasticities for the two step pathway of Scheme 7.1.
(a) Control by the supply pathway with $\varepsilon_M^{supply} = -0.2$: —, C_{supply}^J; · · ·, C_{supply}^M. (b) Control by the demand
pathway with $\varepsilon_M^{demand} = 0.2$: —, C_{demand}^J; · · ·, C_{demand}^M.

M might be a central metabolic intermediate such as acetyl-CoA, in which
case supply would be a catabolic pathway such as glycolysis and the demand
might be further catabolism in the tricarboxylic acid cycle or else fatty acid
biosynthesis.

Jannie Hofmeyr and Athel Cornish–Bowden[106] analysed how regulation of
M interacts with the control of flux by looking at the factors that affect the flux
and concentration control coefficients and their relative values. Their reason for
doing this was that the flux control coefficients show how effective the supply
and demand pathways can be at controlling the flux (assuming the existence
of some mechanism for changing the overall activity of either of these steps).
At the same time, the concentration control coefficients show how much M
will change if control is exerted on either of the steps. The method of deriving
the flux control coefficients of the two steps in terms of the elasticities was
explained in Chapter 5.3.3, p. 120. For Scheme 7.1, the solutions are:

$$C_{supply}^J = \frac{\varepsilon_M^{demand}}{\varepsilon_M^{demand} - \varepsilon_M^{supply}} = \frac{1}{1+Q} \tag{7.1}$$

$$C_{demand}^J = \frac{-\varepsilon_M^{supply}}{\varepsilon_M^{demand} - \varepsilon_M^{supply}} = \frac{Q}{1+Q} \tag{7.2}$$

where Q, which is equal to $-\varepsilon_M^{supply}/\varepsilon_M^{demand}$, has been introduced to emphasize that it is the relative values of the two elasticities that determine the flux
control distribution rather than their absolute values. (The minus sign gives
Q a positive value because ε_{supply}^M, the product inhibition elasticity, is typically

negative.) The control coefficients on M can be derived in a similar fashion (see Chapter 5.8.1, p. 130) to give:

$$C_{supply}^{M} = \frac{1}{\varepsilon_M^{demand} - \varepsilon_M^{supply}} = \frac{1}{\varepsilon_M^{demand}} \frac{1}{1 + Q} \qquad (7.3)$$

$$C_{demand}^{M} = \frac{-1}{\varepsilon_M^{demand} - \varepsilon_M^{supply}} = \frac{-1}{\varepsilon_M^{demand}} \frac{1}{1 + Q} \qquad (7.4)$$

Obviously $C_{supply}^{M} = -C_{demand}^{M}$, but it is not possible to express the concentration control coefficients solely in terms of the elasticity ratio. In fact, the magnitude of the concentration control coefficients are inversely proportional to $(\varepsilon_M^{demand} - \varepsilon_M^{supply})$, the sum of the magnitudes of the two elasticities (because ε_M^{supply} is itself negative).

Why is this important? It is because there are many instances where pathways exhibit large changes in flux accompanied by relatively very much smaller changes in metabolite concentrations. The extreme example is the changes in glycolytic flux in animal muscle on going from the resting to the working state, which can be between 100- and 1000–fold, yet the changes in the concentrations of glycolytic intermediates are trivial.[24, 101, 107, 204] There are significant advantages to metabolite homoeostasis during flux changes.

(1) If pathway intermediates are also participants in other metabolic pathways that are not required to change in rate at the same time as the pathways being controlled, it is evidently better to minimize disturbances in the common intermediate concentrations.

(2) Having to make large changes in intermediate levels slows down the rate at which a pathway can respond to a control signal with a change in flux,[62] so faster responses can be made if metabolite concentrations are kept as near–constant as possible.

(3) Avoiding large concentration changes during large flux changes minimizes the possibility of sudden adverse changes in cellular osmotic strength.[6]

If control is exercised on a metabolic pathway, effective control of the flux combined with good homoeostasis of the intermediates requires that the pathway element acted on by the control mechanisms must have a high flux control coefficient (so it can exhibit a strong response to the effector signal) but low concentration control coefficients, so that the response of the concentrations to the same signal is small. The conditions that have to be met to achieve this are different depending on whether control is exerted in the supply block or the demand block.

In control by the supply block, a high flux control coefficient, C_{supply}^{J}, is obtained if ε_M^{demand} is significantly greater than $|\varepsilon_M^{supply}|$, corresponding to a low value of Q (see Figure 7.1a and Eqn. 7.1). The concentration control coefficient only becomes smaller than the flux control coefficient if ε_M^{demand} is greater than

1 (Figure 7.1a and Eqn. 7.3). The elasticities we are considering are composite elasticities for a block of enzymes rather than those of single enzymes. For single enzymes, elasticities lie mainly in the range -1 to 1 for those showing simple kinetics, or from around -3 to 3 for allosteric enzymes, except where the reaction is near to equilibrium (Chapter 5.3). The way in which the elasticities of the component enzymes combine to give block elasticities generally makes a block elasticity smaller in magnitude than any of its components and, since the blocks we are considering are pathway segments, they would not be near equilibrium. A small (negative) value for ε_M^{supply} would not be difficult to obtain since ε_M^{supply} is a product inhibition elasticity, and these are usually smaller in magnitude than substrate elasticities such as ε_M^{demand} in the case of single enzymes. When we are dealing with a block of enzymes, this difficulty tends to be even worse, since the overall product inhibition elasticity of the block is expected to be much weaker than those of the component enzymes (reflecting a rather poor backward transmission of the signal from the metabolite M). However, too small a value of $|\varepsilon_M^{supply}|$ (e.g. giving $Q < 0.1$) would not be an advantage, since the larger it is, the smaller the concentration control coefficient [Eqn. (7.3)].

If the elasticity of the demand block could be dominated by the elasticity of an enzyme with cooperative substrate kinetics, it might be as large as 3. My investigations of this problem with my colleague Simon Thomas have shown that this may indeed be possible, for example if the cooperative enzyme is the first enzyme in the demand block. The cost of this, though, is poorer metabolite homoeostasis within the demand block. Improving on this probably requires unusual pathway structures not often seen in practice (e.g. sequences of several cooperative enzymes). Thus in spite of the traditional view (Chapter 4.1) that control should be exerted at the beginning of a pathway (i.e. in the supply block), it is not easy to see how this can be implemented with the available components to give a well–regulated pathway, i.e. one that shows good metabolite homoeostasis during flux changes.

What about control by demand? An experimental example where control has been shown to be shifted to the demand end of the pathway is hepatocyte energy metabolism (Chapter 6.3.3.2). The requirement for control by the demand block is that C_{demand}^J exceeds C_{supply}^J, which requires that $|\varepsilon_M^{supply}|$ should be significantly greater than ε_M^{demand}, giving a high value for Q (see Fig. 7.1b and Eqn. 7.2). The concentration control coefficent, C_{demand}^M, only becomes smaller than the flux control coefficient if ε_M^{supply} is more negative than -1 (Fig. 7.1b). A low value of ε_M^{demand} will be obtained if the demand block is approaching saturation with M. This will also make the flux in the demand block relatively insensitive to changes in the level of M, which may well be an advantage if there are other processes that can affect it. The large negative value required for ε_M^{supply} might seem to be a problem, especially as I have just explained that the product elasticity of a block of enzymes tends to be weaker than those of any of its component enzymes. This would create

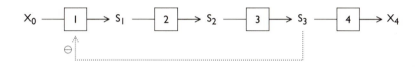

Figure 7.2 A feedback inhibition loop
This is a generalized feedback loop, with the enzymes represented by numbered boxes. Metabolite S_3 inhibits enzyme 1.

an obstacle to efficient homoeostasis in the supply–demand sequence, were it not that metabolism has a solution to this difficulty, as we shall see in the next section.

7.2   Feedback inhibition

7.2.1   Discovery and relationship to allosteric enzymes

If bacteria such as *E. coli* are growing on [^{14}C]glucose together with a nitrogen source, the amino acids incorporated into their proteins are radioactively labelled showing that they are being synthesized from the glucose carbon. If one of these amino acids is added to the medium, it was established in the mid 1950s that the synthesis of this amino acid is selectively discontinued. Part of the mechanism of this effect has been found to involve specific repression of the expression of the synthetic enzymes in the presence of end product, but this cannot provide a complete explanation, since growing bacteria degrade very little of their proteins and therefore repression cannot account for the existing synthetic enzymes not making the amino acid after it has been added to the medium. The other part of the mechanism was discovered in 1956 when Umbarger[250] found that the first enzyme in the pathway to isoleucine, threonine deaminase, is specifically and strongly inhibited by isoleucine. This *feedback inhibition* by the end product of a pathway is highly specific since the structurally similar amino acids leucine and valine are not effective inhibitors of the enzyme.

In the same year, Yates and Pardee[281] also reported feedback inhibition of aspartate transcarbamylase in *E. coli*: this first step in the synthesis of pyrimidine nucleotides from aspartate is inhibited by the end product CTP. Once these two examples had been discovered, further ones followed and it became clear that feedback loops on to the first irreversible enzyme of a pathway are a common structural feature in metabolism. In Chapter 3.5, p. 70, we saw that the unusual inhibition kinetics of these enzymes led to the recognition that they form a special class of *allosteric enzymes*. Although it was clearly established for some of the early examples, particularly in amino acid synthesis, that the feedback does operate to slow the rate of the synthetic pathway, in many other cases it is a presumption that the purpose of the feedback is to regulate the rate of the pathway. In the case of histidine biosynthesis in *E. coli*, the *in*

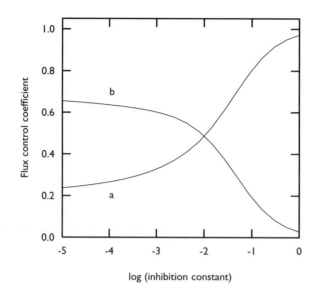

Figure 7.3   Feedback alters the control distribution
The flux control coefficients of enzymes I (curve a) and 4 (curve b) of the pathway in Figure 7.2 are plotted against the inhibition constant for S_3 on enzyme I in this simulated example. The inhibition weakens from left to right.

vivo concentration of histidine is too low to operate feedback inhibition on the first enzyme of the pathway. Again in *E. coli*, mutants do not differ greatly in growth rates and yield when the normal allosteric feedback–regulated phosphofructokinase is replaced by a non–inhibited form.[76] The function of feedback inhibition is therefore not always as simple and obvious as has been assumed.

7.2.2   Feedback inhibition and Control Analysis

It is in the interpretation of feedback inhibition that conventional biochemical thought and Metabolic Control Analysis confront one another with particular force. After all, the concept that there is no single rate–limiting step but instead several steps with varying degrees of influence does not necessarily undermine conventional thinking; superficially it seems that biochemistry can continue as before provided that the label 'rate–limiting' can be replaced by a flux control coefficient that numerically measures the degree of rate limitation. However, Metabolic Control Analysis of feedback inhibition shows that there is a much deeper and more fundamental contradiction between the old and the new.

Right back at the origin of Metabolic Control Analysis, Henrik Kacser & Jim Burns[119] had considered the effects on the flux control coefficients of the pathway caused by feedback inhibition by a metabolite near the end of a linear pathway on to an enzyme near its beginning (e.g. Figure 7.2). They used rather simplified kinetic equations so that the elasticity values could be easily calculated, but were able to show that feedback inhibition makes the flux control coefficient of the regulated enzyme smaller, and the flux control coefficients of the steps following the metabolite exerting feedback larger. This is illustrated by a simulated example in Figure 7.3 where the effect of changing the strength of the feedback inhibition on the control coefficients of the enzymes is shown. (In the example, the first enzyme follows a Monod, Wyman & Changeux allosteric rate law, and the others normal Michaelis–Menten kinetics.) Strong feedback inhibition has the effect of transferring flux control away from the beginning of the pathway, where it would otherwise tend to be, to the enzyme (enzyme 4 in the example) consuming the feedback metabolite (S_3). As the strength of the inhibition weakens, the flux control coefficient of enzyme 1 increases. On the basis of the traditional criteria for the identification of rate–limiting enzymes (Chapter 4), a highly regulated enzyme near the start of a metabolic pathway would be a prime candidate for the rate–limiting step, so the suggestion that it would have a low flux control coefficient was particularly unwelcome and led to considerable resistance to the concepts of Metabolic Control Analysis and the flux control coefficient in particular. However, the Control Analysis interpretation has been vindicated by experiments, such as those quoted in Chapter 6 that showed that substantial increases in the activity of just such an enzyme (phosphofructokinase) has negligible effects on its pathway flux (glycolysis).

The only element of the Kacser & Burns analysis[119] that could be regarded as supporting traditional ideas was their demonstration that the transfer of control by feedback inhibition would be most effective if the enzyme subjected to the inhibition would otherwise have been the rate–controlling step of the sequence up to the feedback metabolite. That is, if the pathway could be terminated at the feedback metabolite and there was some way to keep its concentration constant, then the kinetic and pathway characteristics that would cause the inhibited enzyme to have the largest possible flux control coefficient in this case would also lead to the most effective transfer of flux control in the full pathway with feedback operating. It is therefore a reasonable hypothesis that an enzyme that is subjected to feedback inhibition is the dominant enzyme in rate control in its pathway up to the feedback metabolite, and of course this enzyme would probably have been identified as the 'rate–limiting step' by traditional criteria. However, it is important to note that an experimental test of this hypothesis would be difficult and has not been performed. Furthermore, the hypothesis is little more than a theoretical curiosity that focuses on the point where traditional thought and Metabolic Control Analysis diverge. In practice, the inhibited enzyme will be found to have a small flux control coefficient under the usual circumstances where the feedback metabolite is free to vary in concentration.

An extensive theoretical analysis of the properties of pathways with feedback inhibition was carried out by Michael Savageau in Michigan using his Biochemical Systems Theory.[215–217] This has some differences from Metabolic Control Analysis, but does involve concepts equivalent to elasticities and control coefficients. He showed that feedback inhibition can reduce the concentrations of the feedback metabolite and of all the intermediates between it and the inhibited enzyme. Feedback inhibition also tends to reduce the variation of the feedback intermediate (and that of the other metabolites in the loop) in response to fluctuations in the concentration of the source metabolite. These effects are proportional to the strength of the feedback (as represented by its elasticity on the inhibited enzyme). However, they do depend on how the comparison between the inhibited system and the uninhibited system is made, since there is no obvious single choice for the 'reference state' that is the basis of the comparison. A more generally valid conclusion concerns the effects of feedback on the concentration control coefficients (though he expressed this in terms of his equivalent measures, the *parameter sensitivities of the concentrations*). He showed that feedback inevitably reduces the dependence of the concentrations of the feedback metabolite and the intermediates in the loop upon the enzyme activities, to an extent that depends on the strength of the inhibition. Although Savageau established methods that could examine the effects of feedback on the pathway flux, he did not pursue this aspect of the analysis. He did show though that feedback inhibition causes a pathway to reach a new steady state faster after a perturbation than an uninhibited pathway does;[216] a similar conclusion was also reached by a different theoretical route (the study of the transient times of metabolic pathways) by John Easterby.[63]

Although these results emphasize the stabilizing effects of feedback inhibition, Savageau[215] and many other researchers have identified circumstances where it becomes destabilizing. This happens if the feedback loop is long but the inhibition is strongly cooperative. The pathway then never settles to a steady state but oscillates about it. In intermediate cases, the pathway does reach the steady state relatively rapidly after a perturbation to the rate, but goes through a series of diminishing (or *damped*) oscillations first. Oscillations can be explained by the delay in the transmission of the feedback signal; if the feedback enzyme is running at the wrong rate but the pathway is long, there is a time lag before the concentration of the feedback metabolite changes enough to readjust the rate of the inhibited enzyme. Then, if the adjustment is too severe (because the cooperativity means the rate change is disproportionately much greater than the metabolite change), there is again a delay before this causes a change in the feedback metabolite again, so the rate keeps swinging above and below that required. (The same phenomenon occurs in national economics: there is a delay caused by information gathering and government inertia between some economic imbalance arising and any policy changes being made to counter it; severe measures are then taken to redress the problem, ensuring the inevitable continuation of 'boom' and 'bust' cycles.) Metabolic oscillations have been observed in glycolysis in yeast and muscle as well as in photosynthesis and mitochondrial respiration.[103] Feedback inhibition on phosphofructokinase by ATP (coupled to activation by AMP) can account for the oscillations in glycolysis, which have been studied extensively by Britton Chance and Benno Hess and their colleagues.

Jannie Hofmeyr and Athel Cornish–Bowden[106] used Metabolic Control Analysis to study the effects of feedback inhibition on flux and concentration control coefficients to complement their study of supply and demand structures described earlier (Chapter 7.1). I pointed out there that achieving a high value of the elasticity ratio Q, $-\varepsilon_M^{supply}/\varepsilon_M^{demand}$, presents a difficulty that has to be overcome in order to operate the supply and demand pathways in the domain where there is effective homoeostasis of the intermediate metabolite M. This is because the product inhibition elasticity ε_M^{supply} tends to be weaker than any of the product inhibition elasticities of its component enzymes. However, Hofmeyr & Cornish–Bowden showed that when the supply pathway begins with an enzyme that is feedback–inhibited by M, the algebraic expression for ε_M^{supply} contains a new term that comes from the feedback elasticity on the first enzyme, ε_M^1. Furthermore, the supply block elasticity is approximately equal to this elasticity ($\varepsilon_M^{supply} \approx \varepsilon_M^1$) under conditions where the other contributions are small. (As in the original analysis of Kacser & Burns, this ensures that the inhibited enzyme is the most controlling enzyme in the supply block.) So, if the feedback–inhibited enzyme is an allosteric enzyme that can have large–valued elasticities because of cooperativity (e.g. Figure 5.9), it is possible to achieve the large Q value and large negative value of ε_M^{supply} that are required for effective homoeostasis of M. This implies that feedback inhibition loops function primarily to ensure homoeostasis of metabolite concentrations, whereas conventional biochemical explanations have emphasized their function in rate control.

Hofmeyr and Cornish–Bowden continued their Metabolic Control Analysis of feedback inhibition in a supply–demand pathway to examine just this point. They varied the degree of cooperativity of the feedback of M in a computer–simulated pathway and studied the effects this had on the behaviour of the system as the demand was varied. The changes had relatively little impact on the steady state fluxes and the flux control coefficients, but there was a big difference in the variation of M and its concentration control coefficients, with the smallest range of M and smallest value of C_{demand}^M being achieved with the greatest degree of cooperativity of feedback by M. A high degree of cooperativity in the feedback inhibition generates the risk of oscillations, so its existence implies that it has been selected for in evolution in spite of this disadvantage, and the only demonstrable unique advantage that cooperative feedback inhibition has is the improvement of metabolic homoeostasis.

Putting the theoretical analyses together, our picture of feedback inhibition now looks like this.

(1) Feedback inhibition is an antidote to the tendency of reactions at the start of a pathway to have the greater control of flux. It transfers control to the reactions using the feedback metabolite from the enzyme it inhibits, which is probably the most rate–controlling enzyme in the supply of the metabolite, though this control is of lesser significance in the full pathway.

(2) Feedback inhibition improves homoeostasis of the concentration of the feedback metabolite (and all metabolites in the feedback loop), and increased cooperativity of the inhibition specifically enhances this effect.

(3) Feedback inhibition improves the stability of pathways in that it speeds up the return to a steady state after some random perturbation or the rate of reaching a new steady state when external conditions change.

For the reasons given in the earlier section on supply and demand (Chapter 7.1), the first two effects are in fact inextricably linked. Thus enzymes subjected to inhibition are regulatory enzymes in the sense in which regulation was defined in Chapter 1.1, p. 1; they are not, contrary to common belief, effective control sites for changing the pathway flux because they have small flux control coefficients.

Of course, part of the reluctance to accept this conclusion arises because a regulatory enzyme subjected to feedback inhibition is demonstrably inhibited, and the degree of inhibition does change with metabolic circumstances [as shown by cross-over plots that identify phosphofructokinase as a site of inhibition in glycolysis (Figure 4.5)]. In fact, this confers no special status on the feedback–inhibited enzyme; every enzyme in the pathway has also changed in rate under the same circumstances. The only difference is that the feedback–inhibited enzyme had the potential to have a more dominant role in control, but feedback inhibition has suppressed that and made it subordinate to the steps that utilize the feedback metabolite.

7.2.3   Patterns of feedback inhibition in branched pathways

Because anabolism radiates outwards from a relatively small number of metabolic precursors in the core of metabolism, biosynthetic pathways are usually branched so that the early part of the pathway leads ultimately to two or more end products. The regulation of the pathway then has to be able to cope with differential variations in the net demand for the different end products. For example, if the end products were two different amino acids in a bacterial cell, it might occur that in some circumstances neither is available in the environment and they both have to be synthesized in the amounts required for protein synthesis, but in other circumstances, enough of one of them is present in the medium to require very little synthesis of it whereas the other must be synthesized fully. In both cases, the common part of the pathway must ensure homoeostasis of the common branch–point intermediate. The biosynthetic pathways of bacteria exhibit a variety of different molecular mechanisms employed in the regulation of such branched pathways.[237] However, when Michael Savageau continued his theoretical study of feedback inhibition using Biochemical Systems Analysis,[217] he concluded that there are only two functionally distinct types, though one of them can be implemented by a number of different molecular mechanisms. The two basic forms are *nested* and *sequential* feedback.

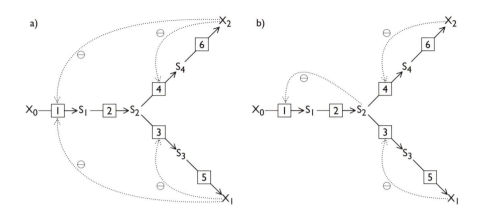

Figure 7.4 Feedback inhibition patterns in branched pathways
(a) Nested inhibition; (b) sequential inhibition. Any step shown above can be regarded as being composed of an arbitrary number of enzyme reactions.

7.2.3.1 Theory of nested and sequential feedback

Savageau's studies of the two basic types of feedback mechanism in branched pathways, illustrated in Figure 7.4, showed that the sequential system seemed to be the more reliable in that it generally behaves as required when the source and end–product metabolites vary, though its degree of effectiveness in ensuring homoeostasis varies with the particular values of the kinetic and inhibition constants of the enzymes involved. The nested pattern can be both better and worse, for the type of behaviour it exhibits varies with the values of the kinetic and inhibition constants. It can give more effective homoeostasis of end–product concentrations in response to variations in the supply of source metabolite and the kinetic characteristics of the enzymes. However, this behaviour is less stable because in some circumstances it changes to one of two undesirable forms. Translating Savageau's results into Control Analysis terminology, the provision of one end product (say, S_2 in Figure 7.5) can cause the concentration and rate of synthesis of the other (S_3) to drop unless:

$$\frac{J_1 \varepsilon_2^1}{J_2 \varepsilon_2^2} < 1 \tag{7.5}$$

Since the flux before the branch point (J_1) is greater than that in the branch (J_2), this requires the product inhibition elasticity of S_2 on its own branch to be significantly stronger (as indicated by the elasticity) than its inhibition of the common pathway. In fact, the equation can be interpreted as a requirement that a given change in the end product, ΔS_2, should potentially cause a bigger change in the rate of the branch than of the common pathway ($\Delta v_2 > \Delta v_1$) if an increase in S_2 is not to cause a fall in S_3. (I say potentially because these are the predictions for the isolated steps, as they are derived from the elasticities, not for the whole system.) Of course, there is an equivalent need for the other

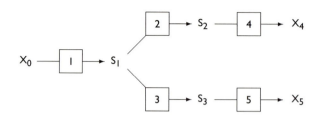

Figure 7.5 A generalized branched pathway
S_2 and S_3 are the end products of the biosynthetic pathways, but are consumed by incorporation into biomass. S_2 and S_3 can exert feedback inhibition of the nested or sequential type.

end product to inhibit its own branch more strongly than the common pathway. Because of the velocity ratio in Eqn. (7.5) and the relatively limited range of inhibition elasticity values, it seems that satisfying both requirements simultaneously will be unlikely unless the two branch fluxes have approximately similar shares of the common feed flux. However, several of the observed molecular mechanisms to be described below may exist to ensure the correct relative relationships of the inhibition strengths. On the other hand, incorrect operation of these systems has been observed experimentally in cases where provision of an excess of one end product (typically an amino acid) results in growth inhibition by causing a deficiency in the synthesis of another.

This requirement on the inhibition strengths has the incipient danger that one of the end products might not inhibit the common pathway sufficiently so that when its concentration is increased, first S_1 and then the other end product start to accumulate excessively. This in fact is Savageau's other undesirable form of behaviour of the nested feedback inhibition pattern: there is the possibility of the breakdown of the steady state if

$$\frac{J_1 \varepsilon_2^1}{J_2 \varepsilon_2^2} \ll 1 \qquad\qquad (7.6)$$

Thus the more effective homoeostasis possible with nested inhibition can only be reliably exploited where the relative inhibition strengths, represented by the inhibition elasticities scaled by the relative fluxes, fall within a restricted range. However, in spite of this apparent unreliability, nested feedback inhibition structures are found in metabolism.

7.2.3.2 Sequential feedback inhibition

Sequential feedback inhibition was discovered in the pathways synthesizing the aromatic amino acids tryptophan, tyrosine and phenylalanine in *Bacillus subtilis* (Figure 7.6). The final common intermediate of this pathway is an equilibrium mixture of chorismate and prephenate. These intermediates can inhibit the

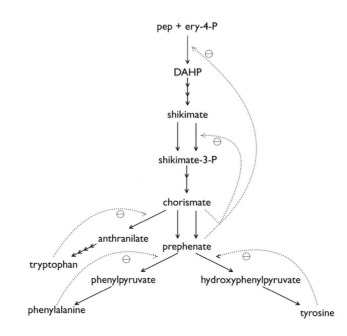

Figure 7.6 Feedback in aromatic amino acid synthesis
The pathways in *Bacillus subtilis* exhibit sequential feedback inhibition.

first step in their synthesis, the joining of the glycolytic intermediate phospho-enolpyruvate and the four–carbon sugar erythrose 4–phosphate catalysed by an enzyme sometimes termed DHAP synthase (because its true name, and that of its product, are too long to be memorable). On the other hand, none of the aromatic amino acids inhibits this enzyme. Each of them specifically inhibits the first step of its own branch.

7.2.3.3 Nested feedback inhibition

As mentioned previously, Michael Savageau regarded a set of apparently different feedback inhibition systems as different molecular mechanisms for implementing a single functional type: nested feedback inhibition (Figure 7.4a). The following examples illustrate the different categories of mechanism.

7.2.3.3.1 Enzyme multiplicity

A common method of ensuring that the inhibited step in the common pathway responds to each of the end products, without any one of them having too powerful an effect (which must be avoided as shown by Savageau's conditions on the effectiveness of nested inhibition), is to have separate isozymes, each of which is inhibited by one of the products. (This is also generally linked to separate controls on synthesis of each of the isoenzymes, such as specific repression by the end product that also inhibits it.) This is seen in the synthesis of threonine and lysine from aspartate in *E. coli* (Figure 7.7) where there are separate

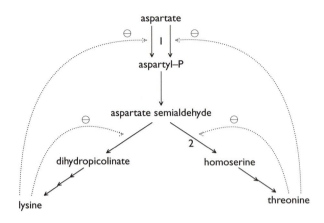

Figure 7.7   Nested inhibition with multiple enzymes in threonine and lysine synthesis
Three aspartate kinase isoenzymes (step 1) occur in this pathway in *E. coli*, though the one repressed
by methionine (which is formed from homoserine) has not been shown here. Step 2 is homoserine
dehydrogenase.

aspartate kinases inhibited by each product. Furthermore, work by Georges
Cohen and his colleagues[41] showed that the isoenzymes aspartate kinase I and
homoserine dehydrogenase I occurred on a single bifunctional molecule and
that both activities were inhibited in parallel by a single threonine inhibitory
site. This seems to fit in with Savageau's theory since it should ensure that the
required degree of relative inhibition of the common and branch-point steps is
ensured by the protein structure. After all, there is no other obvious metabolic
advantage in having these two different activities in a single molecule as they are
not consecutive steps that could transfer their common intermediate between
the sites.

In reality, the regulation of this system is even more complex, since methionine and isoleucine also share parts of this pathway from aspartate, and
there is a third aspartate kinase and a second homoserine dehydrogenase whose
syntheses are repressed by methionine.

Another illustration of the complexity of the patterns of control in branched
biosynthetic pathways is that the aromatic amino acid synthesis pathway cited
above as an instance of sequential control exhibits control by nested feedback
with enzyme multiplicity in *E. coli*. There are three separate DHAP synthases,
each inhibited by one of the products.

7.2.3.3.2   Concerted feedback inhibition
Concerted feedback inhibition (Figure 7.8) is a form of nested feedback inhibition where the enzyme in the common pathway has the property that it is not
inhibited by either of the end products separately. Inhibition by one requires
that the other be present. Like the other versions of nested inhibition listed
below, this is a distinction based on the *in vitro* kinetics, since both products

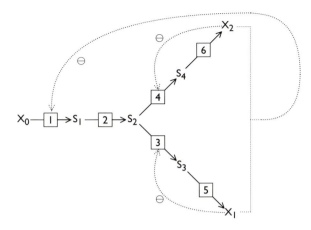

Figure 7.8 Schematic diagram of the concerted form of nested feedback inhibition

would normally be present *in vivo* and therefore both would be inhibitory. This is probably a molecular mechanism for minimizing the chances of the nested inhibition displaying the bad aspects of its behaviour: if the inhibition by the product in excess were stronger than necessary, the consequent tendency of the concentration of the other to drop would be limited by its fall causing a weakening of the inhibition by the one in excess. Conversely, if the inhibition by the product in excess were too weak, the tendency of the other to rise in concentration would cause a strengthening of the inhibition.

This type of inhibition occurs in threonine and lysine synthesis in *Bacillus polymyxa*, which does not have multiple aspartate kinase isoenzymes as *E. coli* does.

7.2.3.3.3 Cumulative feedback inhibition

Cumulative feedback inhibition (Figure 7.9) is effectively just like the standard form of nested feedback inhibition, with the additional property that the inhibition of the common enzyme in the presence of both end products is greater than that caused by either separately. However, this greater inhibition is exactly that expected from the combination of the effects of each when they act independently. For example, if one caused one–half inhibition, and the other caused one–third, the expected outcome for independent effects is the product of the fractional activities, *i.e.* $\frac{1}{2} \times \frac{2}{3} = \frac{1}{3}$, or two–thirds inhibition.

This was first suggested to be the case for the glutamine synthase (glutamate–ammonia ligase) of *E. coli*:

$$\text{ATP} + \text{glutamate} + \text{NH}_3 \longrightarrow \text{ADP} + \text{P}_i + \text{glutamine}$$

Glutamine is the nitrogen donor in the synthesis of a range of end products, and so can be regarded as the common metabolite of a number of diverging pathways (considered in terms of nitrogen flow, rather than carbon flow as

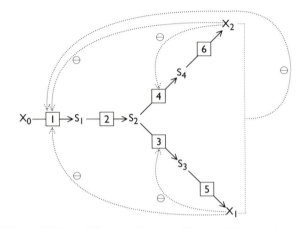

Figure 7.9 Cumulative feedback inhibition
A schematic representation of this form of nested feedback inhibition.

normal), including synthesis of AMP, CTP, histidine, tryptophan, glucosamine 6–phosphate and carbamoyl phosphate. Stadtman and his colleagues[197] established that all of the above (except tryptophan) and alanine and glycine had separate inhibition sites on the enzyme, each of which separately caused only partial inhibition even at saturating concentrations of the inhibitor. Together, the effects were cumulative and all eight together caused almost complete inhibition. However, the original observations were made on enzyme that was a mixture of adenylated and non–adenylated forms, and the interconversion between the two (see Section 7.4.4) causes changes in the inhibition characteristics; from later studies it appears that there may be some interactions between the sites under some circumstances, though probably not enough to change the essential conclusion. (Nor is some uncertainty in the kinetics of an enzyme with six substrates and products, eight inhibitors and a requirement for bivalent cations surprising; Savageau,[217] as quoted in the Introduction, Chapter 1.2.1, pointed out the practical impossibility of a complete kinetic characterization.)

7.2.3.3.4   Synergestic feedback inhibition
Synergestic feedback inhibition is intermediate between concerted and cumulative feedback inhibition. Unlike concerted inhibition, each end product exhibits some partial inhibition on its own account, but the inhibition of both end products together is much greater, and greater than would be expected for cumulative inhibition, *i.e.* there is interaction between the separate inhibition sites. Synergistic inhibition was first observed in purine biosynthesis on the first enzyme of the common pathway to AMP and GMP, amidophosphoribosyltransferase:

$$\text{glutamine} + 5\text{–phosphoribose–1–diphosphate} + H_2O$$
$$\longrightarrow \text{glutamate} + 5\text{–phosphoribosylamine} + \text{pyrophosphate}$$

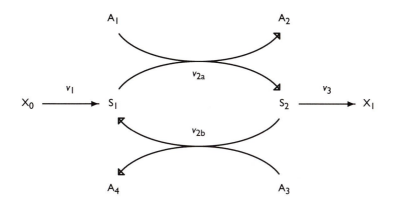

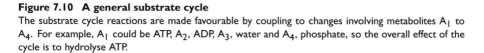

Figure 7.10 A general substrate cycle
The substrate cycle reactions are made favourable by coupling to changes involving metabolites A_1 to A_4. For example, A_1 could be ATP, A_2, ADP, A_3, water and A_4, phosphate, so the overall effect of the cycle is to hydrolyse ATP.

This allosteric enzyme has separate inhibitory sites for AMP and GMP, but both of them together interact to cause greater inhibition than would be expected. Similar synergistic inhibition is seen with the glutamine synthase of *Bacillus lichiniformis*, which is only slightly inhibited by low concentrations of glutamine, histidine or AMP, but almost completely inhibited by AMP plus histidine or glutamine plus histidine.

7.3   Substrate or 'futile' cycles

7.3.1   Definition

Apart from branches, other common network elements in metabolism are the various types of cyclic pathway. Some, like the tricarboxylic acid cycle, are inherently cyclic. In fact, the reactions of the tricarboxylic acid cycle cannot themselves account for the the initial generation of the di– and tricarboxylic acid intermediates, so in the absence of other *anaplerotic* reactions to synthesize them, the intermediates form a *moiety–conserved cycle* in which the total quantity of intermediates is fixed. In other cases, the existence of the cyclic pathway is not inevitable; a circular route can be traced on the metabolic chart, but will only occur if all the reactions are simultaneously active. Amongst these potential cycles are those that appear to be wasteful or unnecessary, and which were therefore termed *futile cycles*. Later, when it was conjectured that these cycles might fulfil certain specific functions, the more neutral term *substrate cycles* came to be preferred.

A substrate cycle could potentially exist in metabolism wherever a reaction (or set of reactions) that converts metabolite S_1 into S_2 is opposed by a second set that reconverts S_2 to S_1. If, under certain circumstances, both sets of reactions are active simultaneously, then there can be a cyclic flux whereby an appreciable proportion, perhaps all, of the S_1 that is converted to S_2 reverts to S_1 (Figure 7.10). Both sets of reactions must be intrinsically favourable (*i.e.* exergonic) even though they link the same two metabolites in opposite directions, and for this to be the case, at least one of the sets must be coupled to some other exergonic process (for example, phosphorylation by ATP). Hence the cyclic flow leads to no net change other than the dissipation of energy by a net flux through the coupled process that drives the cycle. This characteristic — the occurrence of two oppositely directed sets of reactions that would operate to achieve no change other than dissipation of energy — is often given as the definition of a substrate cycle[126, 196, 237] and is the particular justification for the term 'futile cycle'.

The early evidence that cycling was not just a possibility but did actually occur in cells under certain circumstances was provided by:

- Cahill and colleagues[26] in 1959 in respect of cycling between glucose and glucose 6–phosphate in liver;

- Steinberg[241] in 1963 in connection with cycling between fatty acids and triacylglycerol in adipose tissue;

- Newsholme and Underwood[172] in 1966 for cycling between fructose 6–phosphate and fructose 1,6–bisphosphate in kidney cortex.

These specific examples of substrate cycles do, however, illustrate a problem with the definition given above: the definition is too broad and does not represent all the features that are characteristic of actual substrate cycles. Thus the previous definition is applicable to all the types of cycle shown in Figure 7.11, yet:

- only those in Figure 7.11(a) and (f) are indisputably substrate cycles;

- those in Figure 7.11(b) and (e) are possible substrate cycles (though because one of the substrate cycle metabolites is a fixed pool, their properties are essentially those of a simple branched pathway);

- the one in Figure 7.11(c) is a moiety–conserved cycle because the sum of $S_1 + S_2$ remains constant at all times;

- the one in Figure 7.11(d) is a dead–end cycle which cannot affect the steady state properties of the linear pathway.

Definition is important because cycles occur embedded in the highly interconnected network of metabolism where they can be less easy to identify and classify than the idealized cases in Fig. 7.11. Even counting the number of cycles can be difficult.

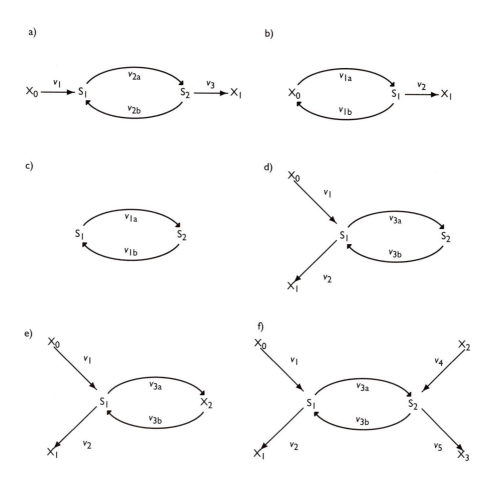

Figure 7.11 Topologies of some cyclic structures in metabolism
Versions of these structures have been referred to as substrate cycles in the literature. Second substrates
used for driving intrinsically endergonic reactions (e.g. ATP) have not been shown. X is used to denote
a pool metabolite, and S to represent a variable metabolite.

Newsholme and Crabtree stated that a distinguishing feature of a system
with a substrate cycle was that there were two distinct fluxes: one a net conversion of S_1 to S_2, matching the rates at which S_1 is produced by input reactions
to the cycle and S_2 is consumed by output reactions, and the other the cyclic
flux itself. This amounts to stating that the pathway must be representable
as Figure. 7.11(a), if necessary by regarding each step as standing for a large
block of reactions. Although their definition arguably covers the 'open futile
cycle' defined by Stein & Blum[240] or Reich & Sel'kov[196] (Figure 7.11f), this
could conceivably have a cyclic flux in the absence of a net flux through the
cycle (when $v_1 = v_2$ and $v_4 = v_5$). I therefore believe their definition should be
generalized as follows. A substrate cycle exists in the following situations.

(1) The flux pattern in the network cannot be fully described as the combination of the minimum number of linear paths needed to account for the mass flows connecting the inputs and outputs. (This can apply to larger, more complex networks such as in Figure 7.11f.)

(2) One of the additional fluxes needed to complete the description is a feasible, internal cyclic route. (All the reactions of the cycle must be exergonic; the requirement that the cycle is internal excludes cycles in Figure 7.11b and 7.11e.)

(3) There is one step of the cycle that can be deleted in principle and still leave a network capable of connecting the observed input fluxes to the observed output fluxes. (This is the criterion that shows the cycle is intrinsically unnecessary; it eliminates conserved cycles such as that in Figure 7.11c and hypothetical oddities such as that in Figure 7.11d.)

There is obviously plenty of scope to disagree with my proposals about which of the cycles in Figure 7.11 is classed as a substrate cycle. The important issue is that there is a number of ways these cycles can be distinguished, and that therefore it is unwise to assume that they all have similar properties.

7.3.2 Evidence for substrate cycling

The obvious difficulty about proving the occurrence of substrate cycles by measuring their rates is that they produce no net change in the amounts of their constituents. This is not true, of course, for the coupling reaction, and cycling can be measured if the formation of products by the coupling reactions can be detected. This is the case for the triacylglycerol:fatty acid cycle in mammalian white adipose tissue during net triacylglycerol storage: glycerol phosphate (derived from glycolysis) is needed for the conversion of fatty acids to triacylglycerol, but the hydrolysis of triacylglycerols to fatty acids releases glycerol. White adipose tissue metabolizes glycerol poorly owing to the virtual absence of glycerol kinase, so the formation of glycerol is a good indicator of the rate of hydrolysis, which can be combined with measurement of the net rate of formation of fatty acids (during net lipolysis) to calculate the degree of cycling.[241] These and similar experiments for studying the glycerol balance can show cycling rates as high as 10–20 times the net rate of lipolysis or lipogenesis in isolated fat tissue. This is so even though there is a potential mechanism for suppressing the cycle *via* control of the hormone–sensitive triacylglycerol lipase, which is activated by protein phosphorylation by the cyclic AMP–dependent protein kinase (Chapter 7.4.3.1).

Several methods for estimating the degree of cycling in the three substrate cycles of glycolysis and gluconeogenesis (Figure 7.12) depend on monitoring the fate of the radioactive hydrogen isotope, tritium (^{3}H). This is because certain of the reactions of the pathway specifically cause the loss of ^{3}H attached to a particular carbon atom of the metabolites. For example, glucose–6–phosphate

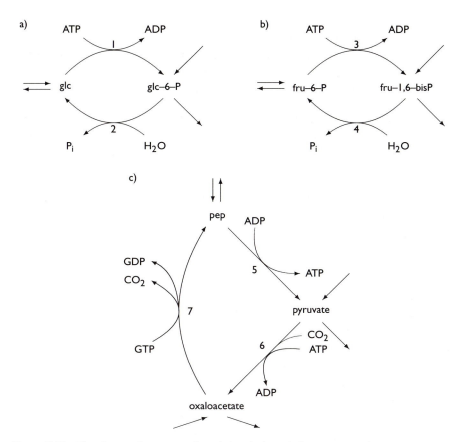

Figure 7.12 The three substrate cycles of glycolysis and gluconeogenesis
(a) The glucose:glucose 6–phosphate cycle catalysed by hexokinase IV (1) and glucose–6–phosphatase
(2); (b) the fructose 6–phosphate:fructose 1,6–bisphosphate cycle catalysed by phosphofructokinase (3)
and fructose–1,6–bisphosphatase (4); (c) the phosphoenolpyruvate:pyruvate cycle catalysed by pyruvate
kinase (5), pyruvate carboxylase (6) and PEPCK (7).

isomerase causes the loss of ^{3}H from [2–^{3}H]glucose 6–phosphate when it is
converted to fructose 6–phosphate; since the ^{3}H enters water and is greatly
diluted, it is not re–incorporated when the reverse reaction occurs. Therefore,
if [2-^{3}H]glucose is supplied to mammalian liver or kidney cortex, the loss of
^{3}H from the 2 position of the glucose can be used as a measure of cycling because it shows that the glucose has been phosphorylated to glucose 6–phosphate
(which rapidly equilibrates with fructose 6–phosphate, losing the ^{3}H, because
of the high rate of the glucose–6–phosphate isomerase reaction), and then dephosphorylated again back to glucose. Because of the other metabolic reactions occurring simultaneously, the relative loss of ^{3}H compared with the ^{14}C
content of a doubly labelled glucose molecule gives a better measure of the
cycling. Interpretation of such experiments is difficult and often controversial; the topic is discussed at length in some of the articles listed under *Further
reading* at the end of the chapter. Randomization of ^{14}C label between dif-

ferent positions of the glucose molecule can also be used. For example, the fructose 6–phosphate:fructose 1,6–bisphosphate cycle can be monitored in this way since, when aldolase splits the latter into two trioses, the fragments can be reassembled at opposite ends of the hexose from their original position.

Measuring metabolic fluxes by monitoring the spread of isotope through a pathway (Chapter 2.5) can give the rates of the component reactions of the cycle. This is because the cycle can give rise to faster migration of the label between intermediates than would be expected from the net pathway flux, just as near–equilibrium reactions do (Figure 4.2, Chapter 4.3). This approach has been used extensively by Jacob Blum's group at Duke University, particularly in connection with the measurement of substrate cycling in rat hepatocytes.[10,58,190] The experiments are much more informative than monitoring isotope loss or rearrangement in a single compound, but involve much more work, both experimentally and computationally.

The results from these measurements differ between the three cycles of glycolysis and gluconeogenesis in rat liver and hepatocytes and between different metabolic states. In general, though, the highest relative rates of cycling are observed with the glucose:glucose 6–phosphate cycle, for which the cycling rate can be many times the net flux of glucose uptake or release.[261] This is consistent with the lack of any obvious mechanism that can suppress the cycle by ensuring that the enzymes are not active simultaneously. In the liver of some mammalian species (including rats, mice and humans) the hexokinase is present as an isoenzyme (hexokinase IV, also commonly but somewhat erroneously known as glucokinase[51]) that is competitively inhibited by the reversible binding of a complex between a specific regulatory protein[256,257] and fructose 6–phosphate, the concentration of which varies in parallel with glucose 6–phosphate. There is, however, no known regulatory mechanism acting on the glucose–6–phosphatase (although it is spatially separated by its location in the endoplasmic reticulum from the cytosolic hexokinase).

The flux round the fructose 6–phosphate:fructose 1,6–bisphosphate cycle can be comparable with net gluconeogenic flux in hepatocytes, though in many cases it is much less.[146] The cycle also occurs in isolated liver, though the results showing that the cycling rate can be several times gluconeogenic flux use a disputed method,[111,127] and other results suggest lower cycling rates, certainly much less than for the glucose:glucose 6–phosphate cycle. There are also a number of regulatory and control mechanisms that act on the cycle enzymes in opposite senses and which could therefore limit cycling. For example, AMP, phosphate and fructose 2,6–bisphosphate activate phosphofructokinase but inhibit fructose bisphosphatase. (The older view that phosphofructokinase is activated by its product fructose 1,6–bisphosphate now seems wrong; the activation observed in assays was because the product binds weakly at the fructose 2,6–bisphosphate activator site but, when the activator is present at physiological levels, product inhibition dominates.[11,186,247,255]) Fructose 2,6–bisphosphate is a *third messenger* of hormone action, since its synthesis and degradation in liver are controlled by glucagon and α–adrenergic agents that change the activity of a bifunctional enzyme, phosphofructo–2–kinase/fructose–2,6–bisphosphatase, by reversible phosphorylation brought about by the cyclic AMP–dependent protein kinase[185] (see Chapter 7.4.3.1). In addition, the cycle enzymes themselves may be phosphorylated by cyclic AMP–dependent protein kinase, but the significance of this is uncertain because the effects of phosphorylation on the kinetics of the enzymes that have been demonstrated to date seem quite small.

Measurements on the phosphoenolpyruvate:pyruvate cycle often show pyruvate kinase fluxes of the same order as gluconeogenic flux, though this has often been in the presence of unphysiologically high levels of gluconeogenic substrates. The gluconeogenic hormone glucagon seems to suppress the cycle by causing inactivation of pyruvate kinase via reversible protein phosphorylation.

7.3.3 Suggested functions

The reason for preferring the term *substrate cycle* to *futile cycle* is the possibility that cycling is intrinsically advantageous, and several different functions have been attributed to cycling:

(1) heat production (*thermogenesis*) in brown adipose tissue of mammals and flight muscle of bumble bees;[168,234]

(2) more sensitive regulation of the net flux through the pathway by regulation of the enzymes carrying the cycle flux,[168,169,171] perhaps involving properties typical of switching and triggering devices;[196]

(3) control of the direction of flow at branch points and in bidirectional pathways;[112,126,169,237]

(4) buffering of metabolite concentrations.[26,112,171]

Of these proposals, (1) is straightforward and capable of experimental confirmation without any theoretical problems, (2) and (3) have been the subject of continuing discussion which will be considered below, and (4) has not been developed in a quantitative manner nor subjected to any extensive theoretical analysis.

7.3.4 Thermogenesis

It seems surprising that the generation of body heat by metabolism should need any special explanation, since catabolism is characteristically exothermic. However, the coupling mechanisms of metabolism create a difficulty, because part of the energy released during catabolic reactions is conserved by the phosphorylation of ADP to ATP and the regulatory mechanisms of catabolism ensure it slows down unless this ATP is hydrolysed. The analyses of the control of supply and demand pathways and feedback inhibition presented earlier (Chapters 7.1–7.2) imply that better homoeostasis of ATP may be obtained if control by demand predominates over control by supply (catabolism), and this expectation is supported by the results of the top–down analysis of hepatocyte energy metabolism (Chapter 6.3.3.2). Therefore, if there is a requirement for extra heat generation, either the demand for ATP must be increased or the coupling of catabolism to ATP production must be weakened. There is evidence that both approaches are adopted, and one of the ways that the demand is increased is by substrate cycling.

Eric Newsholme and Bernard Crabtree suggested that the fructose 6–phosphate:fructose 1,6–bisphosphate cycle is used by bumble bees to raise the temperature of their flight muscles in cold weather.[168] They had made measurements that showed that flight muscles of several species of bumble bees contain unusually high levels of fructose–1,6–bisphosphatase, which is required for the gluconeogenic pathway and is not usually present in significant amounts in a highly glycolytic tissue like muscle. Other species of bee that have relatively little of this enzyme are unable to fly at such low ambient temperatures (10°C) as bumble bees. Even at these temperatures, bumble bees can maintain their thoracic temperature at the 30°C necessary for them (and many other insects) to fly. The hypothesis was supported by measurements made by a different laboratory [39,40] that showed that cycling could be measured in bumble bee muscles at low temperatures, but the cycling decreased with temperature and had disappeared at 27°C. Furthermore, the cycling was prevented in flight, probably by inhibition of the fructose bisphosphatase by the rise in Ca^{2+} that occurs on stimulation of the muscle. However, Newsholme and Crabtree also calculated that the energy yield of this substrate cycle was not enough by itself to account for the total heat generation, so there must be other mechanisms as well.

This also seems to be true of another tissue for which substrate cycling could make a contribution to thermogenesis: brown adipose tissue. Brown adipose tissue is a form of adipose tissue in which the cells have more cytoplasm and mitochondria, and contain several small lipid droplets rather than the single large one found in the more abundant white adipose tissue. Brown adipose tissue is present in neonatal mammals, which generally are less effective than adults at temperature regulation, and in hibernating mammals. In both cases, brown adipose tissue has a significant role in heat generation. The triacylglycerol:fatty acid cycle is active in brown adipose tissue, though calculations imply that it could only account for a small proportion of the heat production by this tissue.[168] The mitochondria of brown adipose tissue contain specific mechanisms that uncouple respiration from ATP synthesis and make a much larger contribution.

7.3.5 Sensitivity of control
Around 1970, Eric Newsholme and his coworkers in Oxford[168,169,171] developed the proposal that substrate cycles could be devices for increasing the sen-

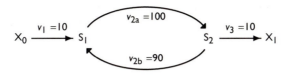

Figure 7.13 Increased sensitivity of control by a substrate cycle
The fluxes shown on each step are illustrative. If stimulation of the forward enzyme of the cycle increases v_{2a} 10% to 110, and the reverse reaction remains unchanged at 90, then v_1 and v_3 must increase 100% to 20.

sitivity of the regulation of pathway flux by an effector acting on one or both of the pathway enzymes. The initial form of their argument[169,171] is shown in Figure 7.13; generalized algebraically, it led to the proposal that an effector that makes a given percentage change in the activity of enzyme 2a will cause a percentage change in the net flux (= v_1 = v_3) that will be larger by a factor $(1 + v_{2b}/v_1)$ than would occur if the pathway were linear with $v_{2b} = 0$.[168] Similarly, the response of the net flux to a change in the activity of enzyme 2b would be amplified by the factor $-v_{2b}/v_1$ (with the minus sign showing that an increase in the enzyme activity produces a decrease in the net flux). If the same effector acted to stimulate one cycle enzyme and to inhibit the other, these effects would be additive. This could be particularly relevant to the fructose 6–phosphate:fructose 1,6–bisphosphate cycle in which AMP and fructose 2,6–bisphosphate activate phosphofructokinase but inhibit fructose–1,6–bisphosphatase.

Stein and Blum[240] pointed out that the basis of the theory was paradoxical since it was derived on the assumption that the concentrations of the intermediates do not change when the flux is altered, yet

- the enzyme 2a dominates the flux control of the pathway, *i.e.* the pathway flux always responds fully to an increase in the activity of this enzyme by matching increases in the rate of enzymes 1 and 3; this requires that S_1 falls and S_2 rises;

- when the flux is increased through 2a, there is no compensating alteration in the flux through the other limb of the cycle, 2b, which requires the assumption of no change in the intermediate concentrations to be true.

They performed three separate computer simulations of open substrate cycles (Figure 7.11f) based on each of those found in carbohydrate metabolism and concluded that the gain in sensitivity of control was small in physiologically feasible conditions and that other functions for the cycles (to be discussed later) seemed more likely.

Crabtree and Newsholme reanalysed their proposal more rigorously with their own form of metabolic sensitivity analysis[54,55] and found that their original equation overstates the gain in sensitivity but that there is still some gain.

Herbert Sauro and I[69] used Metabolic Control Analysis to study the same question (see Appendix 1 to this chapter, *Control Analysis of substrate cycles* for details). We calculated the gain in sensitivity by asking how much the flux control coefficient of the cycle enzyme 2a is increased by cycling, relative to an equivalent pathway with the same net flux and intermediate concentrations. This factor, r, depends on the elasticities of the enzymes and the cycle fluxes in the following way:

$$r = \frac{1}{1 - \dfrac{v_{2b}(\varepsilon_1^1\varepsilon_2^3 - \varepsilon_1^1\varepsilon_2^{2b} - \varepsilon_2^3\varepsilon_1^{2b})}{v_{2a}(\varepsilon_1^1\varepsilon_2^3 - \varepsilon_1^1\varepsilon_2^{2a} - \varepsilon_2^3\varepsilon_1^{2a})}} \tag{7.7}$$

With normal substrate kinetics, where elasticities with respect to substrates are ≥ 0, and with respect to products are ≤ 0, the cycle increases the control coefficient if:

$$\frac{\varepsilon_2^{2b}}{\varepsilon_2^3} + \frac{\varepsilon_1^{2b}}{\varepsilon_1^1} < 1 \tag{7.8}$$

Since each of the two terms on the left of this equation must be less than 1 for the condition to be true, this shows that the output enzyme 3 must be less saturated with S_2 than is enzyme 2b, and that the product inhibition of enzyme 1 by S_1 must be stronger than that of 2b. For r to reach Newsholme and Crabtree's maximum value of $(1 + v_{2b}/v_1)$, it is also necessary that:

$$\left|\frac{\varepsilon_2^{2a}}{\varepsilon_2^3}\right| + \left|\frac{\varepsilon_1^{2a}}{\varepsilon_1^1}\right| \ll 1 \tag{7.9}$$

(The bars around the terms indicate that only their magnitude is considered; any negative signs, such as in the product elasticity ε_1^1, are ignored.) Here the first term on the left shows that the product inhibition of 2a must be much weaker than the elasticity of 3 with respect to its substrate, and the second that the substrate elasticity of 2a must be much smaller in magnitude than the product inhibition of 1 (a condition most likely to be met when 2a is saturated, as noted by Crabtree[54]). These same conditions also maximize the magnitude of the negative flux control coefficient of the reverse limb of the cycle, 2b.

In conclusion, the conditions under which substrate cycles can generate greatly increased flux control coefficients (which are necessary to give increased responsiveness to effectors of the cycle enzymes) are quite restrictive. Also, an effector that acts to increase the net flux through the cycle also reduces the flux control coefficients of the cycle enzymes, and therefore its own response coefficient. At present, there is no indisputable example of the phenomenon; the best candidate is the fructose 6–phosphate:fructose 1,6–bisphosphate cycle in mammalian liver glycolysis/gluconeogenesis, but it is not certain that the cycling rates are high enough and the relevant elasticity values are unknown.

7.3.6   Switching the direction of flux

Figure 7.12 shows that the substrate cycles of carbohydrate metabolism are of the type termed an 'open futile cycle' (Figure 7.11f) and occur at complex metabolic 'crossroads'. The computer simulations carried out by Stein and Blum[240] as mentioned in the previous section certainly suggested that the cycles aided the switching of flux in bidirectional pathways as either the relative flows changed in the inputs and outputs, or modifiers acted on the cycle enzymes. Sel'kov and his colleagues[196] also concluded that a substrate cycle can function as a switch, with a minimum of cycling near the crossover in the direction of the net flux through the cycle. Since the direction of flux does switch direction in these pathways *in vivo*, the proposal seems relatively uncontroversial. What is difficult to quantify is the cost–benefit analysis. The costs are difficult to measure accurately, but in liver cells each of the cycles probably only uses a few percent of the cell's total energy production.[10,146,190] There is no measure for the improvement in switching obtained with a given degree of cycling.

7.3.7   Buffering metabolite concentrations

Cahill's original demonstration[26] of the glucose:glucose 6–phosphate cycle led him to propose that it helped to regulate the blood glucose concentration. Newsholme and Crabtree suggested that the triacylglycerol:fatty acid cycle in adipose tissue could help to buffer the levels of fatty acids in the blood during lipolysis.[168] At one time it was suggested that the cycling of Ca^{2+} between cytosol and mitochondria could buffer the cytosolic Ca^{2+} concentration and allow sensitive control[12,112,174] though nowadays the role of the mitochondria is not thought to be so significant.[155,183] The cycle involves uptake of Ca^{2+} by the mitochondrial matrix driven by the membrane potential component of the protonmotive force and export from the matrix by a $Ca^{2+}/2H^+$ antiport (*i.e.* exchanger) driven by the pH gradient component of the protonmotive force, so both components are exergonic and effectively unidirectional.

The problem with the concept that buffering is a specific property of substrate cycles is revealed by considering the Ca^{2+} cycle, even though this is strictly a conserved cycle (Figure 7.11c) if Ca^{2+} exchange with the endoplasmic reticulum[12] is ignored. If we take the cytoplasmic Ca^{2+}, then its steady state value is that which makes the rate of the supply process (mitochondrial export) equal the rate of the demand process (mitochondrial import). This is true even though the supply and demand processes meet in the mitochondrial matrix to form a cycle, and is in fact a general statement about *any* metabolite at steady state. Any buffering therefore reflects the dynamic equilibrium or non–equilibrium steady state, determined by the specific kinetics of the process. Several conclusions follow.

- Any buffering effect that does exist cannot be a specific function of a substrate cycle.

- There is no specific effect of cycling rate, since the rates of the demand

and supply processes can be multiplied by any arbitrary factor and the same steady state concentration is obtained.

- The question of homoeostasis of the concentration can be addressed by the supply–demand analysis of Hofmeyr and Cornish–Bowden described in Section 7.1. The sensitivity of the control is represented by the concentration control coefficient; the kinetic features of the pathway, but not its flux, will determine whether the sensitivity is high or low.

- If *buffering* is meant to imply the tendency of the system to return to the same steady state after an arbitrary perturbation of the concentrations, then this is a common property of metabolic systems with a dynamically stable steady state, and again the cycling is irrelevant. However, the rate of return to the steady state after a perturbation is related to the turnover rate of the intermediates, and will be shorter if the flux is high.

Another demonstration that substrate cycling does not affect the homoeostasis of metabolites follows from the Metabolic Control Analysis applied to the substrate cycle of Fig. 7.13 in Chapter 7.3.5 and Appendix 1 of this Chapter. I have used the same technique that shows that the flux control coefficients depend on the cycling rate to show that the concentration control coefficients do not.

Is there no truth in the concept that the glucose:glucose 6–phosphate cycle helps to regulate blood glucose concentration? I believe there is, and the computer simulations carried out by Stein and Blum[240] suggest that it is so. The explanation cannot be given just in terms of the effect arising from the cycle. First, if blood glucose was determined solely by the balance of supply by absorption from the intestine and demand by the tissues, it would exhibit poor homoeostasis because the inhibition of absorption by blood glucose is too weak (Chapter 7.1). Through the glucose:glucose 6–phosphate cycle, blood glucose is connected to other supply and demand processes, and the homoeostatic characteristics are now those of the total system. The homoeostasis is therefore related to the switching properties of the cycle, whereby it can bidirectionally connect the input and output processes for blood glucose to liver carbohydrate metabolism. As noted by many authors,[111,171] the steady state level of blood glucose is close to the calculated value at which the rates of liver hexokinase IV and glucose–6–phosphatase would be equal and there would be no net flux through the cycle. This is because the half–saturation value of the sigmoidal hexokinase IV rate curve is in the 1–10 mM range characteristic of mammalian blood glucose levels. When the blood glucose level changes, the substrate cycle automatically operates as a switch with no need for any other mechanism. Thus a rise in blood glucose level, which rapidly equilibrates with liver cytosol glucose causes an increase in the rate of phosphorylation but has no significant effect on the glucose–6–phosphatase rate (since the demand and supply system for glucose 6–phosphate in the liver is fairly effective at ensuring homoeostasis of its concentration), so the cycle switches to cause net phosphorylation and glucose uptake by the liver. The reverse happens when the blood glucose level falls and the rate of phosphorylation drops below that of the phosphatase. Thus the homoeostasis results from the kinetic balance of supply and demand at a complex metabolic crossroads, in which the switching property of the cycle is a relevant factor. There is no need for (and no point in) invoking a specific buffering action of the cycle itself.

7.4 Regulation by covalent modification of enzymes

Much of this book so far has dealt with the extent to which particular enzymes can control metabolic fluxes. Only indirectly does this address the question of what controls metabolism, since it identifies sites at which control might be exerted most effectively, and predicts to some extent the effect that will be produced if the enzyme's activity is changed. The response coefficient (Chapter 5.4) indicates the control that could be exerted via an allosteric enzyme by an allosteric effector external to the pathway; the implication is that this gives a viable method of control, but I can give no example where this has been demonstrated to be quantitatively important in the same way that Keith Snell and I showed that serine could control its rate of synthesis (Chapter 6.3.4.2). Induction and repression of enzyme synthesis, for example in response to nutritional or hormonal signals, are mechanisms of control that can be interpreted in terms of the flux control coefficients of the enzymes involved, and examples of this were given in Chapter 6.1.2. Yet the metabolism of organisms shows substantial and specific responses to signals such as environmental factors, hormones, growth factors and nerve stimulation that precede any effects these signals may have on synthesis and degradation of enzymes, and without direct interactions between the signal molecules and specific pathway enzymes. This is clearly one of the most important aspects of metabolic control. In this section I will present examples that show that many of these controls are exerted via mechanisms that involve post–translational covalent modifications of proteins that affect their enzyme activity. Since the processes involve changes in enzymic activities, they can be interpreted in Metabolic Control Analysis through flux control coefficients.

7.4.1 Irreversible and cyclic cascades

There are many types of post–translational modifications of enzymic proteins that have effects on their activity. Some of these are irreversible and not primarily mechanisms of control. For example, proteolytic cleavage of inactive precursors (or *zymogens*) can be a mechanism for safely synthesizing and storing a potentially hazardous product such as a digestive enzyme until it is released at its site of action. Nevertheless, there is the potential for control in such mechanisms, as illustrated by blood clotting. Here there is a *cascade* of zymogens in which each factor, upon activation, proteolytically cleaves the next zymogen in the sequence, until prothrombin is cleaved to thrombin, which cleaves soluble fibrinogen to yield the clot–forming fibrin fibres. The sequence exhibits great amplification through using catalysts that create catalysts, and converts the minute initiating signal given by tissue injury into a macroscopic response within a few tens of seconds. However, for the enzymes involved, it is a once–only mechanism as the clotting can only be stopped by their proteolytic inactivation.

Another irreversible modification of enzymes, this time intracellular enzymes in metabolic pathways, is the attachment of ubiquitin.[102] This marks the enzyme for energy–dependent degradation by ubiquitin–dependent proteases and may well play a role in metabolic control by adjusting enzyme amounts (Chapter 1.4.1), since different enzymes in the same metabolic pathway often have very different turnover rates in eukaryotic cells. Much remains to be learnt about the role of enzyme degradation in the control of metabolism.

The covalent modifications that play the greatest role in metabolic control are reversible or cyclic, so that the enzyme is interconverted between two forms that differ in activity, either because of effects on the kinetics with respect to substrates or of altered sensitivity to effectors. The first example of such a process was assembled over about 20 years from the combined efforts of several groups of researchers[139,244] studying the enzyme phosphorylase, which breaks down glycogen to form glucose 1–phosphate. The work of the Coris in the 1940s had shown that there were two forms of phosphorylase that differed in activity: phosphorylase *a* was the more active, whereas phosphorylase *b* required AMP activation and was inhibited by glucose 6–phosphate. Furthermore, these two forms were interconverted in some way. In 1950, Sutherland discovered that the activation of phosphorylase in liver brought about by the hormone adrenaline was mediated by a heat–stable factor, though it was not until 1959 that this was identified as cyclic AMP (Figure 7.14). Meanwhile, Edwin Krebs' group was studying phosphorylase in muscle, and in 1955 they discovered that the interconversion was phosphorylation of phosphorylase *b* by ATP, catalysed by an enzyme, phosphorylase kinase. In the same year, Sutherland and Wosilait showed that inactivation of phosphorylase in the liver involved formation of phosphorylase *b* by the action of a phosphatase. Krebs' laboratory went on to establish by 1959 that phosphorylase kinase itself was controlled by phosphorylation and dephosphorylation, showing that the control of a metabolic enzyme could be organized in a cascade fashion. Sutherland's group went on to discover the formation of cyclic AMP by adenylate cyclase in 1962, and in 1965 and 1966 put forward the concept of cyclic AMP as a *second messenger* or intracellular mediator of (extracellular) hormone action.

Since these initial discoveries, it has become clear that there are several types of covalent modification in addition to phosphorylation, and that there are other signals and second messengers apart from cyclic AMP.

Table 7.1   Types of covalent modification of enzymes

Type of modification	Donor	Amino acids modified	No. of targets (approx.)	Comments
Phosphorylation	ATP, GTP	Ser, Thr, Tyr OH–Lys	90	More prevalent in eukaryotes than prokaryotes
ADP–ribosylation	NAD^+	Arg, Glu, Lys	20	
Nucleotidylation	ATP, UTP	Tyr, Ser	4	In prokaryotes
Methylation	S–Adenosyl-methionine	Asp, Glu, Lys, His, Gln	14	Prokaryotes and eukaryotes, but less prevalent in the latter than phosphorylation

Based on data of Schachter et al.,[226] surveyed in 1986.

7.4.2   Types of reversible modification

The description of any reversible covalent modification system involves a target protein, an enzyme for modifying it and one for reversing the modification, and mechanisms (such as allosteric effectors or further covalent modification systems) for controlling the balance of the activities of the two interconverting enzymes. The complexities of classifying the large number of systems now known will become increasingly apparent as this section progresses, but stem from the multiplicity of effects and the many interactions between systems. Thus:

- some modifying enzymes are themselves targets for modification (as implied above), thus forming cascade systems;

- some targets undergo multiple modifications, either of the same type but at different sites by different enzymes, or of different types;

- different signals can have overlapping mechanisms and share a modifying cycle;

- one signal can interfere with or potentiate the actions of another by cross–reactions between the modifying cycles or by interactions between the modified sites on the target.

The principal types of covalent modification known to reversibly affect enzymes are summarized in Table 7.1, based on data of Schachter et al.[226] Phosphorylation is the most common modification in eukaryotic cells and is carried out by several different systems, as will be described below. It is probable that there are many more targets than have been identified currently, since as many as one in four polypeptide chains has been estimated to be phosphory-lated in mouse lymphoma cells[37] (though this average value takes no account of the multiple phosphorylation of some chains, nor the relative abundance of different proteins). In contrast, levels of phosphorylation are much lower in prokaryotic cells,[75] but even so, a significant role for phosphorylation in metabolic control is being discovered.[205] Although there are relatively few identified methylation targets in eukaryotic cells, and it is about 50–fold less extensive than phosphorylation, electrophoresis of radiolabelled mouse lym-phoma cell extracts showed at least 24 different methylated protein bands.[37] To illustrate the reversible modification systems further, I will only deal with phosphorylation and, to a lesser extent, nucleotidylation.

7.4.3   Phosphorylation

It is impossible to know where to start to produce a simple, coherent descrip-tion of such a complex, interacting and interlocking network as the eukaryotic phosphorylation systems. The difficulty is illustrated by the general history of discovery of a system. This usually stems from the observation that a particular target enzyme undergoes phosphorylation. In turn, this leads to the identifica-tion of a kinase that is responsible, and which is known initially by the name of its target (even when this leads to comic names like phosphorylase kinase kinase for the kinase that phosphorylates phosphorylase kinase). Generally, it later emerges that this kinase is similar to, or even identical with, one known by a different name because it has been shown to phosphorylate a different target, and the kinase is named after the signal that stimulates it to act rather than by its target.

The position is even more complicated with the protein phosphatases, since these do not show unique associations with target enzymes, specific protein kinases or signal systems, though they are affected by all of these.

Furthermore, although phosphorylation of an enzyme can lead to activity changes, many enzymes are subject to multiple phosphorylations at different sites, and some of the sites appear to affect ease of phosphorylation or dephos-phorylation at other sites rather than directly affecting activity.

7.4.3.1   Kinases and their control signals

The major groups of protein kinases that affect intermediary metabolism are summarized in Table 7.2, arranged by control signal. Thus for simplicity, phos-phorylation of structural proteins like histones, enzymes of protein synthesis and muscle contractile apparatus have been ignored. Tyrosine protein kinases have not been considered here since these activities seem to be associated with the receptors for certain hormones such as insulin and growth factors and, important as they are, the possible links between phosphorylation and any metabolic effects are only now beginning to be unravelled.[145]

Table 7.2 Protein serine and threonine kinases in metabolism

Signal	Enzyme
Cyclic nucleotides	Cyclic AMP–dependent protein kinases (Types I & II), cyclic GMP–dependent protein kinase
Ca^{2+} and calmodulin	Ca^{2+}/calmodulin multiprotein kinase phosphorylase kinase/glycogen synthase kinase 2
Diacylglycerol	Protein kinase C
AMP	AMP–activated kinase
Metabolic intermediates and other 'local' effectors	Many target–specific kinases, including: pyruvate dehydrogenase kinase; branched–chain ketoacid dehydrogenase kinase; glycogen synthase kinases 3 & 4

Based on the classification by Krebs[139] with the addition of the AMP–activated protein kinase[28,29] characterized by Grahame Hardie's group in Dundee.

7.4.3.1.1 Cyclic AMP

In Chapter 7.4.1 I mentioned the discovery by Sutherland's group that cyclic AMP (Figure 7.14) is an intermediary in the hormonal activation of phosphory-lase. They later showed that it was produced by the enzyme adenylate cyclase, located on the cytoplasmic surface of the plasma membrane of eukaryotic cells:

$$ATP \longrightarrow \text{cyclic AMP} + \text{pyrophosphate}$$

The concentrations of cyclic AMP are generally low, in the region of 0.1–1 μM. It is hydrolysed to AMP by a variety of phosphodiesterase enzymes that differ in their intracellular location, their K_m for cyclic AMP (broadly classified as 'high' and 'low') and the physiological effectors and drugs that modulate their activities. Cyclic AMP is not a metabolic intermediate for the synthesis of any other compound; its function appears to be solely as a signal that controls enzyme activities. Since adenylate cyclase is stimulated by hormones that bind to receptors on the outer surface of cells, causing the intracellular level of cyclic AMP to vary in a hormone–dependent fashion, Sutherland proposed the term *second messenger* to indicate its role in the intracellular relay of a hormonal message.

The hormonal activation of adenylate cyclase is one specific instance of a trans–membrane *signal transduction* pathway, many of the details of which were determined by Martin Rodbell and his colleagues (see ref. [199]). This involves the interactions of three classes of components in the plasma membrane. There are specific receptors at the extracellular surface that can bind stimulatory or

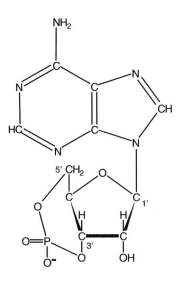

Figure 7.14 Cyclic AMP
Like all adenine nucleotides, cyclic AMP has an adenine ring attached to the 1′ carbon of the ribose sugar. AMP itself has a phosphate on the 5′ carbon atom of the ribose ring, but in 3′,5′–cyclic AMP, this phosphate is bonded to both the 3′ and 5′ positions.

inhibitory signal molecules (R_s and R_i respectively). The interaction of these receptors with the catalytic subunit is mediated by guanine nucleotide-binding regulatory proteins, again of stimulatory and inhibitory types (G_s and G_i). The G–proteins bind GTP when they interact with the receptor–hormone complex, and the G–protein complex with GTP in turn interacts with adenylate cyclase (or other target protein in the general case). The action of the G–protein terminates when it hydrolyses its bound GTP. Hormones that act on adenylate cyclase through a stimulatory G–protein include adrenaline, adrenocorticotropin, thyroid–stimulating hormone (TSH), luteinizing hormone (LH), secretin and glucagon, not necessarily all in the same tissue though those mentioned do all stimulate adenylate cyclase in adipose tissue, eventually causing lipolysis. The action of adrenaline is complex because it acts on adenylate cyclase *via* a class of receptors called β–adrenergic receptors, found particularly in muscle, but *via* α–adrenergic receptors (for example, in liver) it acts to raise intracellular Ca^{2+} concentrations. Adenosine inhibits adenylate cyclase in adipose tissue *via* an inhibitory G–protein.

Stimulation of adenylate cyclase leads to a rise in the intracellular concentration of cyclic AMP, the principal, perhaps only, effect of which is stimulation of cyclic AMP–dependent protein kinase (protein kinase A). The amount by which the cyclic AMP concentration increases must depend on the activity and kinetics of the phosphodiesterase enzymes present in the cells, but since there are phosphodiesterases with K_m values above the intracellular levels of cyclic AMP, it is likely that the concentration changes are at best proportional to the stimulation of the cyclase. Protein kinase A occurs as a set of isoenzymes, but there are two basic classes: Types I and II.[13] Both are tetrameric proteins formed of two regulatory subunits (R) and two catalytic subunits (C) in the inactive state. Activation involves binding of four cyclic AMP molecules by the regulatory subunits and release of free, active catalytic subunits:

$$R_2C_2 + 4 \text{ cyclic AMP} \rightleftharpoons R_2(\text{cyclic AMP})_4 + 2C$$

The two sites for cyclic AMP per regulatory subunit interact cooperatively so that the Hill coefficient for kinase activation with respect to cyclic AMP is about 1.6.[13] The difference between the Type I and Type II kinases is that the latter undergo autophosphorylation of the regulatory subunit, though the physiological significance of this, and the respective physiological roles of the isoenzymes are not very clear.

There is a large number of targets for phosphorylation by protein kinase A. Not all protein serine or threonine residues can be phosphorylated, nor all proteins, so there must be specific sites recognized by the kinase. A common sequence at phosphorylation sites involves two basic amino acids (lysine or arginine) to the N–terminal side, for example Arg-Arg-X-Ser and Arg-Lys-X-Ser. The effects on the target enzyme can be inhibitory or activatory; in general where antagonistic enzymes in potential substrate cycles are phosphorylated, one is activated and one inhibited.[42] Glycogen phosphorylase and glycogen synthase are one such pair, and the evidence is that substrate cycling is not significant between glucose 1–phosphate and glycogen because these two enzymes are not both in their most active forms simultaneously. Philip Cohen,[42] whose group in Dundee has carried out much of the work on the phosphorylation of glycogen synthase and on the phosphoprotein phosphatases, has also suggested that enzymes catalysing biodegradation are generally activated by phosphorylation, and biosynthetic enzymes are inhibited. Phosphorylase, triacylglycerol lipase (in adipose tissue) and phenylalanine 4–mono-oxygenase (in liver) are clearly catabolic enzymes that are activated by phosphorylation. Anabolic enzymes that are inhibited by phosphorylation include glycogen synthase and acetyl–CoA carboxylase (the first enzyme of lipid synthesis). Other instances are less clear cut because of tissue differences both in metabolism and the effects of hormones. Thus whereas in muscle tissue adrenaline promotes glycolysis, in liver, it and glucagon promote gluconeogenesis and here the glycolytic enzyme pyruvate kinase is inhibited by phosphorylation.

Another example of tissue–dependent effects involves phosphofructokinase, which in liver forms a substrate cycle with fructose bisphosphatase (Chapter 7.3.2, p. 218). In mammalian heart[164] and adipose tissue,[206] phosphofructokinase is phosphorylated after adrenaline stimulation (perhaps not by protein kinase A) to give an enzyme that is less sensitive to the action of its inhibitors such as ATP and more sensitive to its activators, in particular fructose 2,6–bisphosphate. As described earlier, fructose 2,6–bisphosphate is a third messenger of hormone action, since it is purely a signal metabolite and its production and consumption by the bifunctional phosphofructo–2–kinase and fructose–2,6–bisphosphatase is affected by cyclic AMP–dependent phosphorylation. However, in heart muscle, it seems that adrenaline causes an increase in the concentration of fructose 2,6–bisphosphate by activation of the 2–kinase,[164] which is the exact opposite of its effect in the liver. Thus in glucose–consuming tissues, it appears that, directly or indirectly, hormone-sensitive phosphorylation activates phosphofructokinase. In liver, glucagon initiates cyclic AMP–dependent phosphorylation of the bifunctional enzyme, causing inhibition of the 2–kinase, activation of the phosphatase and a fall in fructose 2,6–bisphosphate which has the effect of inhibiting phosphofructo-kinase and activating fructose–1,6–bisphosphatase.

Even greater complexity in the cyclic AMP–dependent systems will emerge in the following sections, partly when we encounter the role of the protein phosphatases, but also as the interactions with other covalent modification systems become apparent.

7.4.3.1.2 Ca^{2+} and calmodulin

Even though Ca^{2+} is prevalent in the environment and is present in our blood at 2 mM, the levels of free Ca^{2+} in cells are maintained at an extraordinarily low average level of about 10^{-8} M. Undoubtedly this is necessary in part to avoid the formation of insoluble complexes with the many compounds in the cell that contain phosphate. However, eukaryotic cells have adopted Ca^{2+} as a second messenger in response to a wide variety of external and internal regulatory signals acting on a whole range of cellular activities as well as metabolism. In all eukaryotes, many of these functions are mediated through the regulatory protein *calmodulin*, first discovered in 1970 as a Ca^{2+}–dependent activator of the enzyme cyclic AMP phosphodiesterase by Cheung, Kakiuchi and Yamazaki.[45,266]

Unlike cyclic AMP, which acts exclusively through its protein kinase, the Ca^{2+}/calmodulin system acts through multiple mechanisms, both general and specific, by interaction with particular enzymes of metabolism. The common element is the nature of the interaction with calmodulin. Calmodulin is a single polypeptide chain with four Ca^{2+}–binding domains that have differing Ca^{2+} affinities; its dissociation constants range from 1 to 100 μM. Calmodulin binds to the enzymes it affects, but with substantially higher affinity when it has Ca^{2+} bound than when it is Ca^{2+}–free; by energy conservation principles, this means that formation of the calmodulin–enzyme complex causes an increase in the affinity of the calmodulin in the complex for Ca^{2+} so that the dissociation constants are micromolar or less. At the micromolar levels of calmodulin in the cell, many of the target enzymes will not complex with calmodulin in the absence of Ca^{2+}, but do so in its presence. However, in two Ca^{2+}–activated enzymes, phosphorylase kinase and phosphoprotein phosphatase 2B, calmodulin is present as a permanent subunit in the structure. In virtually all known cases, enzymes that interact with Ca^{2+}/calmodulin are activated.

Ca^{2+}/calmodulin can stimulate phosphorylation *via* a calmodulin–dependent multiprotein kinase,[45] which was previously thought to be a number of separate activities. The target enzymes that this phosphorylates include glycogen synthase in muscle and liver (causing deactivation) and tryptophan 5–mono-oxygenase and tyrosine 3–mono-oxygenase in brain [where they are parts of the pathways to the neurotransmitters dopamine and 5-hydroxytryptamine (serotonin)]. Other enzymes can be phosphorylated by this kinase *in vitro*, but often it is not clear whether this is physiologically significant. Increased Ca^{2+} levels cause glycogen phosphorylase in both muscle and liver to be activated by phosphorylation by phosphorylase kinase, which contains calmodulin as a subunit. In muscle, this links the activation of glycogen breakdown to muscle contraction, since Ca^{2+} is released into muscle cytoplasm from the sarcoplasmic reticulum to activate the contractile apparatus when a nerve impulse arrives. (Ca^{2+}/calmodulin and troponin C, which is related to calmodulin, also have a range of effects on the contractile apparatus and on Ca^{2+} transport which are not of immediate relevance here.)

Apart from the effects that Ca^{2+}/calmodulin has on its own second messenger system through its activation of Ca^{2+} transport, it also interacts with phosphorylation induced by the cyclic AMP system. Thus in brain it stimulates adenylate cyclase, but in most other tissues it stimulates one of the cyclic nucleotide phosphodiesterase isoenzymes. In addition, as will be discussed below, Ca^{2+}/calmodulin specifically activates one of the phosphoprotein phosphatases (2B) that acts on targets phosphorylated by protein kinase A. All this has led to the conclusion that Ca^{2+} can attenuate the actions of cyclic AMP.[44]

7.4.3.1.3 Diacylglycerol

The G–protein signal-transduction system also couples some hormones to membrane phospholipases which break down inositol phospholipids in the membrane to yield inositol triphosphate and diacylglycerol.[199] The inositol triphosphate is involved in promoting the hormone–induced rise in intracellular Ca^{2+}, probably by causing its release from internal stores. The diacylglycerol activates protein kinase C, which also requires Ca^{2+} and phospholipid for activity. Protein kinase C catalyses phosphorylation of a wide range of proteins and influences a range of cellular phenomena including signal transduction itself, hormone release, gene expression, cell proliferation and muscle contraction, but seems less involved in the direct control of intermediary metabolism. It may have roles in steroidogenesis in the adrenal cortex and in glycogen metabolism.

7.4.3.1.4 AMP

The kinases I have described so far respond to external signals; it is therefore particularly significant that David Carling, Grahame Hardie and their

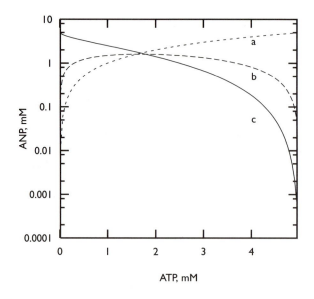

Figure 7.15 The adenylate kinase equilibrium
The curves show the concentrations on a logarithimic scale of ATP (a), ADP (b) and AMP (c) at equilibrium at a given ATP level when the total concentration of adenine nucleotides (ANP) is 5 mM and $K_{eq} = 1.12$.[258]

colleagues in Dundee recently discovered that there is a protein kinase that responds to an internal signal of metabolic state: AMP.[28] There are two fundamental questions about this that need to be answered.

- What is the advantage in having a covalent modification system that responds to an internal metabolite when this is what allosteric enzymes do?

- How does AMP indicate internal metabolic state?

Covalent modification systems can exhibit different responses to effectors compared with allosteric enzymes, as will be discussed in a later section (7.4.5). Even so, many of the advantages that covalent modification has as a transducer of the effect of an external signal present at very low levels would not seem to be relevant for responding to an intracellular metabolite that could bind directly to allosteric sites on enzymes. However, I will argue later (Chapter 8.1) that large changes in a pathway flux require simultaneous and proportional action on a number of the pathway enzymes to avoid disruption of cellular homoeostasis. Activation of a kinase that can operate on a number of enzymes might be one way to achieve this. A common response of several enzymes to the same allosteric effector might be another possibility, but would only work well if the allosteric effects were nearly balanced, and might therefore be difficult to implement reliably. However, ATP and AMP are possible candidates

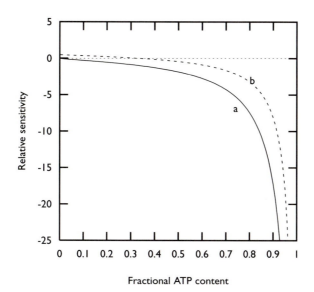

Figure 7.16 Relative sensitivities of the adenine nucleotides to a change in ATP level
The fractional changes in AMP (a) and ADP (b) in response to a fractional change in ATP as a result of the adenylate kinase equilibrium, calculated as described previously.[69] The response of ATP is not shown as it is always 1. Note that the relative sensitivity of ADP changes sign at an ATP fraction of about 0.3, which is the point at which the sensitivity to AMP becomes nearer zero than that to ATP. Again, ANP = 5 mM and K_{eq} = 1.12.

as allosteric signals that operate on a number of enzymes, as they do affect a number of enzymes in carbohydrate metabolism for example.

This leads to the second issue: why AMP is involved in allosteric effects and activation of a protein kinase. It is because AMP amplifies the effects of small changes in ATP concentration, as was explained by Newsholme & Start.[171] The theory involves three general observations about cellular metabolism.

- The total quantity of the adenine nucleotides, ATP, ADP and AMP, is fixed, at least in the short term, by the availability of their common adenosine moiety.

- Cells regulate their energy metabolism so that the concentration of ATP exceeds the other two in nearly all circumstances.

- Cells contain adenylate kinase, which catalyses the reaction:

$$2\,\mathrm{ADP} \rightleftharpoons \mathrm{ATP} + \mathrm{AMP}$$

and maintains the reaction close to equilibrium at all times.

The effect of this is illustrated in Figure 7.15, which shows the equilibrium relationship between the three nucleotides as a function of ATP for an assumed total of 5 mM adenine nucleotides. Measurement of total adenine nucleotide levels in cells commonly shows that ATP can be maintained at over 80% of the total, even in muscle after a 100–fold increase in energy expenditure. Nevertheless, an increase in ATP utilization in the cell does cause a drop in its concentration, however slight measurements show this to be. What the Figure shows is that, in these regions of high relative ATP content, a very slight fall in ATP is accompanied by a rapid rise in AMP from its very low level. It is true that ADP concentrations also show an almost as rapid rise, but ADP has a disadvantage as a signal: any particular ADP concentration could correspond to two different levels of ATP. The qualitative impression of the greater sensitivity of AMP levels to an ATP change is confirmed by my quantitative calculations of the sensitivities[69] shown in Figure 7.16. These show that sensitivity to AMP change is always the greatest provided ATP concentration exceeds that of AMP (*i.e.* for fractional ATP contents greater than about one-third), and that the factor becomes very large indeed when most of the nucleotide exists as ATP. When corrections are made for bound ADP and AMP contents in cells, the ATP increases to as much as 98% of the total free adenine nucleotides.[164,258] This would suggest the possibility of extremely high sensitivities to ADP and AMP, though the exact values are hard to predict as the binding of ADP and AMP affects the graphs (without changing the qualitative picture).

The AMP–dependent protein kinase was discovered to be responsible for the phosphorylation, and inactivation, of acetyl-CoA carboxylase, the first step in the pathways of fatty acid and cholesterol synthesis.[28] It then became apparent that this kinase was the same as that identified as being responsible for the phosphorylation (and inactivation) of hydroxymethylglutaryl-CoA reductase, the first step in the branch to cholesterol and other steroids. It has also been found that the AMP–dependent kinase phosphorylates the hormone–sensitive triacylglycerol lipase of adipose tissue; in this case, the phosphorylation does not affect the enzyme's activity directly, but it prevents its phosphorylation (and activation) by protein kinase A, thus preventing release of fatty acids and cholesterol from the fat stores. The AMP–dependent kinase is activated in two ways by AMP: first, AMP is an allosteric activator of the enzyme, and secondly, AMP makes the enzyme more susceptible to phosphorylation by a kinase (called kinase kinase!) that remains attached to the AMP–dependent kinase throughout nearly all purification steps.[270] Together, the effects cause up to a 50–fold increase in activity of the kinase in response to AMP, providing further amplification of the effect of a change in ATP. The metabolic consequence is that fat metabolism is inhibited in conditions where demand for ATP causes its level to drop, as signalled by the rise in AMP.

The activity of the AMP–dependent protein kinase is also stimulated by very low concentrations of fatty acyl-CoA esters, so it probably also limits the synthesis of fatty acids and cholesterol and the hydrolysis of triacylglycerols under conditions where fatty acyl-CoA is already accumulating. On this basis, it could also be regarded as an example of the next class of protein kinases.

7.4.3.1.5   Metabolic intermediates

The pyruvate dehydrogenase enzyme complex is present in the mitochondrial matrix of eukaryotes and oxidizes pyruvate to acetyl CoA. There is also a similar branched–chain α–keto acid dehydrogenase complex that oxidizes the carbon skeletons from the essential branched chain amino acids (valine, leucine and isoleucine). Both complexes are subject to inactivation by phosphorylation by specific kinases that are tightly bound to the enzyme complexes. The specific phosphatases that activate the enzymes also seem to be tightly bound to the complexes. The kinase activities are allosterically activated by metabolites; for example, in the case of pyruvate dehydrogenase kinase, the phosphorylating activity is stimulated by metabolites that will increase in concentration when mitochondrial oxidative capacity is being stretched, such as acetyl-CoA and NADH, and inhibited by metabolites that indicate a need for more oxidative metabolism, such as ADP. (ADP is present at higher levels in the mitochondria than in the cytoplasm.) The phosphatase is stimulated by Ca^{2+} in the mitochondrial matrix. This may enable the phosphorylation state to respond to this second messenger, since the mitochondria accumulate Ca^{2+} relative to the cytosol, so the dehydrogenase complexes may not be solely regulated by metabolic intermediates.

7.4.3.2 Phosphatases

The action of protein kinases is reversed by the action of phosphoprotein phosphatases. These generally have very broad specificities when tested *in vitro*, which has made classification and determination of their physiological functions difficult. However, Philip Cohen's group in Dundee have assigned the phosphatases into four main groups[42–44] which are generally present in vertebrate and invertebrate animals, and probably in most eukaryotes. The main properties of the four groups are summarized in Table 7.3. (The inhibitor okadaic acid referred to there is useful in distinguishing the physiological roles of the phosphatases and is a toxin produced by marine dinoflagellates. It is also known to accumulate in the shellfish that feed on them and causes diarrhoetic shellfish poisoning.) Table 7.3 shows that there is no simple correspondence between the kinases and the phosphatases. There are some important links though.

(1) Inhibitor–1, which specifically inhibits protein phosphatase 1, only does so when it has been phosphorylated by protein kinase A. Thus activation of this kinase can thereby lead to a reduction in the dephosphorylating activity, so augmenting the increase in phosphorylation that it promotes directly by its kinase action.

(2) Phosphoprotein phosphatase 2B, which is activated by Ca^{2+} and Ca^{2+}/calmodulin, acts specifically on the kinases, phosphatases and Inhibitor–1 that have been phosphorylated by protein kinase A. It therefore forms another link between the cyclic AMP and Ca^{2+} systems. Like the effects

Table 7.3 Phosphoprotein phosphatases

Type	Principal targets	Specific properties
I	Glycogen metabolism, muscle contractility	1. Inhibited by phosphorylated Inhibitor–1 2. Particulate, e.g. attached to glycogen. 3. Inhibited by okadaic acid
2A	Glycolysis, gluconeogenesis, aromatic amino acid catabolism, fatty acid synthesis	1. Cytosolic 2. Inhibited by okadaic acid
2B	Protein kinases, protein phosphatases and Inhibitor–1 which have been phosphorylated by protein kinase A	1. Activity dependent on Ca^{2+} and stimulated 10–fold by Ca^{2+}/calmodulin 2. Poor action on metabolic enzymes 3. May cause Ca^{2+} attenuation of the effects of cyclic AMP
2C	AMP–dependent protein kinase, and possibly its targets in fatty acid and cholesterol metabolism	1. Cytosolic 2. Requires Mg^{2+} for activity

Largely based on information from Cohen and colleagues.[42–44]

of Ca^{2+} on cyclic AMP phosphodiesterase, the result is to cause Ca^{2+} attenuation of the action of cyclic AMP.[42]

In addition, the action of phosphatase 2B in dephosphorylating (and thereby inactivating) Inhibitor–1 will activate phosphatase 1 (by relieving its inhibition) and may be an example of a phosphatase 'cascade'.[42]

Protein phosphatase 1 is found in a variety of forms, mainly associated with cellular structures. For example, in muscle cells it is attached to glycogen, sarcoplasmic reticulum and myofibrils. The glycogen–bound form consists of a complex of the phosphatase with a glycogen–binding subunit. The formation of this complex causes a specific 5–10-fold stimulation in the activity of the phosphatase towards phosphorylase and glycogen synthase, but not towards other substrates. Since phosphatase 1 bound to myofibrils has enhanced activity towards phosphorylated myosin light chains, it seems that the phosphatase is targeted towards its substrates by the binding proteins.

7.4.3.3 Phosphorylation cascades

The activation of glycogen phosphorylase, shown in Figure 7.17, illustrates a covalent modification cascade system where there is more than one stage to the process. Phosphorylase *b*, the unphosphorylated form, only shows signifi-

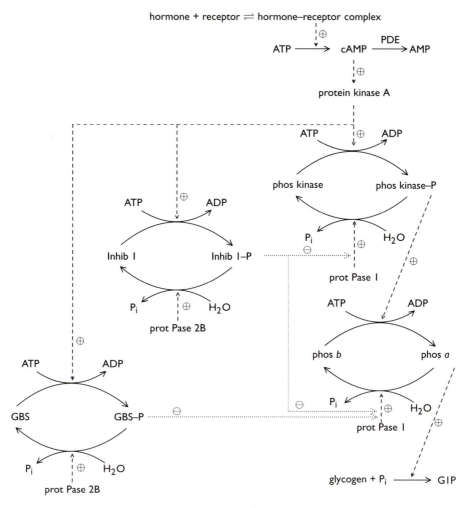

Figure 7.17 The phosphorylase activation cascade in muscle
Abbreviations: PDE, cyclic AMP phosphodiesterase; prot Pase, protein phosphatase; Inhib I, Inhibitor-1; phos, phosphorylase; P_i, inorganic phosphate; GBS, glycogen-binding subunit.

cant enzymic activity towards glycogen when allosterically activated by AMP. Phosphorylase *a* is active without the need for activation by AMP. The phosphorylation of phosphorylase is dependent upon the action of a specific phosphorylase kinase. This itself exists in a less active dephosphorylated form and an active multiply phosphorylated form. Both forms are also activated directly by Ca^{2+} through the calmodulin–like subunit. In muscle this enables phosphorylase activation to occur within about a second of sustained muscular contractions because of the raised cytosolic Ca^{2+} levels. Phosphorylase kinase is phosphorylated by protein kinase A, which in turn is activated by hormones that stimulate the synthesis of cyclic AMP, such as adrenaline. The

activation of phosphorylase by adrenaline in muscle is slower than by contraction.

A further element to the cascade shown in Figure 7.17 has details that are
tissue–specific. The phosphorylated forms of phosphorylase kinase and phosphorylase are primarily dephosphorylated by protein phosphatase 1. In muscle,
this phosphatase is inhibited by the phosphorylated form of Inhibitor-1; since
Inhibitor-1 is phosphorylated by protein kinase A, the cyclic AMP signal acts to
enhance the phosphorylation and inhibit the dephosphorylation of both phosphorylase and its kinase. In addition, the inhibition of dephosphorylation is
further strengthened because protein kinase A phosphorylates the glycogen-
binding subunit that both holds protein phosphatase 1 to the glycogen particle
and prevents Inhibitor-1 acting on it. Phosphorylation of this subunit releases
protein phosphatase 1 from the glycogen, reduces its activity towards phosphorylase and allows Inhibitor-1 to bind. Mechanisms with similar effects operate
in liver and brain.

When cyclic AMP levels fall, phosphorylase will tend to return towards
the dephosphorylated b state. This will in part be caused by the reduced rate
of phosphorylation of phosphorylase kinase, Inhibitor-1 and glycogen-binding
subunit. Inhibitor-1 and glycogen-binding subunit will return more towards
their dephosphorylated state because they are acted on by protein phosphatase
2B, which has not been inhibited. This relieves the inhibition on protein phosphatase 1, so that the rates of dephosphorylation of phosphorylase kinase and
phosphorylase are enhanced.

The same mechanism that activates phosphorylase inactivates glycogen synthase, which in its phosphorylated form is only active when allosterically stimulated by raised concentrations of glucose 6–phosphate. The dephosphorylated form is active without glucose 6–phosphate. Protein kinase A phosphorylates glycogen synthase, but the details of the system are much more
involved than for phosphorylase because glycogen synthase undergoes multiple phosphorylations and a range of protein kinases are responsible. So although it is certainly the case that cyclic AMP–linked hormones inactivate
glycogen synthase, the relative importance of the different components in physiological conditions has been difficult to establish. In liver there is an additional link to the reciprocal relationship between phosphorylase and glycogen synthase: protein phosphatase 1 is inhibited by phosphorylase a, so that
glycogen synthase cannot be dephosphorylated to its active form until virtually all the phosphorylase has been returned to the relatively inactive b
form.

There are a number of points in the phosphorylase cascade where Ca^{2+} can
act. It directly activates phosphorylase kinase, as mentioned above, regardless of phosphorylation state. However, it also activates protein phosphatase
2B, which will lower the amounts of the inhibitory forms of Inhibitor-1 and
glycogen-binding subunit so that protein phosphatase 1 becomes more active.
In addition, by activating one of the cyclic AMP phosphodiesterases, Ca^{2+} will

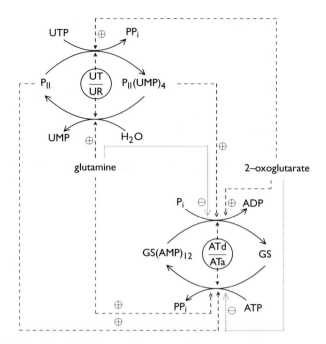

Figure 7.18 The bicyclic glutamine synthase cascade
This system is a central part of the control of nitrogen metabolism in *E. coli*. This figure is based on
one in the paper by Chock et al.[38] but modified so that activation reactions are above deactivations
and enzymically active forms are to the right. Abbreviations: GS, glutamine synthase; UT, uridylyl
transferase; UR, uridylyl removing enzyme; ATa, adenylyl transferase; ATd, the deadenylylating activity of
the transferase; PP_i, inorganic pyrophosphate; P_i, inorganic phosphate.

tend to lower cyclic AMP levels and reduce the degree of activation of protein
kinase A.

7.4.4 Nucleotidylation

Whereas phosphorylase was the mammalian enzyme that led to the discovery of
cyclic covalent modification systems, in bacteria it was the glutamine synthase
(properly glutamate–ammonia ligase) of *E. coli* that furnished the first example.
Glutamine synthase has a central role in nitrogen metabolism, since approximately 12% of cellular nitrogen comes from the amide nitrogen of glutamine,
and most of the remainder largely from the α–amino group of glutamate rather
than directly from ammonia. In bacteria and higher plants, the net synthesis
of glutamate from 2–oxoglutarate and ammonia in turn depends on a cycle
involving both glutamine synthase and glutamate synthase:

$$\text{glutamate} + \text{NH}_3 + \text{ATP} \longrightarrow \text{glutamine} + \text{ADP} + \text{P}_i$$
$$\text{2–oxoglutarate} + \text{glutamine} + \text{NADPH} \longrightarrow 2\,\text{glutamate} + \text{NADP}^+$$
$$\text{Sum: 2–oxoglutarate} + \text{NH}_3 + \text{NADPH} + \text{ATP}$$
$$\longrightarrow \text{glutamate} + \text{NADP}^+ + \text{ADP} + \text{P}_i$$

The problem that organisms have to resolve is the need to maintain appropriate levels of glutamate and glutamine to meet synthetic requirements without withdrawing all the 2–oxoglutarate from the tricarboxylic acid cycle, and to manage to do this across the range from conditions where usable nitrogen is in short supply to those where it is in excess. The enzyme has already been mentioned in Chapter 1.2.1 and earlier in this chapter (Chapter 7.2.3.3.3) because it is an allosteric enzyme affected by eight different feedback inhibitors. (The ninth effector is Mg^{2+}.)

It was Earl Stadtman's group at Bethesda that was largely responsible for establishing that glutamine synthase in *E. coli* was subject to inactivation by *adenylylation* (addition of AMP groups) of tyrosine residues[38] catalysed by an *adenylyltransferase*. Glutamine synthase is composed of 12 identical subunits, and each of these has one modifiable tyrosine. The enzymic activity of a glutamine synthase molecule is inversely proportional to the number of subunits that have been modified. Re-activation of the enzyme is by phosphorolysis of the adenylyl groups to give free enzyme and ADP:

$$12\,ATP + GS_{12} \longrightarrow GS_{12}(AMP)_{12} + 12\,PP_i$$
$$GS_{12}(AMP)_{12} + 12\,P_i \longrightarrow GS_{12} + 12\,ADP$$

(where PP_i is pyrophosphate and P_i is phosphate). The adenylylation is catalysed by glutamine synthase adenylyltransferase (properly glutamate–ammonia ligase adenylyltransferase, EC 2.7.7.42). The de–adenylylation reaction is a phosphorolysis, and is an activity of the same enzyme as the adenylylation, but at a separate active site.

The relative levels of the two activities of the adenylyltransferase are reciprocally modulated by two types of factor (Figure 7.18). First, there are metabolites that affect the activity. Of these, glutamine itself and 2–oxoglutarate (product and substrate of the synthase) have oppositely directed effects with glutamine stimulating the inactivation and inhibiting the activation, whereas 2–oxoglutarate does the opposite. The second factor is the tetrameric regulatory protein P_{II} discovered by Shapiro. This also exists in two forms. The unmodified form is an activator of the adenylylation (inactivation) of glutamine synthase. It is modified by uridylylation (Figure 7.18), and the uridylated form is an activator of the de–adenylylation (activation) of glutamine synthase. The interconversion reactions affecting P_{II} mirror the modification of glutamine synthase itself. The protein–P_{II} uridylyltransferase and the uridylyl–removing enzyme (which this time is a hydrolysis reaction to form UMP) are separate activities on the same polypeptide chain (EC 2.7.7.59). Glutamine stimulates the uridylyl–removing activity, thereby leading to additional activation of the adenylylation of glutamine synthase (in addition to its direct effect on this latter modifying reaction). Again, 2–oxoglutarate has the opposite activity, since it stimulates the uridylyltransferase, forming the modified P_{II} that stimulates the de–adenylylation of glutamine synthase. Thus the control of glutamine synthase involves a cascade system of two cyclic modification reactions, but

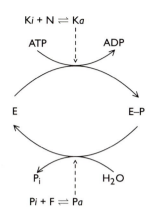

Figure 7.19 Model of a covalent modification scheme
In Stadtman & Chock's model,[238] E is the unmodified enzyme, E–P is its phosphorylated form, K is the kinase and P the phosphatase. i and a indicate the inactive and active forms of the latter. N is the effector of the oN reaction and F is the effector of the oFf reaction.

these cycles are doubly coupled by the reciprocal activities of the two forms of P_{II}. The four modifying activities between them also respond to over 20 other assorted metabolites, including nucleotides and intermediates of the glycolytic pathway and the tricarboxylic acid cycle. (A further layer of complexity is added by the role of P_{II} in modulating the transcription of glutamine synthase. This will not be discussed further here, but is reviewed by Rhee et al.[197])

The detailed properties of a system like this with such a network of interacting effects are not immediately obvious from the structure of the cascade. Stadtman and Chock, and other members of their group, therefore undertook an extensive theoretical analysis of the possible behaviours of cyclic modification cascades. Their conclusions are discussed in the next section, as they are applicable to cyclic modification schemes in general (including phosphorylase) and not just glutamine synthase.

7.4.5 Properties of cyclic modification systems

Stadtman & Chock[226,238] used the basic model shown in Figure 7.19 to investigate how the amount of enzyme in one of the modified forms (say the phosphorylated form) depended at steady state on the effectors of the two modifying reactions. Although a comparison of the model with the examples discussed in this chapter shows that it possesses the fundamental characteristics of covalent modification systems, it is much simplified, in that the converting enzymes are only active when associated with their effector molecules and that the effector binding is simple non–cooperative binding. The model is illustrated as a phosphorylation, but the type of modification is not really important because ATP, ADP and phosphate are not considered as specific variables in the model. Stadtman and Chock derived equations that relate the fraction of the target enzyme in the modified form, when the cycle has reached steady state, to the concentration of one of the effectors of the converting enzymes. From these, they determined the following different aspects of the behaviour of these cycles.

7.4.5.1 Catalytic amplification

Since the modification cycle is catalysed, it is an obvious property that a small amount of converter enzyme can act on a much larger amount of target enzyme. Thus the catalytic power can be amplified in the sense that the limiting rate (V) of the maximally activated target enzyme can be many times greater than that of the modifying enzyme. Of course, if the specific activities of the two enzymes are relatively similar, the catalytic amplification largely reflects the difference in the amounts of the two enzymes. This is undoubtedly an important aspect of many modification cycles, such as cases where small amounts of hormones (at perhaps 10^{-9} M) combine with relatively few receptors to act eventually on relatively abundant enzymes (perhaps at concentrations around 10^{-5} M). Another example is in the irreversible modification cascade of blood clotting, where the initial signal is tiny but a macroscopic blood clot is formed.

Important as it may be, there is little mystery about catalytic amplification. It should be noted that a high degree of catalytic amplification is only obtained at a price that is not evident in steady state studies: the larger the amount of target enzyme relative to modifying enzyme, the longer the system will take to respond to a change in the amount of an effector.

7.4.5.2 Signal amplification

A very significant feature of cyclic modification schemes is that the degree of activation of converting enzyme by an effector does not correspond directly to the amount of modified target enzyme that it forms. This is illustrated in Figure 7.20 with some theoretical curves calculated with Stadtman & Chock's model. Curve a has the parameters of the model set so that half-conversion of the enzyme to the phosphorylated form is achieved at the same concentration of effector (N) that gives half–saturation of the kinase (curve c). Curve b has a 16–fold greater kinase/phosphatase activity ratio and a 2.5–fold decrease in the activation of the phosphatase by its effector F. This causes the concentration of N at half-conversion to have fallen to nearly 10^{-2}, or nearly 100-fold lower than the concentration of N required to half–activate the kinase, which is unchanged at 1. Since N is the signal that initiates phosphorylation, the modification cycle shows *signal amplification*. In this case it can be quantified as:

$$\frac{N \text{ required for half-activation of kinase}}{N \text{ required for half-phosphorylation of target}} \qquad (7.10)$$

The signal amplification arises because the cycle is catalysed and therefore a small amount of kinase can convert a larger amount of target, but it is not the same as the catalytic amplification referred to above. The significance of signal

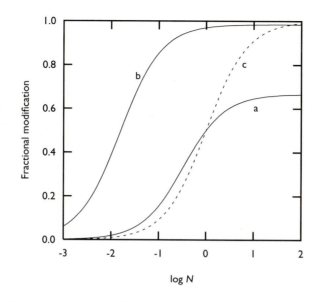

Figure 7.20 Degree of activation of the target enzyme
Curve c shows the fraction of the kinase activated by binding its effector, N (see Figure 7.19). Curves a and b show the fraction of the target enzyme phosphorylated for different values of the parameters in Stadtman & Chock's model.

amplification is that it allows the system to produce an effect on the target enzyme at a signal concentration that is well below the dissociation constant for the binding of the signal to the enzyme it activates.

7.4.5.3 Amplitude

Figure 7.20 also shows that the modification cycle cannot necessarily produce complete conversion of the target to its phosphorylated form. The symmetry of the cycle implies that there will also be circumstances where there cannot be complete conversion to the dephosphorylated form. The *amplitude* is the range of fractional modification that is covered in going from zero level of an effector to saturating levels. For curve b of Figure 7.20 it is nearly 1.0, whereas for curve a it is only 0.67. Variation of the parameters of the model can produce amplitudes anywhere from 0 to 1.

7.4.5.4 Sensitivity

Stadtman & Chock were concerned to know whether their model of a covalent modification cycle produced a curve that was steeper or less steep than the familiar rectangular hyperbola for enzyme kinetics and ligand binding. To measure this they introduced a measure of *sensitivity*. They took as their reference the change in ligand concentration required to go from 10% to 90% saturation for a normal rectangular hyperbolic binding curve. From Eqn. (3.10), Chapter 3.4, it is possible to calculate that this requires an increase in the ligand concentration equal to 8.89 times the dissociation constant (or ligand concentration that gives 50% binding). They therefore defined sensitivity, S, as:

$$S = \frac{8.89\,N_{0.5}}{N_{0.9} - N_{0.1}} \tag{7.11}$$

where $N_{0.5}$ is the concentration of the effector N that gives 50% of the maximal amplitude of modification. This sensitivity function differs from those defined in Metabolic Control Analysis (*i.e.* control coefficients and elasticities) in that it is measured over a finite interval rather than from the gradient of a curve, but it does share the properties of being dimensionless and of measuring the steepness of response. It is actually more like the Hill coefficient (Chapter 3.4, p. 68) in that values of S greater than 1 indicate that the curve relating the fractional modification to effector concentration is steeper than a rectangular hyperbola, whereas values less than 1 show it is less steep. As it happens, Stadtman & Chock's relatively simple model for the modification cycle gives sensitivity values equal to 1 unless an effector acts at more than one site. For example, if N activates the kinase and inhibits the phosphatase, then the sensitivity is greater than 1. (The result is similar to that seen in curves a and c of Figure 7.21, though these were calculated for a different model.) This is equivalent to positive cooperativity in its outcome, though it is obtained without any cooperative effects in the binding of the effector. An example of an effector that acts in opposite directions on the two converting enzymes of the cycle is glutamine in the modification of glutamine synthase (Figure 7.18). There are other ways which the sensitivity can be altered that will be discussed further below.

7.4.5.5 Biological integration

Cyclic modification systems involve more enzymes and therefore naturally create more sites at which effectors can act. This is well illustrated by glutamine synthase, which responds directly as an allosteric enzyme to about 15 ligands, but indirectly to about another 20 that act through one or more of the converting enzymes. In addition, Figure 7.19 represents just one pattern of effector action in a covalent modification system; as mentioned above, the sensitivity of the response is changed if one effector acts on both converting reactions. Thus these systems have the potential to show a range of behaviours and to integrate a wide range of signals. The phosphorylase system is a particularly good example of signal integration, since hormones, via cyclic AMP, and other hormones or nerve impulses via Ca^{2+}, can separately activate phosphorylase, but when they occur together, the responses do not simply multiply together because there is interaction between the signals.

7.4.5.6 Multiple cyclic cascades

One of the ways in which covalent modification is often more complex than the simple cyclic scheme shown in Figure 7.19 is that multiple cycles can form a cascade. These can either be *open* like the phosphorylase cascade (Figure 7.17), where a cascade at one level has only a single point of action on the next level, or *closed*, like the glutamine synthase cascade (Figure 7.18) where the two interconverted forms of the enzyme at one level both act on the next level, but on opposite sides.

In essence, the properties of a single modification cycle become even more pronounced in the multiple cycles. Thus the model of Stadtman & Chock shows that the signal amplification can increase dramatically with the number of cycles in the cascade, basically because the amplifications of each stage multiply together. Similarly, the sensitivity increases in proportion to the number of stages that the effector N modulates (see Figure 7.21, curve c).

Another property that is affected by the number of cycles is the rate of modification of the final target enzyme. If the initiating effector N is increased in concentration, there is a lag before the target enzyme is modified. This lag increases with the number of cycles in the cascade, not unreasonably as this increases the number of stages through which the signal has to be transmitted. However, the rate of modification is increased at each stage, corresponding to *rate amplification*. The rate amplification is cumulative in multiple cycle cascades so, after a lag, there is an almost explosive increase in the amount of the modified target enzyme. With realistic estimates of the kinetic constants, Stadtman & Chock's models show that it is feasible for covalent modification cascades to operate in the millisecond to second time span. Indeed, measurements of the rate of formation of phosphorylase *a* in frog sartorius muscle upon electrical stimulation, carried out by C F Cori and his colleagues in the 1960s, showed that the half-time of activation was 700 ms. Similar measurements on mouse muscle gave a half-time of 1 s.[101] However, since phosphorylase is activated on muscle contraction by a single cycle cascade (Ca^{2+} activation of phosphorylase kinase), and the effects of adrenaline on phosphorylase in muscle are slower, even though they involve a multistage cascade, these experiments are not an indubitable illustration of rate amplification.

7.4.5.7 Ultrasensitivity

The next development in the theoretical understanding of covalent modification systems came from Albert Goldbeter of the Free University of Brussels and Daniel Koshland of the University of California. Whereas the analysis described above had used simple chemical kinetics for the modification reactions, Goldbeter and Koshland represented them as true enzymic reactions with the dependence of rate on the concentration of their substrates (the unmodified and modified forms of the target enzyme) described by the Michaelis–Menten equation.[88] For their sensitivity measure, they used the measure earlier developed by Koshland and his colleagues for describing the steepness of cooperative binding curves in allosteric enzymes.[137] For a factor N that affects the degree of modification, their sensitivity R_N is defined as:

$$R_N = \frac{N_{0.9}}{N_{0.1}} \tag{7.12}$$

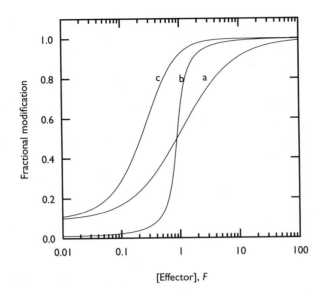

Figure 7.21 Zero–order ultrasensitivity
Curve a, Fractional phosphorylation of the target enzyme according to Goldbeter & Koshland's[88] model with unsaturated modifying enzymes and F, a non–competitive inhibitor of the phosphatase (Figure 7.19). Curve b, as curve a, but showing ultrasensitivity with the target enzyme 10–fold higher than the K_m values of both modifying enzymes. Curve c, as curve a, except F activates the kinase and inhibits the phosphatase.

N could be either the concentration of an effector or the ratio of limiting rates of the two converting enzymes. Unlike Stadtman and Chock's sensitivity measure [Eqn. (7.11)], or the Hill coefficient, this value decreases with increasing steepness of the curve, from a value of 81 for a rectangular hyperbolic curve to a minimum of 1 for an infinitely steep transition. The use of the different definitions means that neither the equations derived by the two groups nor the numerical measures of sensitivity are exactly comparable, though in qualitative terms they are referring to the same concept. (Such differences in the operational definition of sensitivity, of which these are merely two instances, were the main reason that Kacser and Burns abandoned their original term *sensitivity* for the flux control coefficient.) The analysis carried out by Goldbeter and Koshland showed that the sensitivity was much more variable than in Stadtman and Chock's studies, where it only changed in response to the number of steps at which an effector acted.

    Their novel finding was that, if one or both of the converting enzymes is operating close to saturation, the fractional modification of the target enzyme can become an extremely sensitive function of the ratio of the limiting rates of the converting enzymes. They termed this *zero-order ultrasensitivity*, since a saturated enzyme shows near-zero-order kinetics in the terminology of chemical kinetics, and it was possible to show theoretical curves with a steepness equivalent to a Hill coefficient, h, of 13 or more. The effect is illustrated in

Figure 7.21, where curve a has been calculated with their model for concentrations of the target enzyme well below the K_m values of the modifying kinase and phosphatase. Curve b is far steeper, but the only change is that the total amount of target enzyme has been increased to 10 times the level of both K_m values. For comparison, the smaller increase in steepness obtained with an effector that acts on both kinase and phosphatase is shown in curve c. Goldbeter and Koshland also showed that the ultrasensitivity can be amplified in a multi-cycle cascade if each component cascade exhibits ultrasensitivity. Furthermore, a non–competitive inhibitor of a modifying enzyme shows a greater degree of ultrasensitivity than a competitive inhibitor, since the latter increases the apparent K_m of the modifying enzyme and moves it from the zero–order region towards the first-order region.

Unlike the comparable conjecture for increased sensitivity in substrate cycles (Section 7.3.3), there is some experimental support for the occurrence of ultrasensitivity in covalent modification. A reconstituted, *in vitro* system of phosphorylase plus protein phosphatase and phosphorylase kinase showed a response that could be fitted by the equations derived by Goldbeter and Koshland at phosphorylase concentrations comparable to those found in muscle.[156] The degree of ultrasensitivity is roughly equivalent to a Hill coefficient of 2.3. The only problem with this interpretation was that the activation of phosphorylase kinase (whether by Ca^{2+} or by phosphorylation) was believed at the time to be caused by a decrease in the K_m for phosphorylase, which would not be an effective stimulus in the zero–order sensitivity region of operation. However, a subsequent re–investigation of the kinetics of phosphorylase kinase has shown that the predominant action of these effectors is to increase the limiting rate.[173]

7.4.5.8 Control Analysis

So far, the analysis of the properties of cyclic modification cascades has not made use of the concepts of Metabolic Control Analysis. However, there are three reasons why it is important to apply Control Analysis to covalent modification.

(1) Covalent modification represents an important class of control mechanisms, and therefore Control Analysis would not be complete if it did not take account of it.

(2) The analyses presented above have been very dependent on the particular types of molecular mechanism used in the model, which need not be the case with Control Analysis.

(3) The analyses have only considered whether the degree of activity of a single pathway enzyme can be changed substantially, and not whether this will have a significant effect on pathway flux.

María Luz Cárdenas and Athel Cornish–Bowden[27] in Marseilles used the response coefficient of Metabolic Control Analysis [Eqn. (5.21), Chapter 5.4] as a measure of the dependence of the fraction of a modifiable target enzyme in the active form upon the concentration of an effector of the modifying enzymes. The advantage of this is that a value of the response coefficient greater than 1 can be regarded as useful enhanced sensitivity, on the basis that a value up to 1 could be achieved by the direct action of an effector on an enzyme without the need for additional enzymes and the energy expenditure involved in a covalent modification cycle. On this basis, they were able to show that an effector that acts only on the K_m values of the modifying enzymes can only generate enhanced sensitivity if it acts on both enzymes and if it inhibits the deactivating enzyme at lower concentrations than are required to stimulate the activating enzyme. Otherwise, the response to the effector is actually poorer than would be obtained by direct action of the effector on the target enzyme.

They also carried out a numerical search on a general model of a covalent modification cycle to determine the circumstances under which the model showed the maximum attainable ultrasensitivity, with the effector acting on both modifying enzymes. This confirmed Goldbeter and Koshland's observation that the modifying enzymes should both be as near to saturation with target enzyme as possible. In addition, the actions of the effector on the limiting rates of the enzymes must predominate over its effects on the K_m values. Again, they also found that it was important that the inhibition of one modifying enzyme occurred at much lower concentrations of effector than were required to activate the other. Under the most favourable combination of circumstances, the sensitivity of the target enzyme to the effector could be equivalent to a Hill coefficient as high as 800. This represents the potential of the system, since there is no experimental evidence for a system showing an effect as large as this.

At about the same time, Rankin Small and I were also applying the concepts of Metabolic Control Analysis to covalent modification of an enzyme embedded in a metabolic pathway, so that we could consider the effects on the pathway flux rather than just on the amount of activated enzyme.[231] One conclusion we reached was that the flux control coefficient of the modifiable enzyme (defined in terms of the total amount of that enzyme) could be increased, decreased or unchanged by the occurrence of the modification cycle. For it to be increased, the modifying enzymes would have to have small elasticities with respect to the target enzyme; this is equivalent to the requirement for zero–order ultrasensitivity, except that it has been reached for the pathway flux, and it is general in that it does not depend on any particular assumptions about the kinetic equations of the modifying enzymes. It is also a reminder of an important factor that has been almost lost sight of: whatever the effect of the modification cycle on the activity of the target enzyme, there will be no effect on flux unless the enzyme has a non–zero flux control coefficient. We also extended the concept of the response coefficient to define the response of pathway flux (J) to an effector (N) that acts on a modifying enzyme (a) of a target enzyme (t) as:

$$R_N^J = C_t^J C_a^{t^*} \varepsilon_N^a \qquad (7.13)$$

where $C_a^{t^*}$ is the concentration control coefficient of the modifying enzyme a on the concentration of the active form t^* of the target enzyme. This confirms that an enhanced response of the pathway flux to the effector cannot be guaranteed by a large value for one of the terms, such as $C_a^{t^*}$ (which does have a large value under the conditions favourable for ultrasensitivity). Small values of the other coefficients can nullify the advantage. Again, algebraic analysis of the term $C_a^{t^*}$ shows that it will be less than 1 if the modifying enzymes are unsaturated with the target enzyme, and hence under these circumstances, the covalent modification cycle actually acts to reduce the response of the flux to the effector. We were also able to confirm and extend the conclusions reached by Cárdenas and Cornish–Bowden about the conditions that would lead to ultrasensitivity, with the advantage that many of our arguments depend on relative values of elasticities, and not on the molecular mechanisms underlying them.

Our overall conclusions were that only a quite restricted set of conditions generate ultrasensitivity and ensure it is translated into a more sensitive response of pathway flux to an effector. This is even more so in multicyclic cascades, where additional terms appear in the response coefficient, but each of these with a value less than 1 contributes to an unavoidable attenuation of the sensitivity of the flux to the signal. Nevertheless, the actual examples of covalent modification cycles presented above show that the theoretical models studied so far are relatively simple and that there is plenty of potential for complex properties to emerge from covalent modification cascades. Also, most of the analysis has been concerned with steady state behaviour, but the transient behaviour in the change between metabolic states is almost certainly very important as well. However, the weakest link in all the studies, whether practical or theoretical, has been that little attention has been paid to the link between the change in modification state and the effect on the metabolic pathway of which the target enzyme is part. (Modular Control Analysis is a recent development of Control Analysis that deals more systematically with this problem.[123]) Metabolic Control Analysis has shown that enzymes that are truly rate–limiting, with flux control coefficients of 1, are not generally found. It has also shown that for an enzyme with a flux control coefficient less than 1, the scope for increasing flux by activating the enzyme is relatively limited (see Chapter 5.2.2). How then, can we explain covalent modification mechanisms that only appear to exist to cause a significant change in flux by making large changes in the amount of active enzyme in response to small changes in signal molecules, when the evidence suggests this cannot be effective? The traditional paradigm of covalent modification systems was that they control metabolism by acting on rate–limiting enzymes. This is no longer tenable; a new view of how control of metabolism is actually exerted in the light of the analyses presented in this Chapter will be developed in the next and final chapter.

7.5   Summary

(1) Traditional theories of metabolic control assumed there were obvious advantages of controlling the rate of a pathway near its start. Analysis of the control of supply of and demand for a metabolite shows that better homoeostasis of metabolite concentrations is achieved when the greater flux control is exerted by the demand reactions, *i.e.* towards the end.

(2) Feedback inhibition loops are common regulatory structures in metabolic pathways. Analysis of their properties suggests their primary effect is homoeostasis of metabolite concentrations rather than flux control, as previously believed. This is because feedback loops transfer control to the demand reactions after the metabolite exerting feedback.

(3) In branched pathways, both sequential and nested patterns of feedback inhibition are found. Sequential feedback inhibition is the more reliable, though nested feedback inhibition can give better homoeostasis over a limited range of conditions.

(4) Cyclic pathways that dissipate energy potentially exist in metabolism, and measurements confirm that some of these routes are indeed active. Such substrate or futile cycles could fulfil a number of functions, of which thermogenesis and switching fluxes at complex metabolic crossroads are the best established.

(5) Covalent modification cycles are another common control structure in metabolism, linking it to a range of internal and external signals. They amplify the effects of small initial signals in a variety of ways and allow metabolism to integrate a range of different, possibly conflicting, signals. Theoretical analysis reveals the possibility that they show ultrasensitivity, where the response to a stimulus becomes sharpened, and there is evidence that the activation system for glycogen phosphorylase exhibits this.

7.6   Appendix 1: Control Analysis of substrate cycles

For the substrate cycle pathway shown in Figure 7.13, the following theorems of Metabolic Control Analysis apply. There is a summation theorem:

$$C_1^J + C_{2a}^J + C_{2b}^J + C_3^J = 1$$

There are two connectivity theorems with respect to S_1 and S_2:

$$C_1^J \varepsilon_{S_1}^1 + C_{2a}^J \varepsilon_{S_1}^{2a} + C_{2b}^J \varepsilon_{S_1}^{2b} = 0$$
$$C_{2a}^J \varepsilon_{S_2}^{2a} + C_{2b}^J \varepsilon_{S_2}^{2b} + C_3^J \varepsilon_{S_2}^3 = 0$$

Finally, as explained in Chapter 5.3.3, p. 119, there is a need for an additional theorem, the substrate cycle summation relationship, originally developed by myself and Herbert Sauro.[69] Its form varies depending on the choice of which flux is used in the flux control coefficients, but for $J = J_1 = J_3$ it is:

$$\frac{C_{2a}^J}{v_{2a}} + \frac{C_{2b}^J}{v_{2b}} = 0$$

These relationships form a set of four simultaneous equations that can be expressed in matrix form[69] as:

$$
\begin{bmatrix}
1 & 1 & 1 & 1 \\
\varepsilon_{S_1}^1 & \varepsilon_{S_1}^{2a} & \varepsilon_{S_1}^{2b} & 0 \\
0 & \varepsilon_{S_2}^{2a} & \varepsilon_{S_2}^{2b} & \varepsilon_{S_2}^3 \\
0 & 1/v_{2a} & 1/v_{2b} & 0
\end{bmatrix}
\cdot
\begin{bmatrix}
C_1^J \\
C_{2a}^J \\
C_{2b}^J \\
C_3^J
\end{bmatrix}
=
\begin{bmatrix}
1 \\
0 \\
0 \\
0
\end{bmatrix}
$$

Algebraic solution of these equations gives each of the flux control coefficients in terms of the elasticities and the rates of the cycle enzymes.[69] The flux control coefficient of enzyme 2a is:

$$C_{2a}^J = \frac{\varepsilon_1^1 \varepsilon_2^3 (1 + v_{2b}/v_1)}{D}$$

where

$$
\begin{aligned}
D &= \varepsilon_1^1 \varepsilon_2^3 - (1 + v_{2b}/v_1)(\varepsilon_1^1 \varepsilon_2^{2a} + \varepsilon_2^3 \varepsilon_1^{2a}) \\
&\quad + (v_{2b}/v_1)(\varepsilon_1^1 \varepsilon_2^{2b} + \varepsilon_2^3 \varepsilon_1^{2b})
\end{aligned}
$$

The factor, r, by which cycling increases the flux control coefficient of enzyme 2a is obtained by comparing two cases with the same net flux and intermediate concentrations, except that in the reference state, the cycling rate, v_{2b}, is zero:

$$r = \frac{1}{1 - \dfrac{v_{2b}(\varepsilon_1^1 \varepsilon_2^3 - \varepsilon_1^1 \varepsilon_2^{2b} - \varepsilon_2^3 \varepsilon_1^{2b})}{v_{2a}(\varepsilon_1^1 \varepsilon_2^3 - \varepsilon_1^1 \varepsilon_2^{2a} - \varepsilon_2^3 \varepsilon_1^{2a})}} \tag{7.14}$$

Further reading

Stadtman, E. R. (1970) *Mechanisms of enzyme regulation in metabolism.* In The Enzymes (Boyer, P. D., ed.), 3rd edn. vol. 1, pp. 397–459, Academic Press, New York

Katz, J. & Rognstad, R. (1976) *Futile cycles in the metabolism of glucose.* Curr. Top. Cell Regul. **10**, 237–289

Hue, L. (1981) *The role of futile cycles in the regulation of carbohydrate metabolism in the liver.* Adv. Enzymol. **52**, 247–331

Hue, L. (1982) *Futile cycles and regulation of metabolism.* In Metabolic Compartmentation (Sies, H., ed.), pp. 71–97, Academic Press, London

Boyer, P. D. & Krebs, E. G. (eds.) (1986) *Control by phosphorylation, parts A & B.* In The Enzymes, vols. XVII and XVIII, Academic Press, New York

Shaltiel, S. & Chock, P. B. (eds) (1985) *Modulation by covalent modification.* Curr. Top. Cell Regul. **27**

8

Conclusion

At first glance, the impact of Metabolic Control Analysis on conventional approaches to biochemical control can appear limited and benign: the concept of a single rate–limiting step is replaced by the concept that a number of steps could share control without any of them being fully rate–limiting. On this interpretation, the search for rate–limiting enzymes is replaced by the measurement of flux control coefficients to determine which enzymes have the coefficients with the largest values, as illustrated in Chapter 6. However, once a rigorous approach to the systematic analysis of metabolic control is embarked upon, it becomes increasingly clear that the whole edifice of conventional biochemical thinking about metabolic control is very shaky, in spite of the very impressive level of knowledge about the molecular properties of the underlying components. One after another, cherished ideas have been found to be untenable.

First were the conventional criteria used to identify rate–limiting enzymes (Chapter 4). These have been shown to be a poor guide to identifying enzymes with large flux control coefficients (e.g. Chapter 5.5.1). In fact, they are an inconsistent mix of criteria, since some of them identify enzymes with regulatory properties that can be shown (in the study of feedback inhibition effects, Chapter 7.2.2) to result in those enzymes being poor sites of flux and concentration control. In this case the properties relate to improved regulation, showing that regulation and control can be distinguished. To the surprise of critics of the theory, the experimental results on phosphofructokinase (Chapter 6.1.1.3) have confirmed that the theoretical view is correct: the enzyme is regulatory but cannot be used to control flux.

Another doubtful conventional concept is that the allosteric control of regulatory enzymes is responsible for rapid responses in flux control on shorter time scales than either covalent modification or enzyme synthesis and degradation.[5,139] However, the transition time for pathways to reach a steady state flux is typically in the region of seconds to minutes,[63,196,249] which is the time scale on which covalent modification works (as mentioned in Chapter 7.4.5).

Thus there is no obvious 'functional gap' in flux control that allosteric effects have to fill so long as covalent modification mechanisms are operating.

Even the teleological principle, that it is advantageous to control a pathway near its beginning, is open to doubt. The study of supply and demand pathways (Chapter 7.1), combined with the effects of feedback inhibition, shows that metabolic control structures exist to give good regulation (*i.e.* strong flux control combined with relatively weaker effects on metabolite concentrations) if flux control is concentrated at the demand end of the pathway. It is not known at present whether there are equivalent control structures to ensure such good regulation if control is exerted near the beginning of the pathway, but the evidence is against it. In this context, it is most remarkable that control of flux in cells is often achieved with so little change in metabolite concentrations. For example, when a 1000–fold increase in the glycolytic rate of rat muscle was obtained by stimulating the muscle, the measured metabolites increased less than 10–fold in concentration.[107] These and similar experiments led Bücher and Rüssmann[24] to speculate that metabolic pathways are controlled at more than a single enzyme in order to ensure homoeostasis of metabolite concentrations, as mentioned in Chapter 1.4.3. Similarly, Helmreich and Cori[101] noted the constancy of metabolite levels with large glycolytic flux changes in vertebrate muscle and also concluded that glycolysis must be controlled as a unit, particularly as they could not account for the changes in rates of several of the enzymes by the small changes in concentrations of their substrates and effectors.

Metabolic Control Analysis has confirmed these authors' suspicions that there was a problem still to be solved about the control of glycolysis. Even if the fallacy of the rate–limiting step is made apparently more respectable by supposing that control is exerted by action at the enzyme with the largest flux control coefficient, control at a single site has a clear problem: Small and Kacser's theory of large changes (Chapter 5.2.2) shows that it is impossible to achieve anything other than small total changes in the flux in response to massive changes in an enzyme's activity if its flux control coefficient is only slightly less than 1. Therefore, if large changes in flux occur in cells (such as in glycolytic flux in muscle upon changes in mechanical activity, or in photosynthesis in plants upon changes in illumination) they cannot be achieved by controls acting at a single site; there must be widespread sites of action of any control signal. Furthermore, even though the covalent modification of phosphorylase apparently provides an obvious mechanism for flux control of muscle glycolysis, the analysis of homoeostasis and regulation makes it unlikely that control of flux solely from the beginning of the pathway can explain such good homoeostasis of metabolite concentrations as is observed.

Thus although this book has covered a systems theory of the control of metabolism and has examined the range of control and regulatory mechanisms available in metabolism, we have arrived at its final chapter without a satisfactory answer to the question: how is the flux of a metabolic pathway controlled

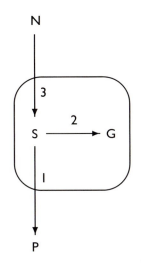

Figure 8.1 Schematic cell metabolism for the Universal Method
The metabolic inputs are grouped as N, the desired product is P, and all the other products and cell biomass are G. S is the metabolite at which synthesis of P branches from the rest of metabolism. Each arrow represents a complex metabolic network.

in vivo? In the next section, I will suggest an answer, developed with my colleague Simon Thomas,[72] that is consistent with the theory and the experimental evidence.

8.1 A new view of the physiological control of flux

The unresolved problem of metabolic control is how to achieve a large change in metabolic flux in response to some environmental or hormonal signal without disruption of other areas of metabolism and whilst maintaining metabolite levels relatively stable. In fact, Henrik Kacser found an answer to this problem, not by studying control systems *in vivo* but by asking how a biotechnologist could stimulate a pathway that makes a useful product (such as an amino acid or the antibiotic penicillin). Practical attempts to do this by using genetic engineering techniques to increase the amount of a particular enzyme in a pathway have tended to be unsuccessful. In part, this is because the genetic engineers have selected enzymes that are likely to have small flux control coefficients, such as feedback–inhibited enzymes. (The example of phosphofructo-kinase in yeast has been mentioned previously.) In any case, the predictions that Rankin Small and Henrik Kacser have made of the effects of large changes in a single enzyme show that this procedure is likely to give disappointing results.

Therefore in 1993 Kacser and Luis Acerenza studied how biotechnologists could design a change in metabolism to cause an arbitrarily large flux increase in a specific pathway, whilst leaving all concentrations and most other fluxes unperturbed.[117,118] They termed their result the 'Universal Method', since it does not depend on the details of the kinetics and should be possible, at least in principle, under most circumstances. (Whether it is universally practicable remains to be seen.) To illustrate their method, assume the target pathway is one producing an end product of metabolism, P (Figure 8.1). The method proposes making proportional increases in *all* the enzymes leading directly to this output from the input(s), with the largest changes in activity being made in all the enzymes in the final linear sequence to the output, and with progressively smaller changes being made in each preceding branch so that the fluxes in colateral branches remain unchanged. In Figure 8.1, suppose that the rate of production of P (J_1) is to be increased 5–fold. All the enzymes along that branch would have to be increased by a factor of 5. This creates an additional consumption of S equal to $4J_1$. To ensure that the concentration of S, and hence the rate of synthesis of G, remain constant, the rate of production of S has to be increased by the same amount. That is J_3 has to be increased to $J_3 + 4J_1$. The fractional increase required in the enzymes synthesizing S is therefore $4J_1/J_3$. Since J_1 is much less than J_3, the change required in J_3 is quantitatively less significant, and probably the need to change enzyme levels dies away as the pathway is traced back to the inputs. In effect, the method exploits the different behaviour of fluxes and concentrations when the activities of a sequence of enzymes are all increased in the same proportion. According to the summation theorem for flux control coefficients (Chapter 5.2.3), the flux will increase in proportion to the enzyme activities, whereas the metabolite concentrations will remain constant in accordance with the summation theorem for concentration control coefficients (Chapter 5.8.1). It might not be necessary to increase every enzyme along each branch affected provided that any enzymes omitted have flux control coefficients very near zero.

The potential for success of this strategy of multiple enzyme manipulations, compared with the failure of manipulating single enzymes in a pathway, has been illustrated by Peter Niederberger and his colleagues for the tryptophan biosynthesis pathway of yeast.[117,175] There are five enzymes from chorismate, the common precursor of the amino acids tryptophan, tyrosine and pheny-lalanine, to tryptophan itself, encoded by the genes *TRP1* to *TRP5*. The ap-proximate control coefficients of these five enzymes were estimated from mea-surements of tryptophan synthesis flux in mutant/wild–type heterozygotes in tetraploid yeast. None of the enzymes had a large control coefficient, and the sum of the five was 0.26. The five enzymes were overexpressed in yeast by incorporating their genes, either singly or in combination, into a yeast plasmid. As might have been expected from the low flux control coefficients, overex-pression of any of the enzymes singly, even up to 50–fold, had barely any effect on the flux. The more interesting result was the demonstration that the flux increase achieved when all the enzymes were changed together was far greater than the product of the flux changes obtained by increasing each enzyme sep-

Table 8.1 Metabolic engineering of tryptophan synthesis in yeast

Genes overexpressed					Mean fold	Relative
TRP2	TRP4	TRP1	TRP3	TRP5	increase	flux to Trp
-	-	-	-	-	1	1.0
-	-	+	+	-	58	2.0
+	+	-	+	-	35	2.4
+*	-	+	+	-	34	1.2
+*	+	+	+	-	30	2.1
+	+	-	+	+	19	8.2
+*	+	+	+	+	23	8.8

Results are from Niederberger et al.[175] The genes are arranged in order of their enzymes between chorismate and tryptophan (see Figure 7.6). Each row represents a separate experiment where '+' indicates the enzyme was overexpressed from plasmid–borne genes; '-' indicates wild–type level. For *TRP2*, '+*' indicates that a mutant allele, resistant to feedback inhibition by tryptophan, was overexpressed. The mean fold increase column gives the average overexpression of the engineered genes.

arately. The results are summarized in Table 8.1, where it is clear that the best increase in flux is obtained when all five enzymes are overexpressed. Even so, an average 23–fold excess of the enzymes still only produces a 9–fold increase in flux because no changes have been made to increase the supply of chorismate. Incidentally, the experiments also show that abolishing the allosteric feedback on anthranilate synthase (*TRP2*) does not significantly stimulate tryptophan synthesis.

The Universal Method is a theoretical proposal for engineering a desired change in metabolic flux. Although the experiments on tryptophan synthesis are not a complete implementation of it, the results indicate that relatively large changes of flux can be obtained by activating all the enzymes in a pathway. Whilst writing this book, it occurred to me to examine the possibility that cells had already implemented this method in the control of their own metabolism.

8.1.1 Evidence for multisite modulation in cells

If cells do control their metabolism by simultaneously changing the activities of many enzymes (*multisite modulation*), then it should be possible to see the principles of the Universal Method being implemented *in vivo*. For example:

(1) When enzyme amounts change in response to physiological or environmental signals, the relative proportions of pathway enzymes would remain constant.

(2) The common factor by which the amounts of the pathway enzymes change would be equal to the factor by which the flux changes.

(3) The levels of change would be greatest in the main branch of the pathway being controlled, although coordinated, but smaller, changes would occur in more distal branches.

(4) In addition to enzyme induction, other control mechanisms that act on the pathway would also operate on a similar set of multiple target sites.

The first point is well illustrated by the organization of the genes for pathway enzymes in operons (*i.e.* as adjacent genes with a common control of expression) and also in *regulons*[152] where the genes are not all adjacent and do not share control elements yet still respond to the same signals. Srere[236] has recently noted that the concept of control by rate–limiting steps is contradicted by the many examples (glycolysis, the tricarboxylic acid cycle, photosynthesis and the syntheses of fatty acids, urea, nucleotides and amino acids) where environmental or physiological signals cause coordinated induction of all the enzymes in a pathway. I shall therefore concentrate on some examples that illustrate the other three characteristics listed above.

8.1.1.1 Lipogenesis

Lipogenesis, or triacylglycerol synthesis (Figure 8.2), exemplifies all three. One type of genetic obesity in mice maps to a single locus, the *obese* gene. This codes for a secreted protein, specifically made by adipose tissue, that appears to have signalling functions and the absence of which causes profound obesity.[282] The obese phenotype is linked to the alteration of enzyme levels in adipose tissue and liver relative to wild–type levels[25] as summarized in Table 8.2. The mutant mouse appears to be capable of a rate of lipid synthesis per unit lean tissue some 3-fold higher than normal mice.[25] This is consistent with the 2–4-fold activation of eight of the major enzymes of lipid and carbohydrate metabolism as shown in Table 8.2 (point 2). (Effectively it is more enzymes than this, because fatty acid synthase is itself a multienzyme complex of the seven enzymes needed to add malonyl–CoA to a growing acyl–CoA chain.) In connected parts of carbohydrate metabolism, Table 8.2 shows that four enzymes are elevated by about 50%, and two adipose tissue lipases are significantly depressed[25] (point 3). Of the enzymes in this Table, acetyl-CoA carboxylase, fructose–1,6–bisphosphatase, hormone–sensitive lipase, phosphofructokinase and pyruvate kinase are known to be subject to control, directly or indirectly, by protein phosphorylation and dephosphorylation reactions that respond to dietary status[105] (point 4).

Two lines of evidence suggest that this is not an odd result from a particular type of mutant mouse. First, Bulfield and his colleagues obtained essentially similar results in a later study of the differences in enzyme contents between lean and fat lines of mice that had been selected over 26 generations from the same base population.[4] For most of the enzymes in Table 8.2, there is good evidence that the controls on their levels of expression respond to starvation, refeeding or high-carbohydrate diets[105] in rats. On the other hand, there is a lack of

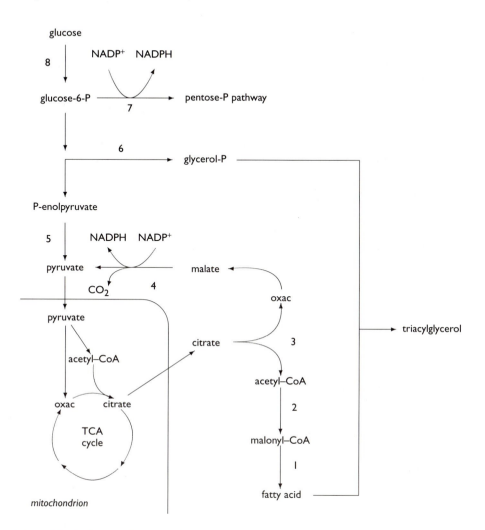

Figure 8.2 Pathways of lipogenesis
The numbered enzymes are: 1, fatty acid synthase; 2, acetyl–CoA carboxylase; 3, ATP citrate-lyase; 4, 'malic' enzyme; 5, pyruvate kinase; 6, glycerol–3–phosphate dehydrogenase; 7, glucose–6–phosphate dehydrogenase; 8, hexokinase. oxac, oxaloacetate; TCA, tricarboxylic acid.

experimental evidence supporting any system–wide role for allosteric effectors in physiologically significant control of lipogenesis by dietary factors.[105]

8.1.1.2 Urea cycle

The rate of urea synthesis in rats responds proportionately to the amount of protein in the diet, and over a range of protein intakes, the amounts of all four of the urea cycle enzymes and carbamoyl–phosphate synthase also vary proportionately.[221] A comparison of the enzyme contents of rats on diets that

Table 8.2 Relative enzyme levels in the obese mouse

Tissue	Enzyme	Change (%)
Group 1: elevated		
Adipose	Glycerol kinase	371
Liver	Hexokinase IV	357
Liver	Acetyl–CoA carboxylase	335
Liver	Fatty acid synthase	267
Liver	Malic enzyme	254
Liver	ATP citrate-lyase	231
Liver	Fructose–1,6–bisphosphatase	213
Liver	Glycerol–3–phosphate dehydrogenase	210
Group 2: slightly elevated		
Liver	Glucose–6–phosphatase	163
Liver	Phosphofructokinase	160
Adipose	Glucose–6–phosphate dehydrogenase	151
Liver	Pyruvate kinase	150
Liver	Glucose–6–phosphate dehydrogenase	139
Group 3: depressed		
Adipose	Hormone–sensitive lipase	73
Adipose	Monoacylglycerol lipase	20

The percentage change in activity represents the amount in obese mice relative to lean controls; data from Bulfield.[25] Hexokinase IV is also known as glucokinase.[51] 'Malic' enzyme is malate dehydrogenase (oxaloacetate–decarboxylating) (NADP⁺) (EC 1.1.1.40).

can cause a 4–fold difference in urea outputs showed that eight of the enzymes measured increased significantly. All the enzymes of the urea cycle increased 2–3-fold in activity, which is sufficient to account for the flux change if there is also a slight stimulation by increased substrate supply (point 2 above). There were also large increases in alanine transaminase and glucose–6–phosphate dehydrogenase.

8.1.1.3 Carbohydrate metabolism

George Weber and his colleagues carried out extensive investigations in the 1960s into the effects of dietary changes, starvation and hormone treatments on carbohydrate metabolism in rat liver. The hormones investigated included glucocorticoid steroids, which stimulate gluconeogenesis, and insulin, which suppresses it.[268,269] They concluded that the liver enzymes fall into three groups: the exclusively gluconeogenic enzymes (in the left-hand column of Table 8.3), the exclusively glycolytic enzymes (those in the right-hand column of Table 8.3 except aldolase) and the dual–function enzymes (the rest). The amounts of the members of a group change coordinately, but the directions and magnitudes of the changes differ between the groups, exemplifying points

Table 8.3 Control of expression of enzymes of gluconeogenesis and glycolysis in mammalian liver

Expression inhibited by insulin, stimulated by cyclic AMP	Expression stimulated by insulin or glucose, inhibited by cyclic AMP
Glucose–6–phosphatase	Hexokinase IV (glucokinase)
Fructose–1,6–bisphosphatase	Phosphofructo–1–kinase
Phosphoenolpyruvate carboxykinase	Phosphofructo–2–kinase / fructose–2,6–bisphosphatase
	Aldolase
	Pyruvate kinase

See Figure 6.17 for the positions of most of these enzymes in gluconeogenesis. The effects shown are ones for which the molecular mechanisms have recently been established.[147] However the existence of these two groups of oppositely regulated enzymes has been known for 30 years.[268]

1 and 3 above. For several of these enzymes, the molecular mechanisms of control of enzyme amount have been shown to include the actions of insulin, cyclic AMP and glucocorticoids on transcription.[147,184] Some support for a similar pattern of control by other mechanisms (point 4) comes from the effects of protein phosphorylation. The actions of glucagon and α–adrenergic agents in stimulating gluconeogenesis in rat liver involve the inhibition of pyruvate kinase by phosphorylation, and the activation of fructose–1,6–bisphosphatase and the inhibition of phosphofructo–1–kinase by changes in the level of fructose 2,6–bisphosphate brought about by protein phosphorylation. As it is possible that as many as one in four mammalian cell proteins can be reversibly phosphorylated,[37] it is even conceivable that there are more undiscovered sites of phosphorylation involved in the stimulation of gluconeogenesis.

In other tissues, protein phosphorylation stimulates glycolysis. For example, in the different types of animal muscle, stimulation of contraction may be associated with activation of some or all of phosphorylase, phosphofructo–1–kinase, pyruvate dehydrogenase and myosin ATPase.

8.1.1.4 Steroid synthesis

The synthesis of the several corticosteroid hormones in the adrenal cortex (Figure 8.3) can be stimulated by adrenocorticotropic hormone (ACTH; corticotropin) both in the short term (seconds to minutes) and over periods of several days[181,267] increasing production up to 10–fold relative to basal rates.[138,191] Cyclic AMP is involved on both time scales. The pathway provides another example of parallel multisite changes both in the rapid–acting modulation of activity (by mechanisms including protein phosphorylation) and the control of enzyme amounts. The rapid acting effects increase the availability of cholesterol at the mitochondrial site of cytochrome P–450_{SCC} (where SCC signifies side

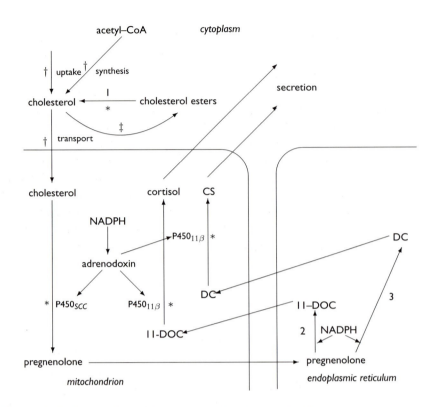

Figure 8.3 Pathways of steroidogenesis in adrenal cortical cells
Key: 11–DOC, 11–deoxycortisol; DC, deoxycorticosterone; CS, corticosterone; 1, cholesterol ester hydrolase; 2, 3–β–hydroxysteroid dehydrogenase + P–450_{C21} + P–$450_{17\alpha}$; 3, 3–β–hydroxysteroid dehydrogenase + P–450_{C21}; *, ACTH activates *via* cyclic AMP; †, ACTH stimulated, mechanism unclear; ‡, possibly inhibited by ACTH. Enzymes involved in NADPH production are also activated.

chain cleavage). Cholesterol is stored in the cells largely as cholesterol esters, and the cholesterol esterase is activated by protein phosphorylation induced by cyclic AMP. However, uptake of cholesterol into the cell and its transfer from the cytoplasm into the mitochondrial matrix are also both rapidly stimulated by mechanisms that are not entirely understood. Esterification of cholesterol is possibly also inhibited by ACTH, but this is controversial. Both mitochondrial P–450 enzymes involved in the pathway (P–450_{SCC} and P–$450_{11\beta}$) appear to be rapidly activated by ACTH, the latter by a mechanism involving cyclic AMP, the former by a mechanism that is still unknown but might involve cyclic AMP.

The longer-term effects of ACTH involve action on all aspects of metabolism that affect the amount of the common precursor steroid, cholesterol, its conversion to the common intermediate pregnenolone, and many sites in the final formation of the various products by oxidation.[181,267] The synthesis rates are increased of the four cytochrome P–450 enzymes (P–450_{SCC}, P–$450_{11\beta}$, P–$450_{17\alpha}$ and P–450_{C21}) and of their associated electron-transport elements: the FeS protein adrenodoxin; the enzyme adrenodoxin reductase which catalyses its reduction by NADPH in the mitochondria, and NADPH–cytochrome *P*–450 reductase in the endoplasmic reticulum. ACTH also exerts long–term activation of the uptake of cholesterol into the cell and increases the amounts of cholesterol esterase. In other related branches of metabolism, esterification of cholesterol for storage in lipid droplets is inhibited whilst increased amounts of isocitrate dehydrogenase ($NADP^+$), 'malic' enzyme and glucose–6–phosphate dehydrogenase provide NADPH for the hydroxylation reactions.[138] The synthesis of cholesterol from acetate is also stimulated over about 36 h; increased activity of one of the early enzymes of the pathway, hydroxymethylglutaryl–CoA reductase, has been demonstrated but does not match the time course of the stimulation of the pathway flux, which could be evidence that synthesis of other enzymes is required as well.[191] Significantly, hydroxymethylglutaryl–CoA reductase is an enzyme known to be controlled by reversible phosphorylation (Chapter 7.4.3.1.4).

8.1.1.5 Photosynthesis

Finally, light–dependent activation of plant photosynthesis in the chloroplasts and associated metabolism in the plant cytoplasm illustrates rapid control mechanisms acting at multiple sites throughout a metabolic network (point 4). As well as the diurnal cycle, plants are subject to continual fluctuations in illumination from light flecks (shifting patches of sunlight filtering through the leaf canopy) and changing orientations of their leaves as they bend and shake in the wind. These transient increases in illumination can be responsible for a significant fraction of daily carbon fixation and can cause sudden increases in assimilation of CO_2 of the order of 10–fold on a time scale of a few seconds.[180]

There are several components to plant photosynthesis. For the C_3 plants typical of temperate regions these are:

- the *light reactions* in the chloroplast, where photosystems I and II harness the light energy on the thylakoid membranes and generate ATP and NADPH;

- the so–called *dark reactions* in the chloroplast which use the ATP and NADPH to fix CO_2 with ribulose–bisphosphate carboxylase (rubisco), regenerate the ribulose bisphosphate by the Calvin cycle and store photosynthate as starch;

- the processing of photosynthate in the cytosol, by the formation and export primarily of sucrose but also of amino acids.

Short–term variations in the rate of the light reactions largely follow the availability of light; however, the balance between the production of ATP and NADPH is kept by regulating the ratio between non–cyclic photophosphorylation (which uses both photosystems and produces both products) and cyclic photophosphorylation, which uses only photosystem I and produces

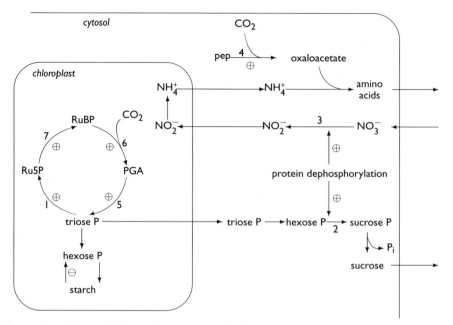

Figure 8.4 Effects of light on photosynthesis in C₃ plants
Key: ⊕, light activation by a variety of mechanisms; ⊖, light inactivation. Abbreviations: pep, phospho-enolpyruvate; PGA, phosphoglycerate; Ru5P, ribulose 5–phosphate; RuBP, ribulose 1,5–bisphosphate. Enzymes: 1, pentose pathway — activatable enzymes are fructose bisphosphatase and sedoheptulose bisphosphatase; 2, sucrose phosphate synthase; 3, nitrate reductase; 4, phosphoenolpyruvate carboxy-kinase; 5, glyceraldehyde–3–phosphate dehydrogenase; 6, rubisco; 7, ribulose–5–phosphate kinase.

only ATP. This regulation involves reversible phosphorylation of the light–harvesting component of photosystem II by a protein kinase that responds to the redox state of the intermediate electron transport chain between the two photosystems,[15] but is not the aspect I wish to focus on here. Rather, I want to look at how the assimilation of carbon in the chloroplast and cytoplasm (Figure 8.4) is controlled in accordance with the fluctuations in the supply of ATP and NADPH from the light reactions. The levels of ATP and NADPH change relatively little during the day, so there is obviously control on the de-mand reactions (*i.e.* the dark reactions) in accordance with the requirement for effective homoeostasis in supply–demand pathways.

The activation state of four of the enzymes of the Calvin cycle was dis-covered by Buchanan to depend on light–mediated reduction carried out by small proteins called thioredoxins.[3] This is a covalent modification reaction involving the oxidation state of cysteine thiol groups in the enzymes. When they are oxidized to form disulphide linkages, the enzymes are inactive; when they are reduced to the thiol form, the enzymes are active. Thioredoxins are abundant in chloroplasts and themselves contain adjacent thiol groups that can be oxidized to disulphides. They are oxidized by atmospheric oxygen, but are reduced by ferredoxin, the electron-transport component that is itself reduced by photosystem I and that in turn reduces $NADP^+$ to NADPH. Thus the redox state of thioredoxin senses the activation of the light reactions and transmits this to activate phosphoribulokinase, glyceraldehyde–3–phosphate dehydrogenase, fructose–1,6–bisphosphatase and sedoheptulose bisphosphatase. The system can also respond to the state of the Calvin cycle because the susceptibility of the enzymes to reduction is also modulated by levels of the Calvin cycle intermediates.[80] Ribulose–bisphosphate carboxylase itself, the enzyme that actually fixes the CO_2, is controlled by multiple effects including a covalent modification: an activation by carbamoylation of a lysine group promoted by rubisco activase, which is itself activated by light.[80] In some plants, rubisco is inhibited by carboxyarabinitol 1–phosphate, which is synthesized in the dark and degraded in the light;[180] again, rubisco activase is involved in releasing rubisco from this inhibition. Calvin cycle enzymes also respond to the light–induced changes in stromal pH and Mg^{2+} concentration[277] that occur as the light reactions pump protons out of the stroma into the thylakoid space. In C_4 plants, such as tropical grasses, the activity of one of the key enzymes in their alternative mode of CO_2 fixation, pyruvate phosphate dikinase, is controlled by phosphorylation in a light–dependent manner.[110] In addition, light–dependent changes in protein phosphorylation activate enzymes of the assimilatory pathways in the cytoplasm (Figure 8.4), including sucrose phosphate synthase, nitrate reductase and phosphoenolpyruvate carboxykinase,[110] presumably so that the relative amounts of starch, sucrose and amino acids being synthesized are kept in balance both with one another and with the amount of CO_2 being fixed.

Much remains to be learnt about the molecular mechanisms underlying the several different light–activated control systems operating in photosynthesis. There are also differences between different types of plant, such as C_3 and C_4 plants. However, even though the account given above is not exhaustive in terms of the enzymes whose activities are controlled by light, it is sufficient to demonstrate that the rate of carbon assimilation is very far from being controlled by a single enzyme such as rubisco. Indeed, the measurements of the flux control coefficient of rubisco, made by Mark Stitt's group and described in Chapter 6.1.1.5, p. 145, reveal how unlikely this would be: under most circumstances the control coefficient is not large enough to allow significant stimulation of carbon assimilation by activation of rubisco alone.

8.1.2 Implications of multisite modulation

As seen from the examples, there are undoubtedly cases where environmental or physiological signals that induce large changes in metabolic flux do so by acting on many, or even all, of the enzymes in a pathway. It is difficult to find examples of the negative case, *i.e.* large changes in flux indubitably initiated solely by action on a single enzyme. One possible contradictory example is the stimulation of tryptophan catabolism by nutritional or hormonal induction of tryptophan dioxygenase, as discussed in Chapter 6.1.2. Here the catabolic flux does seem to be stimulated by a selective increase in the amount of this pathway enzyme alone; on the other hand, the degree of stimulation of the flux is relatively small and the pathway is short and soon enters the main areas of catabolism which are of far higher capacity. So if, as the theory suggests, multi-site modulation is the only effective way to achieve large changes in metabolic flux in the majority of cases, some uncomfortable conclusions follow.

(1) The rate–limiting step concept is more misguided than even Metabolic Control Analysis initially suggested. Under its influence, biochemists have searched for a single or a small number of key control points when the important control mechanisms are those that have multiple sites of action in metabolism.

(2) If control is exerted by multisite modulation, the effects are synergistic. There will be deleterious effects from interfering with the response at any of the control sites, and the response from a single control site operated in isolation will always be relatively poor. Characterizing the importance of individual steps to an overall flux response will be very difficult since the overall response is a property of the system itself, not of its components.

(3) If the physiological control mechanisms are interlinked throughout a pathway, experiments in Metabolic Control Analysis will not be easy to design because it will be difficult to find ways of perturbing a specific point in the pathway without the possibility that the control mechanisms will transmit the perturbation to other parts of the pathway by routes that have not been taken into account.

Addressing these problems is not a simple issue, even within Metabolic Control Analysis. Its suitability to take on this challenge is discussed in the next section.

8.2   Limitations of Control Analysis

I have presented neither all aspects of Metabolic Control Analysis nor its full complexity in this book. This would obviously have been inappropriate in an introductory text. Nevertheless, I believe I have presented enough of the central aspects of the theory for the reader to consider, and form a judgement on, some of the criticisms of Metabolic Control Analysis as I have described it here. I shall consider these criticisms in two groups:

- objections to the formulation and general approach of Control Analysis as a whole;

- criticisms of over–simplifications in Control Analysis, which have led to changes and extensions to the theory.

8.2.1   Objections to Control Analysis

There have been arguments against both the name and the concept of the control coefficients. Some of the principal grounds cited have been that:

(1) enzyme concentration is not a parameter that is particularly relevant to metabolic control, e.g.[8,56], compared with the action of effectors that bind to allosteric enzymes;

(2) the sensitivity of a flux to an enzyme concentration is not a measure of whether that enzyme is a *control* or a *regulatory* enzyme,[8,56,218] so the term is misleading;

(3) the flux control coefficient has limited predictive value because it is only valid under the conditions of measurement, and as the state of the system changes, the values of the flux control coefficients change.[56,259]

The first of these criticisms has been made particularly forcefully by both Eric Newsholme and Dan Atkinson. Newsholme, with Bernard Crabtree, has developed an alternative theoretical approach to metabolic control which involves characterizing the *net sensitivity* of a pathway to an effector of an enzyme.[55] If necessary, a hypothetical effector is assumed to exist in order to allow definition of the net sensitivity. In Metabolic Control Analysis, the equivalent measure is the response coefficient (Chapter 5.4), so the key difference between the approaches is that in Control Analysis the flux control coefficient is separated out as an individual entity that can be combined with different elasticities to indicate the responses of the pathway flux to a range of effectors whereas in Newsholme's theory the net sensitivity is the primary entity. Atkinson[8] objected that the key feature in control of metabolism is the action of effectors of allosteric enzymes which frequently change the affinity of an enzyme for its substrates, not the catalytic activity. Again, the response coefficient of the flux to the effector, formed from the flux control coefficient of the enzyme and the elasticity of the enzyme to the effector, provides a measure of the strength of the response. Thus it is the belief of the advocates of Metabolic Control Analysis, admittedly not shared by the objectors, that the measures they seek are provided in Control Analysis. A more fundamental rebuttal of their objection would be that control by allosteric effectors is not the only control mechanism; the equally important effects of genes, DNA manipulation, environment, diet and hormones on metabolism can be mediated through the change in the concentration of the active form of an enzyme, and the flux control coefficient indicates what the effect of such a change will be.

The second objection returns to a theme that has run through this book. There is no doubting that regulatory enzymes are often predicted by Control Analysis to have small flux control coefficients, and the argument is therefore that there is little use in a measure that does not identify the important characteristics of an enzyme. The reasons why regulatory enzymes subjected to feedback regulation have small flux control coefficients have been considered at length in the Chapter on feedback inhibition (Chapter 7.2). I have sympathy for the concept that there ought to be a measure of the strength of the regulatory role of an enzyme; in fact, some measures have been suggested but have not been widely adopted. However, as long as molecular biologists are overexpressing regulatory enzymes in the expectation of altering metabolic flux and are being disappointed by the results, I believe the priority is to emphasize the distinction between regulation and control and to persuade molecular biologists to pay more attention to the flux control coefficient, which could have been used to predict their disappointment.

There is truth in the third objection, made by Newsholme & Crabtree and Savageau & Voit. The flux control coefficient is only valid under the conditions of its measurement, and therefore it can make only limited predictions about what will happen if circumstances change greatly. Everybody would be happier if it was possible to make accurate predictions about the effects of large perturbations induced by factors such as hormonal stimulation, but this is extremely difficult. If we had complete models of metabolism, it would be possible, but the information needed to build completely accurate models is not, and may never be, available. If it were, we would not need Metabolic Control Analysis. Henrik Kacser was sensitive to the force of this criticism and his response to it was expressed in his characteristically entertaining way in the last article he completed[117] before his death in March 1995. In response, he cited his work on the relationship between flux control coefficients and large changes in enzyme activity (summarized in Chapter 5.2.2), and also the Universal Method, referred to earlier in this chapter (Chapter 8.1) for obtaining large changes in flux. As he pointed out, these go beyond the realm where Metabolic Control Analysis is strictly valid, but have depended on the insights from Control Analysis. Savageau's criticism reflects the different aims he had in developing his Biochemical Systems Theory, which is intended as a complete tool for the modelling and analysis of stability and sensitivity.[217] Furthermore, he claims that Metabolic Control Analysis is only a limited subset of his theory;[218,219] I accept that it is possible to view the two theories in this light, but I and other advocates of Control Analysis feel that our theory avoids some of the aspects of Biochemical Systems Theory that we regard as undesirable.[48]

There have also been criticisms of the roles of the theorems, such as the summation and connectivity theorems, in Metabolic Control Analysis. Kacser & Burns[119] gave them a central role in the development of the theory, and I have used them to provide the explanations in this book. Savageau and colleagues[219] have claimed that they are unnecessary because they are implicit in the mathematical description of a metabolic system at steady state. It is also true that Christine Reder in Bordeaux, Marta Cascante in Barcelona and Christoph Giersch in Darmstadt have shown that pathways can be analysed in terms of Metabolic Control Analysis without assuming the existence of the theorems,[31,32,83,195] and that the theorems then emerge from the analysis. This is extremely useful work because it provides deeper mathematical foundations for Control Analysis. It is not the same as saying the theorems have no use; they summarize important properties that assist in explanations of how control is distributed and make a link to a biochemical interpretation of the mathematics. But at this stage, I am content to abide by the reader's judgement: take a look at some of the papers cited in this section, and see if you prefer their approach.

8.2.2 Extensions of Control Analysis

Only the simplest and most straightforward aspects of Metabolic Control Analysis have been presented in this book. However, over the last 10 years there has been considerable development of the theory. Much of this has been driven by the urge to examine claims that Metabolic Control Analysis would not be able to deal with metabolic pathways containing particular features that have not been taken into account during the development of the theory. In most cases it has proved possible to use the definitions and formalisms of Metabolic Control Analysis to incorporate these features, but at the expense of greater complexity in the mathematics and a loss of validity of the theorems. There are three main areas where potential problems could arise:

- the degree of connectedness of the metabolic network;

- the relationship between enzyme amount and catalytic activity;

- the validity of metabolite concentration measures.

I shall briefly summarize the complications to which each of these can lead.

8.2.2.1 Connectedness of metabolic networks

In the treatment of Metabolic Control Analysis given in this book I did not choose to show the proof that the summation theorem applies over a network that is fully connected by mass flows; in other words, it is a statement about a reaction network where the material flowing in can be traced all the way to the outputs, and every reaction in the network is carrying some of that flow. On this basis, two pathways occurring simultaneously that involve completely separate metabolites and have uncorrelated fluxes should be completely independent and each should have its own summation theorem with respect to the enzymes that catalyse its reactions. But what if the metabolites from one influence the rates of the other, even though they do not appear as substrates or products of its reactions? It is not difficult to find examples: covalent modification cascades consist of a hierarchy of pathways where the substrates and products of one pathway are the catalysts of the next pathway down, but do not participate in the flux of that pathway. Transcription and translation of genes to form enzymes, which then catalyse pathways, is another example where the mass flows at the protein synthesis level might be weakly coupled to the mass flows at pathway level, but again there is a catalytic relationship between them, and even the possibility of influence in the reverse direction through effects of metabolites from the pathway on the transcription and translation of the enzymes.

One possible solution in simple cases is to define the response of the pathway to events occurring at a higher level in an *ad hoc* way. An example is the treatment that Rankin Small and I gave to covalent modification reactions, described in Chapter 7.4.5. However, Daniel Kahn in Toulouse and Hans Westerhoff in Amsterdam have developed a Modular (or hierarchical) Control Analysis which uses the same mathematical formulation as Metabolic Control Analysis, but which can handle these problems systematically.[123,224] In essence, the solutions contain terms that represent the standard Control Analysis of the separate pathway components, but these are modified by interaction terms between the pathways. The approach has much potential, but is not for the mathematically faint–hearted; experimental applications are under way, but are not yet concluded.

8.2.2.2 Enzyme properties

As was briefly mentioned in Chapter 5.7 in the Appendix *More about flux control coefficients*, the simple form of Metabolic Control Analysis presented here has defined flux control coefficients in terms of the relative change in flux for a relative change in enzyme concentration. A hidden assumption is that the rate of an enzymic process is proportional to the enzyme concentration, and that one enzyme acts uniquely on a single metabolic step. There are a number of conceivable cases where this assumption is not obeyed:

- where an enzyme catalyses more than one step in the same metabolic pathway,[30] as occurs in purine metabolism and the pentose phosphate pathway;

- where the enzyme undergoes association equilibria, either with other molecules of the same enzyme or molecules of a different enzyme, and the aggregates have different catalytic properties from the free enzymes;[122,212] in the first case, the relationship between the enzyme concentration and the rate of the step is not linear; in the second, the two enzymes involved could each affect the rate of the other's step;

- where the enzyme is subject to covalent modification,[231] unless the enzyme concentration is defined in terms of the active form only, rather than the total.

The effects of most of these are as follows:

- The value of the flux control coefficient will depend on whether it is defined relative to enzyme concentration or to some other parameter that does affect enzymic rate linearly.

- Different experimental approaches could give different results for the flux control coefficient.[223] For example, a genetic manipulation that changes the total amount of an enzyme might not give the the same result as an inhibitor titration that changes the activity of the enzyme.

- The summation theorem may be invalidated.

However, each of these difficulties can be formulated in terms of Metabolic Control Analysis; it is just that the resulting analysis becomes more complex than the cases illustrated in this book. Are these potential problem cases frequent enough and severe enough to invalidate the application of Metabolic Control Analysis? They have not shown up in any of the experimental applications studied so far, but this might be because it is difficult to do the experiments with sufficient accuracy to detect the small deviations that might occur. My subjective impression is that until the accuracy and precision of the methods for measuring flux control coefficients have been improved substantially, these problems will remain a minor issue.

8.2.2.3   Metabolite concentrations

The third and most difficult of the problems is the appropriateness of metabolite concentration measures. Here I am not referring to the experimental difficulties in making meaningful measurements discussed in Chapter 2.3, since these are neither better nor worse for Control Analysis than for any other mode of interpreting metabolic control and regulation. This is a deeper problem relating to the underlying assumption in Metabolic Control Analysis that there exists a single value for the concentration of a metabolite that enters the equations and determines the values of coefficients such as the elasticity coefficients. In other words, the concentration must be adequately represented by a single value that is equally applicable to all the enzyme molecules. Again, the problem here does not come from the possibility of compartmentation in the cell, provided that a unique value can be assigned to the concentration in each compartment. It is more the possibility that the concentration of a metabolite varies with its position within a single compartment. This could happen in a system where the reactions do not occur uniformly throughout the space, and the rate of diffusion is not sufficiently fast relative to the reaction rates to cause completely uniform mixing. I have calculated that this could occur with cyclic AMP in some cells, for it is synthesized only at the plasma membrane but is hydrolysed throughout the cell, and this could give rise to cyclic AMP concentration gradients in the cell.[68] Such systematic spatial variation in metabolite concentration has not been taken into account in Control Analysis. On the other hand, diffusion of metabolites is a fast process on the scale of cellular dimensions, and is likely to be able to keep concentration gradients in the aqueous compartments small in most cases.

A related problem, but one that also involves aspects of enzyme–enzyme interaction is the effect of *channelling*. This refers to cases where the common metabolite between two enzymes is not released into the medium but is directly transferred between them, either in a static channel (one that involves a relatively permanent association of the enzymes) or a dynamic channel (one where the metabolite is transferred in a transient association between the enzymes). This is a controversial area (see, for example, the paper by Ovadi[178] and the papers in the same issue of that journal), with respect to the frequency of occurrence, the mechanisms involved, and the effects (if any) that channelling has on metabolite concentrations in the bulk medium. Again, it is possible to modify the theory of Metabolic Control Analysis to cover this case[131,132,210] but the question remains how often any effects will be large enough to be detectable with current experimental techniques.

One final worry about metabolite concentrations has turned out not to be a great cause for concern at all. In some pathways where the enzymes are relatively abundant (glycolysis and rubisco in photosynthesis for example), the enzyme concentrations can be higher than the metabolite concentrations.[1] Some people were concerned that if the enzyme levels were not negligible compared with the metabolites, the theory would be invalidated. In fact, there should be no problem in terms of the steady state behaviour of the pathway provided that it is the free and not the total metabolite concentrations that appear in any of the equations. With Herbert Sauro, I identified one case where the effect might matter,[70] and this was where an enzyme present at relatively high concentration was binding a significant fraction of a moiety–conserved grouping (e.g. the adenosine of the adenine nucleotides or the $NAD^+/NADH$ pair). Even so, deviations in the summation theorems and discrepancies between different definitions of the flux control coefficients only become significant if the amount of complexed metabolite on the enzyme is a significant fraction of the total of the metabolites in the conserved pool (not of a single member of the group). This circumstance is likely to be much rarer than simple comparability between enzyme and metabolite concentrations, and again there are no experiments suggesting a problem at the moment.

8.3 Applications of Metabolic Control Analysis

Finally, what is the use of Metabolic Control Analysis? I hope that by now I have persuaded you that Metabolic Control Analysis provides a framework within which it is possible to carry out a rational and quantitative examination of the regulation and control of metabolism. This can be by the design and execution of appropriate experiments, as described in Chapter 6, or by theoretical analysis of common metabolic structures as illustrated in Chapter 7 and this chapter. Either way, the results have been a challenge to much traditional thinking in biochemistry and the debate will undoubtedly continue.

Because this is a biochemistry book, it would be easy to overlook the important implications of Metabolic Control Analysis for genetics, which were mentioned in Chapter 5.2.2 in connection with its relevance to the phenomenon of dominance. Putting biochemistry and genetics together links Metabolic Control Analysis with the evolution of metabolic pathways and even with population ecology. These aspects are again more theoretical than practical, but Jean–Pierre Mazat's group in Bordeaux has been using Metabolic Control Analysis to diagnose and understand the genetic disorders known as mitochondrial cytopathies.[149,150] These are a diverse group of inborn errors of metabolism with variable symptoms. They are caused by mutations in the mitochondrial genome, but the variability arises because there are multiple copies of the mitochondrial DNA in every human cell, so that the proportion of mutant to wild–type genes can be almost continuously variable, in contrast with nuclear genes where there are generally just two copies per cell. The variability in the symptoms reflects the non–linear relationship between the amount of an enzyme and the pathway flux. For many of the enzymes, the content can be reduced significantly with limited effects on flux, and therefore with little in the way of symptoms, but beyond a certain point (an apparent threshold), the flux decreases more rapidly with enzyme content, and the respiration rate of the mitochondria becomes progressively more limited by the step with the mutation.

Another potential area of application of Control Analysis in medicine is the identification of particularly suitable sites for the manipulation of metabolism with drugs. This is not a new idea; Hans Krebs[141] advocated it in 1957, but he considered that the answer would be to find the *pacemaker* enzymes. The concept has been reformulated in Metabolic Control Analysis terms by Chris Pogson and his group at the Wellcome pharmaceutical company.[208] They reasoned that even though it is unlikely that true pacemaker, or rate–limiting, enzymes exist, it would nevertheless still be worth while in the drug–discovery process to target the enzymes with the highest flux control coefficients. Very often, the aim with a drug is to inhibit a metabolic process, such as an essential pathway in a parasite or cancer cell, and in this case, any enzyme in the process is a potential target because every enzyme in a sequence is essential for the sequence to work. Even so, the effects on metabolism are likely to be obtained with lower concentrations of drug if an enzyme with a high flux control coefficient is being inhibited, rather than one with a low coefficient.

The area where Metabolic Control Analysis could make the biggest impact in the near future is the area of biotechnology known as *metabolic engineering*. Modern genetic engineering techniques have the potential to sidestep the traditional genetic approaches of selective breeding for organisms with a desired characteristic by permitting directed rational changes that could modify the metabolism of organisms in a desired direction. Generally, increasing the flow in a specific pathway is the more usual goal, and as discussed earlier in this Chapter, increasing the flux is a more difficult problem than decreasing it. In this area, Metabolic Control Analysis is already winning the argument over traditional concepts of metabolic control, because so–called rate–limiting enzymes have already been overexpressed in cells with little effect. Identifying enzymes with large flux control coefficients would allow a more rationally targeted approach, but the two limitations of this approach have already been discussed:

- It is conceivable that no enzyme in a pathway has a large flux control coefficient.

- Even where an enzyme has a moderately large flux control coefficient, the theory of finite changes in enzyme amounts predicts that the effects on metabolic flux of overexpressing it may be very modest.

There is no doubting the incentives to solve these problems. For example, plant metabolism might be manipulated to allow sustainable production from renewable resources of alternative raw materials to those currently derived from oil (such as plastics from starch). Advocates of Metabolic Control Analysis should not expect to be popular for suggesting that our knowledge of metabolic control shows such goals may be much more difficult to attain than is commonly thought. This was one of the problems that Henrik Kacser's 'Universal Method'[118] (discussed earlier in Chapter 8.1) was designed to solve, but the procedures it predicts to be necessary in order to change flux will not be simple to carry out. There is much scope here for further work.

8.4   Summary

(1) Control of flux cannot be exerted by one or a few enzymes at the beginning of a pathway when large changes in pathway flux are seen to be associated with much smaller relative changes in metabolite concentrations.

(2) In biotechnological applications, to ensure a significant increase in a metabolic flux without a marked change in metabolite concentrations, Kacser's Universal Method predicts that it is necessary to simultaneously activate many, even most, of the pathway enzymes.

(3) Examples of significant flux changes in a number of pathways provide evidence that these too are achieved by multisite modulation, *i.e.* the parallel activation of several, many, or even most of the enzymes of the pathway.

(4) Control Analysis alone may not be able to tackle all conceivable problems in regulation and control. Nevertheless, it is a better starting point

for acquiring a deeper understanding than the qualitative principles of conventional biochemistry.

Further reading

Fell, D. A. (ed.) (1995) *The control of flux: 21 years on.* Biochem. Soc. Trans. **23**, 341–391

References

1. Albe, K. R., Butler, M. H. and Wright, B. E. (1990) J. Theor. Biol. **143**, 163–195
2. Albe, K. R. and Wright, B. E. (1994) J. Theor. Biol. **169**, 243–251
3. Anderson, L. E. (1986) Adv. Bot. Res. **12**, 1–46
4. Asante, E. A., Hill, W. G. and Bulfield, G. (1991) Genet. Res. Camb. **58**, 123–127
5. Ashworth, J. M. and Kornberg, H. L. (1963) Biochim. Biophys. Acta **73**, 519–522
6. Atkinson, D. E. (1969) Curr. Top. Cell. Regul. **1**, 29–43
7. Atkinson, D. E. (1977) Cellular Energy Metabolism and its Regulation, Academic Press, New York
8. Atkinson, D. E. (1990) in Control of Metabolic Processes, (Cornish-Bowden, A. and Cárdenas, M. L., eds.), pp. 3–11, Plenum Press, New York
9. Babul, J., Clifton, D., Kretschmer, M. and Fraenkel, D. G. (1993) Biochemistry **32**, 4685–4692
10. Baranyi, J. M. and Blum, J. J. (1989) Biochem. J. **258**, 121–140
11. Bartrons, R., Van Schaftingen, E., Vissers, S. and Hers, H.-G. (1982) FEBS Lett. **143**, 137–140
12. Becker, G. L., Fiskum, G. and Lehninger, A. L. (1980) J. Biol. Chem. **255**, 9009–9012
13. Beebe, S. J. and Corbin, J. D. (1986) Enzymes, 3rd edn., **27**, 43–111
14. Benevolensky, S. V., Clifton, D. and Fraenkel, D. G. (1994) J. Biol. Chem. **269**, 4876–4882
15. Bennett, J. (1991) Annu. Rev. Plant. Physiol. Plant Mol. Biol. **42**, 281–311
16. Berry, M. N. and Friend, D. S. (1969) J. Cell Biol. **43**, 506–520
17. Berthon, H. A., Bubb, W. A. and Kuchel, P. W. (1993) Biochem. J. **296**, 379–389
18. Blackman, F. F. (1905) Ann. Bot. **19**, 281
19. Blum, J. B. and Stein, R. B. (1982) in Biological Regulation and Development, vol. 3A, (Goldberger, R., ed.), pp. 99–125, Plenum Press, New York
20. Brand, M. D. (1993) in Surviving Hypoxia: Mechanisms of Control and Adaptation, (Hochachka, P. W., Lutz, P. L., Sick, T., Rosenthal, M. and van den Thillart, G., eds.), pp. 295–309, CRC Press, Boca Raton
21. Brand, M. D., Hafner, R. P. and Brown, G. C. (1988) Biochem. J. **255**, 535–539
22. Brindle, K. M. (1988) Biochemistry **27**, 6187–6196
23. Brown, G. C., Lakin-Thomas, P. L. and Brand, M. D. (1990) Eur. J. Biochem. **192**, 355–362
24. Bücher, T. and Rüssmann, W. (1964) Angew. Chem. Int. Ed. **3**, 426–439. (Originally published as Angew. Chem. **73**, 881 in 1963).
25. Bulfield, G. (1972) Genet. Res. Camb. **20**, 51–64
26. Cahill, G. F., Ashmore, J., Renold, A. E. and Hastings, A. B. (1959) Am. J. Med. **26**, 264–282
27. Cárdenas, M. L. and Cornish-Bowden, A. (1989) Biochem. J. **257**, 339–345
28. Carling, D. J., Zammit, V. A. and Hardie, D. G. (1987) FEBS Lett. **223**, 217–222
29. Carling, D. J., Clarke, P. R., Zammit, V. A. and Hardie, D. G. (1989) Eur. J. Biochem. **186**, 129–136
30. Cascante, M., Canela, E. I. and Franco, R. (1990) Eur. J. Biochem. **192**, 369–371
31. Cascante, M., Franco, R. and Canela, E. I. (1989) Math. Biosci. **94**, 271–288
32. Cascante, M., Franco, R. and Canela, E. I. (1989) Math. Biosci. **94**, 289–309
33. Chance, B., Holmes, W., Higgins, J. J. and Connelly, C. M. (1958) Nature (London) **182**, 1190–1193
34. Chance, B. and Williams, G. R. (1955) J. Biol. Chem. **217**, 409–427
35. Chance, B., Williams, G. R., Holmes, W. F. and Higgins, J. (1955) J. Biol. Chem. **217**, 439–451
36. Chance, E. M., Seeholzer, S. H., Kobayashi, K. and Williamson, J. R. (1983) J. Biol. Chem. **258**, 13785–13794

37. Chelsky, D., Ruskin, B. and Koshland Jr., D. E. (1985) Biochemistry **24**, 6651–6658
38. Chock, P. B., Shacter, E., Jurgensen, S. R. and Rhee, S. G. (1985) Curr. Top. Cell. Regul. **27**, 3–12
39. Clark, M. G., Bloxham, D. P., Holland, P. C. and Lardy, H. A. (1973) Biochem. J. **134**, 589–597
40. Clark, M. G., Kneer, N. M., Bosch, A. L. and Lardy, H. A. (1974) J. Biol. Chem **249**, 5695–5703
41. Cohen, G. N. (1969) Curr. Top. Cell. Regul. **1**, 183–231
42. Cohen, P. (1985) Curr. Top. Cell. Regul. **27**, 23–37
43. Cohen, P. (1989) Annu. Rev. Biochem. **58**, 453–508
44. Cohen, P. and Chen, P. T. W. (1989) J. Biol. Chem. **264**, 21435–21438
45. Cohen, P. and Klee, C. B. (eds.) (1988) Calmodulin. Molecular Aspects of Cellular Regulation, vol. 5. Elsevier, Amsterdam
46. Cohen, S. M. (1987) Biochemistry **26**, 573–580
47. Cornish, A., Greenwood, J. A. and Jones, C. W. (1988) J. Gen. Microbiol. **88**, 3111–3122
48. Cornish-Bowden, A. (1989) J. Theor. Biol. **136**, 365–377
49. Cornish-Bowden, A. (1995) Fundamentals of Enzyme Kinetics, 2nd edn., Portland Press, London
50. Cornish-Bowden, A. and Cárdenas, M. L. (1987) J. Theor. Biol. **124**, 1–23
51. Cornish-Bowden, A. and Cárdenas, M. L. (1991) Trend Biochem. Sci. **16**, 218–282
52. Cornish-Bowden, A. and Hofmeyr, J.-H. S. (1991) Comp. Appl. Biosci. **7**, 89–93
53. Cornish-Bowden, A. and Hofmeyr, J.-H. S. (1994) Biochem. J. **298**, 367–375
54. Crabtree, B. (1976) Biochem. Soc. Trans. **4**, 999–1002
55. Crabtree, B. and Newsholme, E. A. (1985) Curr. Top. Cell. Regul. **25**, 21–76
56. Crabtree, B. and Newsholme, E. A. (1987) Biochem. J. **247**, 113–120
57. Crabtree, B. and Newsholme, E. A. (1987) Trends Biochem. Sci. **12**, 4–12
58. Crawford, J. M. and Blum, J. J. (1983) Biochem. J. **212**, 585–598
59. Davies, S. E. C. and Brindle, K. M. (1992) Biochemistry **31**, 4729–4735
60. Denton, R. M. and Pogson, C. I. (1976) Metabolic Regulation, Chapman & Hall, London
61. Dykhuizen, D. E., Dean, A. M. and Hartl, D. L. (1987) Genetics **115**, 25–31
62. Easterby, J. S. (1981) Biochem. J. **199**, 155–161
63. Easterby, J. S. (1986) Biochem. J. **233**, 871–875
64. Easterby, J. S. (1990) Biochem. J. **269**, 255–259
65. Eisenthal, R. and Cornish-Bowden, A. (1974) Biochem. J. **139**, 715–720
66. El-Yassin, D. I. and Fell, D. A. (1982) J. Mol. Biol. **156**, 863–889
67. Endrenyi, L. and Chan, F.-Y. (1981) J. Theor. Biol. **90**, 241–263
68. Fell, D. A. (1980) J. Theor. Biol. **84**, 361–385
69. Fell, D. A. and Sauro, H. M. (1985) Eur. J. Biochem. **148**, 555–561
70. Fell, D. A. and Sauro, H. M. (1990) Eur. J. Biochem. **192**, 183–187
71. Fell, D. A. and Snell, K. (1988) Biochem. J. **256**, 97–101
72. Fell, D. A. and Thomas, S. (1995) Biochem. J. **311**, 35–39
73. Fiegelson, M. and Fiegelson, P. (1965) Adv. Enzyme Regul. **3**, 11–27
74. Flint, H. J., Tateson, R. W., Bartelmess, I. B., Porteous, D. J., Donachie, W. D. and Kacser, H. (1981) Biochem. J. **200**, 231–246
75. Forsberg, H., Zetterqvist, O. and Engström, L. (1969) Biochim. Biophys. Acta **181**, 171–175
76. Fraenkel, D. G. (1992) Annu. Rev. Genet. **26**, 159–177
77. Galazzo, J. L. and Bailey, J. E. (1990) Enzyme Microb. Technol. **12**, 162–172
78. Garfinkel, D. (1971) Comput. Biomed. Res. **4**, 18–42
79. Garfinkel, D. (1981) Trends Biochem. Sci. **6**, 69–71
80. Geiger, D. R. and Servaites, J. C. (1994) Annu. Rev. Plant Physiol. Plant Mol. Biol. **45**, 235–256
81. Gellerich, F. N., Kunz, W. S. and Bohnensack, R. (1990) FEBS Lett. **274**, 167–170
82. Gerhart, J. C. (1970) Curr. Top. Cell. Regul. **2**, 275–325
83. Giersch, C. (1988) J. Theor. Biol. **134**, 451–462
84. Giersch, C. (1994) J. Theor. Biol. **169**, 89–99
85. Giersch, C. (1995) Eur. J. Biochem. **227**, 194–201

86. Giersch, C., Lämmel, D. and Farquhar, G. (1990) Photosynth. Res. **24**, 151–165
87. Giersch, C., Lämmel, D. and Steffen, K. (1990) in Control of Metabolic Processes, (Cornish-Bowden, A. and Cárdenas, M. L., eds.), pp. 351–361, Plenum Press, New York
88. Goldbeter, A. and Koshland, D. E. (1981) Proc. Natl. Acad. Sci. U.S.A. **78**, 6840–6844
89. Groen, A. K. (1984) Quantification of Control in Studies on Intermediary Metabolism, Ph.D. thesis, University of Amsterdam
90. Groen, A. K., van der Meer, R., Westerhoff, H. V., Wanders, R. J. A., Akerboom, T. P. M. and Tager, J. M. (1982) in Metabolic Compartmentation (Sies, H., ed.), pp. 9–37, Academic Press, London
91. Groen, A. K., van Roermund, C. W. T. Vervoorn, R. C. and Tager, J. M. (1986) Biochem. J. **237**, 379–389
92. Groen, A. K., Wanders, R. J. A., Westerhoff, H. V., van der Meer, R. and Tager, J. M. (1982) J. Biol. Chem. **257**, 2754–2757
93. Haber, J. E. and Koshland, D. E. (1967) Proc. Natl. Acad. Sci. U.S.A. **58**, 2087–2093
94. Hafner, R. P., Brown, G. C. and Brand, M. D. (1990) Eur. J. Biochem. **188**, 313–319
95. Hales, C. N. (1967) in Essays in Biochemistry, (Campbell, P. N. and Greville, G. D., eds.), vol. 3, pp. 73–104, The Biochemical Society/Academic Press, London
96. Heinisch, J. (1986) Mol. Gen. Genet. **202**, 75–82
97. Heinrich, R. (1985) Biomed. Biochim. Acta **44**, 913–927
98. Heinrich, R. (1990) in Control of Metabolic Processes (Cornish-Bowden, A. and Cárdenas, M. L., eds.), pp. 329–342, Plenum Press, New York
99. Heinrich, R. and Rapoport, T. A. (1974) Eur. J. Biochem. **42**, 89–95
100. Heinrich, R. and Rapoport, T. A. (1974) Eur. J. Biochem. **42**, 97–105
101. Helmreich, E. and Cori, C. F. (1965) Adv. Enzyme Regul. **3**, 91–107
102. Hershko, A. and Ciechanover, A. (1992) Annu. Rev. Biochem. **61**, 761–807
103. Hess, B. (1977) Trends Biochem. Sci. **2**, 193–195
104. Higgins, J. (1963) Ann. N. Y. Acad. Sci. **108**, 305–321
105. Hillgartner, F. B., Salati, L. M. and Goodridge, A. G. (1995) Physiol. Rev. **75**, 47–76
106. Hofmeyr, J.-H. S. and Cornish-Bowden, A. (1991) Eur. J. Biochem. **200**, 223–236
107. Hohorst, H. J., Reim, M. and Bartels, H. (1962) Biochem. Biophys. Res. Commun. **7**, 137–141
108. Holzhütter, H.-G., Jacobasch, G. and Bisdorff, A. (1985) Eur. J. Biochem. **149**, 101–111
109. Holzhütter, H.-G., Schuster, R., Buckwitz, D. and Jacobasch, G. (1990) Biomed. Biochim. Acta **49**, 791–800
110. Huber, S. C., Huber, J. L. and McMichael, R. W. (1994) Int. Rev. Cytol. **149**, 47–98
111. Hue, L. (1981) Adv. Enzymol. Relat. Areas Mol. Biol. **52**, 247–331
112. Hue, L. (1982) in Metabolic Compartmentation, (Sies, H., ed.), pp. 71–97, Academic Press, London
113. Jensen, P. R., Michelsen, O. and Westerhoff, H. V. (1993) Proc. Nat. Acad. Sci. U.S.A. **90**, 8068–8072
114. Jensen, P. R., Westerhoff, H. V. and Michelsen, O. (1993) EMBO J. **12**, 1277–1282
115. Jensen, P. R., Westerhoff, H. V. and Michelsen, O. (1993) Eur. J. Biochem. **211**, 181–191
116. Kacser, H. (1983) Biochem. Soc. Trans. **11**, 35–40
117. Kacser, H. (1995) Biochem. Soc. Trans. **23**, 387–391
118. Kacser, H. and Acerenza, L. (1993) Eur. J. Biochem. **216**, 361–367
119. Kacser, H. and Burns, J. A. (1973) Symp. Soc. Exp. Biol. **27**, 65–104 (reprinted in Biochem. Soc. Trans. **23**, 341–366, 1995)
120. Kacser, H. and Burns, J. A. (1979) Biochem. Soc. Trans. **7**, 1149–1160.
121. Kacser, H. and Burns, J. A. (1981) Genetics **97**, 639–666
122. Kacser, H., Sauro, H. M. and Acerenza, L. (1990) Eur. J. Biochem. **187**, 481–491
123. Kahn, D. and Westerhoff, H. V. (1991) J. Theor. Biol. **153**, 255–285
124. Kantrowitz, E. R. and Lipscomb, W. N. (1990) Trends Biochem. Sci. **15**, 53–59

125. Kashiwaya, Y., Sato, K., Tsuchiya, N., Thomas, S., Fell, D. A., Veech, R. L. and Passonneau, J. V. (1994) J. Biol. Chem. **269**, 25502–25514

126. Katz, J. and Rognstad, R. (1976) Curr. Top. Cell. Regul. **10**, 237–289

127. Reference deleted

128. Katz, J., Wals, P. A. and Rognstad, R. (1978) J. Biol. Chem. **253**, 4530–4536

129. Kell, D. B. and Westerhoff, H. V. (1986) FEMS Microbiol. Rev. **39**, 305–320

130. Kelly, P. J., Kelleher, J. K. and Wright, B. E. (1979) Biochem. J. **184**, 589–597

131. Kholodenko, B. N., Cascante, M. and Westerhoff, H. V. (1993) FEBS Lett. **336**, 381–384

132. Kholodenko, B. N., Cascante, M. and Westerhoff, H. V. (1994) Mol. Cell Biochem. **133**, 313–331

133. King, E. L. and Altman, C. (1956) J. Phys. Chem. **60**, 1375–1378

134. Klotz, I. M. (1985) Q. Rev. Biophys. **18**, 227–259

135. Kohn, M. (1983) Ann. Biomed. Eng. **11**, 533–549

136. Kohn, M. C. and Chiang, E. (1983) J. Theor. Biol. **100**, 551–565

137. Koshland, D. E., Némethy, G. and Filmer, D. (1966) Biochemistry **5**, 365–385

138. Kowal, J. (1970) Recent Prog. Horm. Res. **26**, 623–687

139. Krebs, E. G. (1986) Enzymes, 3rd edn. **27**, 1–20

140. Krebs, H. A. (1946) Enzymologia **12**, 88–100

141. Krebs, H. A. (1957) Endeavour **16**, 125–132

142. Krebs, H. A. (1963) Adv. Enzyme Regul. **1**, 385–400

143. Kruckeberg, A. L., Neuhaus, H. E., Feil, R., Gottlieb, L. D. and Stitt, M. (1989) Biochem. J. **261**, 457–467

144. Lagunas, R. and Gancedo, C. (1983) Eur. J. Biochem. **137**, 479–483

145. Lawrence, J. C. (1992) Annu. Rev. Physiol. **54**, 177–193

146. Leiser, J. and Blum, J. J. (1985) Cell Biophys. **11**, 123–138

147. Lemaigre, F. P. and Rousseau, G. G. (1994) Biochem. J. **303**, 1–14

148. Letellier, T. (1992) Contrôle du Métabolisme Cellulaire: Application aux Oxydations Phosphorylantes Normales et Pathologiques., Ph.D. thesis, Université de Bordeaux II

149. Letellier, T., Heinrich, R., Malgat, M. and Mazat, J.-P. (1994) Biochem. J. **302**, 171–174

150. Letellier, T., Malgat, M. and Mazat, J.-P. (1993) Biochim. Biophys. Acta **1141**, 58–64

151. Low, S. Y., Salter, M., Knowles, R. G., Pogson, C. I. and Rennie, M. J. (1993) Biochem. J. **295**, 617–624

152. Maas, W. K. and Clark, A. J. (1964) J. Mol. Biol. **8**, 365–370

153. Makins, R. A., Drynan, L. F., Zammit, V. A. and Quant, P. A. (1995) Biochem. Soc. Trans. **23**, 288S

154. Mayorek, N., Grinstein, I. and Bar-Tana, J. (1989) Eur. J. Biochem. **182**, 395–400

155. McCormack, J. G. and Denton, R. M. (1986) Trends Biochem. Sci. **11**, 258–262

156. Meinke, M. H., Bishop, J. S. and Edstrom, R. D. (1986) Proc. Natl. Acad. Sci. U.S.A. **83**, 2865–2868

157. Meléndez-Hevia, E., Torres, N. V., Sicilia, J. and Kacser, H. (1990) Biochem. J. **265**, 195–202

158. Mendes, P. (1993) Comp. Appl. Biosci. **9**, 563–571

159. Middleton, R. J. and Kacser, H. (1983) Genetics **105**, 633–650

160. Monod, J., Changeux, J.-P. and Jacob, F. (1963) J. Mol. Biol. **6**, 306–329

161. Monod, J., Wyman, J. and Changeux, J.-P. (1965) J. Mol. Biol. **12**, 88–118

162. Morgan, H. E., Randle, P. J. and Regen, D. M. (1959) Biochem. J. **73**, 573–579

163. Murphy, M. P. and Brand, M. D. (1987) Biochem. J. **243**, 499–505

164. Narabayashi, H., Lawson, J. W. R. and Uyeda, K. (1985) J. Biol. Chem. **260**, 9750–9758

165. Neuhaus, H. E., Kruckeberg, A. L., Feil, R. and Stitt, M. (1989) Planta **178**, 110–12

166. Neuhaus, H. E., Quick, W. P., Siegl, G. and Stitt, M. (1990) Planta **181**, 583–592

167. Neuhaus, H. E. and Stitt, M. (1990) Planta **182**, 445–454

168. Newsholme, E. A. and Crabtree, B. (1976) Biochem. Soc. Symp. **41**, 61–109

169. Newsholme, E. A. and Gevers, W. (1967) Vitam. Horm. **25**, 1–87

170. Newsholme, E. A. and Randle, P. J. (1964) Biochem. J. **93**, 641–651

171. Newsholme, E. A. and Start, C. (1973) Regulation in Metabolism, Wiley and Sons, London

172. Newsholme, E. A. and Underwood, A. H. (1966) Biochem. J. **99**, 24C–26C

173. Newsholme, P. and Walsh, D. A. (1992) Biochem. J. **283**, 845–848

174. Nicholls, D. G. and Crompton, M. (1980) FEBS Lett. **111**, 261–268

175. Niederberger, P., Prasad, R., Miozzari, G. and Kacser, H. (1992) Biochem. J. **287**, 473–479

176. Norby, J. G., Ottolenghi, P. and Jensen, J. (1980) Anal. Biochem. **102**, 318–320

177. Orr, H. A. (1991) Proc. Natl. Acad. Sci. U.S.A. **88**, 11413–11415

178. Ovadi, J. (1991) J. Theor. Biol. **152**, 1–22 (see also the following discussion by various authors on pp. 23–141)

179. Page, R. A., Kitson, K. E. and Hardman, M. J. (1991) Biochem. J. **278**, 659–665

180. Pearcy, R. W. (1990) Annu. Rev. Plant Physiol. Plant Mol. Biol. **41**, 421–453

181. Pedersen, R. C. and Brownie, A. C. (1986) Biochem. Action Horm. **13**, 129–166

182. Pettersson, G. and Ryde-Pettersson, U. (1988) Eur. J. Biochem. **175**, 661–672

183. Pietrobon, D., Di Virgilio, F. and Pozzan, T. (1990) Eur. J. Biochem. **193**, 599–622

184. Pilkis, S. J. and Claus, T. H. (1991) Annu. Rev. Nutr. **11**, 465–515

185. Pilkis, S. J., Claus, T. H. and El-Maghrabi, M. R. (1988) Adv. Second Messenger Phosphoprotein Res. **22**, 175–191

186. Przybylski, F., Otto, A., Nissler, K., Schellenberger, W. and Hofmann, E. (1985) Biochim. Biophys. Acta **831**, 350–352

187. Quant, P. A. and Makins, R. A. (1994) Biochem. Soc. Trans. **22**, 441–446

188. Quant, P. A., Robin, D., Robin, P., Girard, J. and Brand, M. D. (1993) Biochim. Biophys. Acta **1156**, 135–143

189. Quick, W. P., Schurr, U., Scheibe, R., Schulze, E.-D., Rodermel, S. R., Bogorad, L. and Stitt, M. (1991) Planta **183**, 542–554

190. Rabkin, M. and Blum, J. J. (1985) Biochem. J. **255**, 761–786

191. Rainey, W. E., Shay, J. W. and Mason, J. I. (1986) J. Biol. Chem. **261**, 7322–7326

192. Randle, P. J., England, P. J. and Denton, R. M. (1970) Biochem. J. **117**, 677–695

193. Rapoport, T. A., Heinrich, R., Jacobasch, G. and Rapoport, S. (1974) Eur. J. Biochem. **42**, 107–120

194. Rapoport, T. A., Heinrich, R. and Rapoport, S. M. (1976) Biochem. J. **154**, 449–469

195. Reder, C. (1988) J. Theor. Biol. **135**, 175–201

196. Reich, J. G. and Sel'kov, E. E. (1981) Energy Metabolism of the Cell, Academic Press, London

197. Rhee, S. G., Chock, P. B. and Stadtman, E. R. (1989) Adv. Enzymol. Relat. Areas Mol. Biol. **62**, 37–92

198. Rigoulet, M., Leverve, X. M., Plomp, P. J. A. M. and Meijer, A. J. (1987) Biochem. J. **245**, 661–668

199. Rodbell, M. (1992) Curr. Top. Cell. Regul. **32**, 1–47

200. Rognstad, R. (1979) J. Biol. Chem. **254**, 1875–1878

201. Rolleston, F. S. (1972) Curr. Topics Cell Regul. **5**, 47–75

202. Rudolph, F. B. and Fromm, H. J. (1971) J. Biol. Chem. **246**, 6611–6619

203. Ruijter, G. J. G., Postma, P. W. and van Dam, K. (1991) J. Bacteriol. **173**, 6184–6191

204. Sacktor, B. and Wormser-Shavit, E. (1966) J. Biol. Chem. **241**, 624–631

205. Saier, M. H., Wu, L.-F. and Reizer, J. (1990) Trends Biochem. Sci. **15**, 391–395

206. Sale, E. M. and Denton, R. M. (1985) Biochem. J. **232**, 897–904

207. Salter, M., Knowles, R. G. and Pogson, C. I. (1986) Biochem. J. **234**, 635–647

208. Salter, M., Knowles, R. G. and Pogson, C. I. (1994) in Essays in Biochemistry (Tipton, K. F., ed.), vol. 28, pp. 1–12, Portland Press, London

209. Sauro, H. M. (1993) Comput. Appl. Biosci. **9**, 441–450

210. Sauro, H. M. (1994) Biosystems **33**, 55–67

211. Sauro, H. M. and Fell, D. A. (1991) Mathl. Comput. Modelling **15**, 15–28

212. Sauro, H. M. and Kacser, H. (1990) Eur. J. Biochem. **187**, 493–500

213. Sauro, H. M., Small, J. R. and Fell, D. A. (1987) Eur. J. Biochem. **165**, 215–221

214. Savageau, M. A. (1971) Arch. Biochem. Biophys. **145**, 612–621

215. Savageau, M. A. (1974) J. Mol. Evol. **4**, 139–156

216. Savageau, M. A. (1975) J. Mol. Evol. **5**, 199–222
217. Savageau, M. A. (1976) Biochemical Systems Analysis: a Study of Function and Design in Molecular Biology, Addison–Wesley, Reading, MA
218. Savageau, M. A., Voit, E. O. and Irvine, D. H. (1987) Math. Biosci. **86**, 127–145
219. Savageau, M. A., Voit, E. O. and Irvine, D. H. (1987) Math. Biosci. **86**, 147–169
220. Schaaff, I., Heinisch, J. and Zimmerman, F. K. (1989) Yeast **5**, 285–290
221. Schimke, R. T. (1962) J. Biol. Chem. **237**, 459–468
222. Schuster, R., Holzhütter, H.-G. and Jacobasch, G. (1988) Biosystems **22**, 19–36
223. Schuster, S. and Heinrich, R. (1992) Biosystems **27**, 1–15
224. Schuster, S., Kahn, D. and Westerhoff, H. V. (1993) Biophys. Chem. **48**, 1–17
225. Serrano, R., Gancedo, J. M. and Gancedo, C. (1973) Eur, J, Biochem. **34**, 479–482
226. Shacter, E., Chock, P. B., Rhee, S. G. and Stadtman, E. R. (1986) Enzymes, 3rd edn., **27**, 21–42
227. Shalwitz, R. A., Beth, T. J., MacLeod, A. M. K., Tucker, S. J. and Rolison, G. G. (1994) Am. J. Physiol. **266**, E433–E437
228. Small, J. R. (1988) Theoretical Aspects of Metabolic Control, Ph.D. thesis, Oxford Polytechnic
229. Small, J. R. (1993) Biochem. J. **296**, 423–433
230. Small, J. R. (1994) Microbiology **140**, 2439–2449
231. Small, J. R. and Fell, D. A. (1990) Eur. J. Biochem. **191**, 405–411
232. Small, J. R. and Fell, D. A. (1990) Eur. J. Biochem. **191**, 413–420
233. Small, J. R. and Kacser, H. (1993) Eur. J. Biochem. **213**, 613–624
234. Smith, R. E. and Horwitz, B. A. (1969) Physiol. Rev. **49**, 330–425
235. Snell, K. and Fell, D. A. (1990) Adv. Enzyme Regul. **30**, 13–32
236. Srere, P. A. (1993) Biol. Chem. Hoppe–Seyler **374**, 833–842
237. Stadtman, E. R. (1970) Enzymes 3rd edn., **1**, 397–459
238. Stadtman, E. R. and Chock, P. B. (1978) Curr. Top. Cell. Regul. **13**, 53–95
239. Stanley, J. C., Salter, M., Fisher, M. J. and Pogson, C. I. (1985) Arch. Biochem. Biophys. **240**, 792–800
240. Stein, R. B. and Blum, J. J. (1978) J. Theor. Biol. **72**, 487–522
241. Steinberg, D. (1963) Biochem. Soc. Symp. **24**, 111–143
242. Stitt, M. (1989) Philos. Trans. R. Soc. London. B **323**, 327–338
243. Stitt, M., Quick, W. P., Schurr, U., Schulze, E.-D., Rodermel, S. R. and Bogorad, L. (1991) Planta **183**, 555–566
244. Sutherland, E. W. (1972) Science **177**, 401–408
245. Thomas, S. and Fell, D. A. (1993) Biochem. J. **292**, 351–360
246. Thomas, S. and Fell, D. A. (1994) J. Theor. Biol. **167**, 175–200
247. Tornheim, K. (1985) J. Biol. Chem. **260**, 7985–7989
248. Torres, N. V., Mateo, F., Melendez-Hevia, E. and Kacser, H. (1986) Biochem. J. **234**, 169–174
249. Torres, N. V. and Meléndez-Hevia, E. (1992) Mol. Cell. Biochem. **112**, 109–115
250. Umbarger, H. E. (1956) Science **123**, 848
251. Umbarger, H. E. (1978) Annu. Rev. Biochem. **47**, 533–606
252. Utter, M. F. and Scrutton, M. C. (1969) Curr. Top. Cell. Regul. **1**, 253–296
253. Van Schaftingen, E., Hue, L. and Hers, H. G. (1980) Biochem. J. **192**, 887–895
254. Van Schaftingen, E., Hue, L. and Hers, H. G. (1980) Biochem. J. **192**, 897–901
255. Van Schaftingen, E., Jett, M.-F., Hue, L. and Hers, H.-G. (1981) Proc. Natl. Acad. Sci. U.S.A. **78**, 3483–3486
256. Vandercammen, A. and Van Schaftingen, E. (1990) Eur. J. Biochem. **191**, 483–489
257. Vandercammen, A. and Van Schaftingen, E. (1993) Biochem. J. **294**, 551–556
258. Veech, R. L., Lawson, J. W. R., Cornell, N. W. and Krebs, H. A. (1979) J. Biol. Chem. **254**, 6538–6547
259. Voit, E. O. and Savageau, M. A. (1987) Biochemistry **26**, 6869–6880
260. Waley, S. G. (1964) Biochem. J. **91**, 514–517

261. Wals, P. A. and Katz, J. (1994) J. Biol. Chem. **269**, 18343–18352
262. Walsh, K. and Koshland Jr., D. E. (1985) Proc. Natl. Acad. Sci. U.S.A. **82**, 3577–3581
263. Walsh, K., Schena, M., Flint, A. J. and Koshland Jr., D. E. (1987) Biochem. Soc. Symp. **54**, 183–195
264. Walter, R. P., Morris, J. G. and Kell, D. B. (1987) J. Gen. Microbiol. **133**, 259–266
265. Wanders, R. J. A., van Roermund, C. W. T. and Meijer, A. J. (1984) Eur. J. Biochem. **142**, 247–254
266. Wang, J. H., Pallen, C. J., Sharma, R. K., Adachi, A. M. and Adachi, K. (1985) Curr. Top. Cell. Regul. **27**, 419–436
267. Waterman, M. R. and Simpson, E. R. (1989) Recent Prog. Horm. Res. **45**, 533–566
268. Weber, G., Singhal, R. L. and Srivastava, S. K. (1965) Adv. Enzyme Regul. **3**, 43–75
269. Weber, G., Singhal, R. L., Stamm, N. B., Lea, M. A. and Fisher, E. A. (1966) Adv. Enzyme Regul. **4**, 59–81
270. Weekes, J., Hawley, S. A., Corton, J., Shugar, D. and Hardie, D. G. (1994) Eur. J. Biochem. **219**, 751–757
271. Welch, G. R. (1985) J. Theor. Biol. **114**, 433–446
272. Westerhoff, H. V. and Chen, Y.-D. (1984) Eur. J. Biochem. **142**, 425–430
273. Westerhoff, H. V., Groen, A. K. and Wanders, R. J. A. (1984) Biosci. Rep. **4**, 1–22
274. Westerhoff, H. V. and Kell, D. B. (1987) Biotechnol. Bioeng. **30**, 101–107
275. Wilkinson, G. N. (1961) Biochem. J. **80**, 324–332
276. Woodrow, I. E. (1986) Biochim. Biophys. Acta **851**, 181–192
277. Woodrow, I. E., Murphy, D. J. and Latzko, E. (1984) J. Biol. Chem. **259**, 3791–3795
278. Wright, B. E. and Albe, K. R. (1994) J. Theor. Biol. **169**, 231–241
279. Wright, B. E., Butler, M. H. and Albe, K. R. (1992) J. Biol. Chem. **267**, 3101–3105
280. Wright, B. E. and Reimers, J. M. (1988) J. Biol. Chem. **263**, 14906–14912
281. Yates, R. A. and Pardee, A. B. (1956) J. Biol. Chem. **221**, 757–770
282. Zhang, Y., Proenca, R., Maffei, M., Barone, M., Leopold, L. and Friedman, J. M. (1994) Nature (London) **372**, 425–432
283. Zuurendonk, P. F. and Tager, J. M. (1974) Biochim. Biophys. Acta **333**, 393–399
284. Zuurendonk, P. F., Tischler, M. E., Akerboom, T. P. M., van der Meer, R., Williamson, J. R. and Tager, J. M. (1979) Methods Enzymol. **56**, 207–233

Index